GASTRIC CANCER

Edited by **Gyula Mózsik** and **Oszkár Karádi**

Gastric Cancer
http://dx.doi.org/10.5772/65828
Edited by Gyula Mózsik and Oszkár Karádi

Contributors

Ilze Strumfa, Andrejs Vanags, Tatjana Bogdanova, Roberts Rumba, Inese Drike, Arnis Abolins, Arvids Jakovlevs, Dainis Balodis, Dzeina Mezale, Boriss Strumfs, Ander Matheu, Estefania Carrasco-Garcia, Mikel Garcia-Puga, Nicolas Sampron, Manuel Moreno, Sara Arevalo, Alejandro H. Corvalan, Petra Hudler, Radovan Komel, Shouji Shimoyama, Alexander Quaas, Alfredo J. A. Barbosa, Vitězslav Marek, Daniela Lazar, Francis Megraud, Marta Vitola, Gyula Mozsik

Published by InTech

Janeza Trdine 9, 51000 Rijeka, Croatia

Publishing Process Manager Teo Kos
Technical Editor SPi Global
Cover InTech Design team

First published September, 2017
Printed in Croatia
Legal deposit, Croatia: National and University Library in Zagreb

Additional hard copies can be obtained from orders@intechopen.com

Gastric Cancer, Edited by Gyula Mózsik and Oszkár Karádi
p. cm.
Print ISBN 978-953-51-3527-2
Online ISBN 978-953-51-3528-9

For EU product safety concerns:
IN TECH d.o.o., Prolaz Marije Krucifikse Kozulić 3, 51000 Rijeka, Croatia,
info@intechopen.com or visit our website at intechopen.com.

Meet the editors

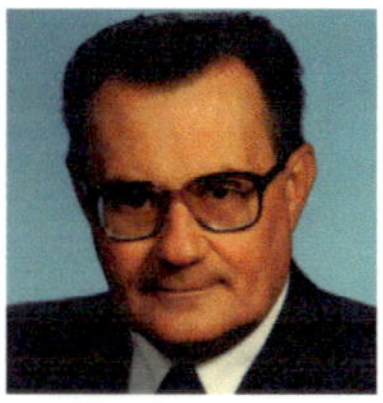

Gyula Mózsik, MD, PhD, ScD (Med.) is a professor emeritus of Medicine at the First Department of Medicine, University of Pécs, Hungary. He was the head of this department from 1993 to 2003. His specializations are internal medicine, gastroenterology, and clinical pharmacology. His research fields are biochemical and pharmacological studies in the gastrointestinal tract, experimental and clinical gastroenterology, clinical pharmacology, experimental and clinical nutrition and dietetics, innovative pharmacological and nutritional (dietetical) researches, and new drug and food productions. He published more than 400 papers in peer-reviewed journals and 20 monographs and edited 31 books. He received an Andrés Robert award from the International Union of Pharmacology, Gastrointestinal Section (2014). Fourteen of his students were appointed as full professors in Cuba, Egypt, and Hungary.

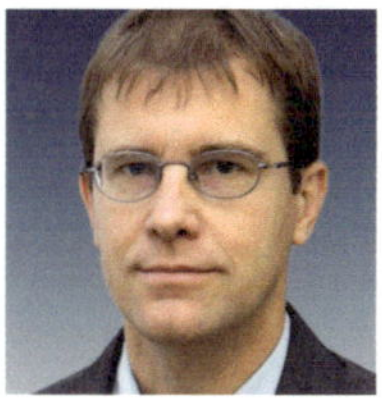

Oszkár Karádi acquired a general medical qualification at the University Medical School of Pécs, Hungary, in 1992. He had worked at the First Department of Medicine in the Medical University of Pécs between 1992 and 2008. He was specialized as an internalist in 2000, as a clinical oncologist in 2002, and as a gastroenterologist in 2004. He received his PhD degree in the year 1998. The topic of dissertation was the role of vagal nerve in the gastrointestinal mucosal lesions caused by nonsteroidal anti-inflammatory drugs. Since 2008, he is working in the Institute of Oncotherapy, University of Pécs as an associate professor. He is a member of the National Society of Oncology in Hungary. His field of interest is the gastrointestinal tumors.

Contents

Preface

Gastric cancer remains an important issue in the world of oncology. In 2013, it ranked fifth by global incidence and second by mortality. It is true that the death rates have decreased significantly in the USA and Europe over the last 100-year period; meanwhile, gastric cancer is characterized by poor prognosis and high mortality, except in early diagnosed cases.

The basic and clinical oncological research increased extremely in the last years, and our knowledge from this field is changing from day to day.

The same applies to the field of gastric cancer.

This book deals with details of the results of the most recently carried out basic and clinical observations (as the possible role of Epstein-Barr virus in tumor genesis, gastric carcinoma stem cells, molecular heterogeneity of gastric cancer, a summary of prognostic factors, treatment strategies, the actualities in targeting therapy, the key role of teamwork in the diagnosis and therapeutic decisions, etc.).

The authors of 12 different book chapters, apart from the Introductory Chapter, are basic and clinical researchers from Chile, Spain, France, Slovenia, Romania, Japan, Slovakia, Latvia, Germany, and Brazil, and they together give an excellent cross section of our updated basic and clinical research in the field of gastric cancer.

The conclusions of these abovementioned observations fall between the results of classical prospective, randomized, multiclinical, multinational (and meta-analyzed) generally accepted studies (in accordance with the presently applied and internationally accepted protocols) and the scientifically-based (however individual) molecular targeting organ therapies.

Gyula Mózsik, MD, PhD, ScD (Med.)
Professor Emeritus of Medicine
First Department of Medicine
University of Pécs, Hungary

Oszkár Karádi, MD, PhD
Associate Professor
Institute of Oncotherapy,
University of Pécs, Hungary

Section 1

Introductory Chapter

Chapter 1

Introductory Chapter: Gastric Cancer in the Past and Our Days

Gyula Mózsik and Oszkár Karádi

Additional information is available at the end of the chapter

http://dx.doi.org/10.5772/intechopen.70203

1. Introduction

The medicine went over extremely increased developmental process in the last century. The early decades of twentieth century can be characterized by the descriptive medicine, when the different clinical entities were separated from each other on the basis of symptomatology of different diseases, and the role of classical physical examinations was emphasized. These years, we practically can't speak on the curative medical therapy (the surgery was an exception in this term).

From the mid of last century, different methods such as X-ray examinations, ultrasonography, and other iconographic methods (including a computer tomography, MRI examination methods, and radioisotope examinations) and different laboratory examinations (including the general approaching parameters, later the specific parameters to infection diseases, immunological disorders, and radioimmunoassays) entered into the different medical activities of the physicians. These above-mentioned changes in the medical practice resulted in an extremely strong development in making a correct diagnosis of the patients.

In the 1970s appeared the "problem-orientated medicine" both in the teaching and in the clinical practice. The aims of this period can be characterized by the logical planning and carrying out of examinations of patients with different disorders aimed at the correct diagnosis for patients. The medical therapy was not well emphasized as the diagnostics (of course, we have relatively little knowledge on the therapeutic possibilities).

The pharmacological research started very actively from the second part of the last century. Some of the physicians recognized the facts that the results obtained in animal observations can't be applied directly in the human therapy (without some human observations). The human clinical pharmacology (as a very important branch of practical medical research) appeared from 1960s. The established clinical pharmacology introduced the "evidence-based medicine" from 1980s. This period covered the correct diagnosis and scientifically based (proved) therapy in terms of medicine. In the early years of this period, the drug actions were observed (later tested) on healthy human beings and in patients with different diagnosis. Following the first years appeared the randomized, prospective, multicentric, and multiclinical studies, and thereafter these studies were carried out in huge number of patients suffering from the same disorders.

The international organization of human drug research has been absolutely required the involvement of different nations from the different continents in the same studies (multinational) studies. One of the many factors the selections of patients including the same study other problems (age, body weight, correct diagnosis, the same stadiums of the disease, correct laboratory parameters, genders, nutritional habits, used drugs, etc.). The selections of the patients into the different drug therapies had been carried out randomly. Physicians (who actively participated in carrying out these observations) were not informed on therapeutically applied drugs (similarly to the patients), because these studies were done in accordance to previously permitted protocol(s).

These observations were done absolutely in accordance to earlier and the strictly prepared protocols (time of drug administration, collection of biological samples (blood and urine), relevant examinations, food and fluid consumption, etc.), and the protocols were previously permitted by the national authorities (respecting the ethical and medical aspects, cost and benefit, dangers of treated patients, etc.).

The critical evaluation of efficiencies of different drugs (or drug combinations) included the very complicated computer participation in the pharmacological research. Meanwhile, the detailed therapeutic effects resulted in the "meta-analysis" of drug (or drug-combination) actions.

The results of these examinations led us to plan a "generally accepted therapeutically used form" of drug therapy in the everyday medical treatment (guidelines).

Medically, we have to understand that these studies depended on the results obtained in huge number of human observations; however, an actually present patient was only one from the patients participated in whole ones of the big studies. Surprisingly, the results obtained in one patient differed from those obtained in big randomized studies. Of course, the physicians recalled the insufficient complaints of patients or some other causes. Later on, many other possibilities existed to explain the insufficient medical therapies, and their became to be clear by the new results of molecular biology, genetics, immunology, immunohistochemistry, and of new development of medical science (molecular pharmacology, biochemical pharmacology pharmacogenetics, etc.).

In this century, the development of medical sciences has been in an extremely high speed in different fields (including the basic research and clinical research), which produced an abnormally increased quantity and quality of our knowledge.

We have to realize that oncology is one of these fields indicating rapid changes from day to day. Consequently, the diagnostic and therapeutic possibilities in our hand are changing day to day. This is an absolutely new challenge to physicians and this offers new possibilities for the patients.

http://dx.doi.org/10.5772/intechopen.70203

Gastric cancer remains an important issue in the world of oncology. In 2013, it was ranked fifth by the global incidence and second by mortality. It's true that the death rates have decreased significantly in the USA and Europe over the near one hundred year period; meanwhile, gastric cancer is characterized by poor prognosis and high mortality, except in early diagnosed cases. The well-known histology of gastric cancer clearly indicates the correct diagnosis of disease, and the National Comprehensive Cancer Network (NCCN) indicates therapeutic guidelines to treat the patients with gastric cancer (recently Gastric Cancer, Version I.2017 – March 21, 2017. www.NCCN.org).

The oncological research in gastric cancer covers the classical clinical examinations, genetics, iconography, molecular biology, biochemical pharmacology, modern immunohistochemistry, clinical pharmacology, immunology, medicine, gastroenterology, surgery, oncology, nutrition, chemical toxicology, modern bacteriology, and virology.

The book gives an excellent cross section of the different oncological studies done in the last years and offers absolutely new knowledge both for basic and clinical researchers (role of Epstein-Barr virus in tumor genesis, gastric carcinoma stem cells, molecular heterogeneity, prognostic factors, treatment strategies, the actualities in the targeting therapy, responsibility of pathologists in the diagnosis and therapeutic decisions) and these together indicate clearly the change in our therapeutic strategies in the field of malignant disease.

The present book contains 11 excellent book chapters, which indicate the most recently obtained results in the fields of researches on gastric cancer. The participants of this book are basic and clinical researchers from Chile, Spain, France, Slovenia, Romania, Japan, Slovakia, Latvia, Germany, and Brazil.

The results of these above-mentioned observations are going on the border existing between the results of classical multiclinical, randomized, prospective, and multinational studies (including the presently applied and internationally accepted protocols) vs. the scientifically based (however individual) molecular targeting organ therapies (respectively the updated new results of molecular biological, immunological, immunohistochemical observations, etc.). These scientific and medical challenges a priori suggest the fruitful cooperation between the different research and medical treatment centers all over the world and offer new era of therapies of malignant disorders (including gastric cancer).

Acknowledgements

The editors thank very much the excellent cooperations of the contributors in this book at the time of book edition.

The editors are especially thankful for the excellent support given by Ms. Ana Pantar (Senior Commissioning Editor) and by Ms. Mirena Čalmić (Publishing Process Manager) and Mr. Teo Kos (Publishing Process Manager) from Intech Open Access Publisher; without their help, the publication of this book would not be possible.

Author details

Gyula Mózsik[1*] and Oszkár Karádi[2]

*Address all correspondence to: gyula.mozsik@gmail.com

1 First Department of Medicine, University of Pécs, Hungary

2 Institute of Oncotherapy, University of Pécs, Hungary

Section 2

Already Known and Recently Verified Etiologies of Gatric Cancer

Chapter 2

Epstein-Barr Virus–Associated Gastric Carcinoma: The Americas' Perspective

Alejandra Alarcón, Ursula Figueroa,
Bastian Espinoza, Alejandra Sandoval,
Gonzalo Carrasco-Aviño, Francisco R. Aguayo and
Alejandro H. Corvalan

Additional information is available at the end of the chapter

http://dx.doi.org/10.5772/intechopen.70201

Abstract

Epstein-Barr virus (EBV) infection has been associated with different malignancies, and compelling evidence has shown that it may have a causative or at least contributing role in gastric carcinogenesis. EBV-associated gastric cancers have a unique molecular signature, which has defined this group of tumors as a distinctive molecular subtype of gastric cancer. This subtype has shown a greater incidence in the Americas than in the Asian countries. This chapter discusses about possible factors underlying these differences and the emerging roles of epigenetics in the pathogenesis of Epstein-Barr virus–associated gastric cancer.

Keywords: gastric cancer, Epstein-Barr virus, strains, phylogeographic diversity, epigenetic abnormalities

1. Introduction: an overview of the Epstein-Barr virus

Epstein-Barr virus (EBV) belongs to the human gammaherpesvirus and is a 175 kbp double-stranded linear DNA virus. EBV infection is associated with the development of different malignancies, including several lymphoid neoplasms like Burkitt's lymphoma, Hodgkin's lymphoma, and immunosuppression-related B-cell lymphoma; in addition, epithelial malignancies like nasopharyngeal carcinomas (NPC) and gastric carcinomas have also been associated with the EBV [1]. Primary EBV infection is most of the time asymptomatic, and like other members of the herpesvirus family, the EBV maintains its genome as extrachromosomal circular episomes with repression of genes involved in virus replication. If latent persistent infection is established, viral reactivation may occur with the expression of specific EBV genes defining the type of latency in the infected cell. Genes involved in these patterns are shown in **Figure 1** and include the EBV-encoded RNAs (EBERs), the EBV nuclear antigens (EBNAs), the BamH1-A rightward transcripts (BARTs) and the latent membrane protein (LMP)-1, 2A and 2B [3]. These latency-associated patterns have been associated with specific malignancies and in the case of gastric cancer, the virus shows a latency type I/IIab. The EBERs 1 and 2 genes are the most abundant small noncoding RNAs that interact with proteins of the host and are the standard target for EBV detection by in situ hybridization (ISH) [4]. The EBNA-1 and -2 genes are exclusive nuclear proteins expressed in latent infected gastric carcinoma cells and related to the disruption of promyelocytic leukemia nuclear bodies [5]. EBNA-1 is a DNA-binding protein that lacks enzymatic activity although it can interact with some cellular proteins such as CK2 and P32/TAP [6]. Interestingly, EBNA-1 is expressed in all of the EBV-associated tumors and is involved in viral DNA replication, mitotic segregation and transcriptional activation [7]. BART genes encode highly expressed multispliced RNAs whose protein-coding function is controversial [8]. Although some BARTs open reading frames (ORFs) have been predicted, currently it is not clear if any of them can be endogenously translated. In addition, BART genes, small as well as long noncoding RNAs, are highly expressed and associated with oncogenic transformation and immune evasion

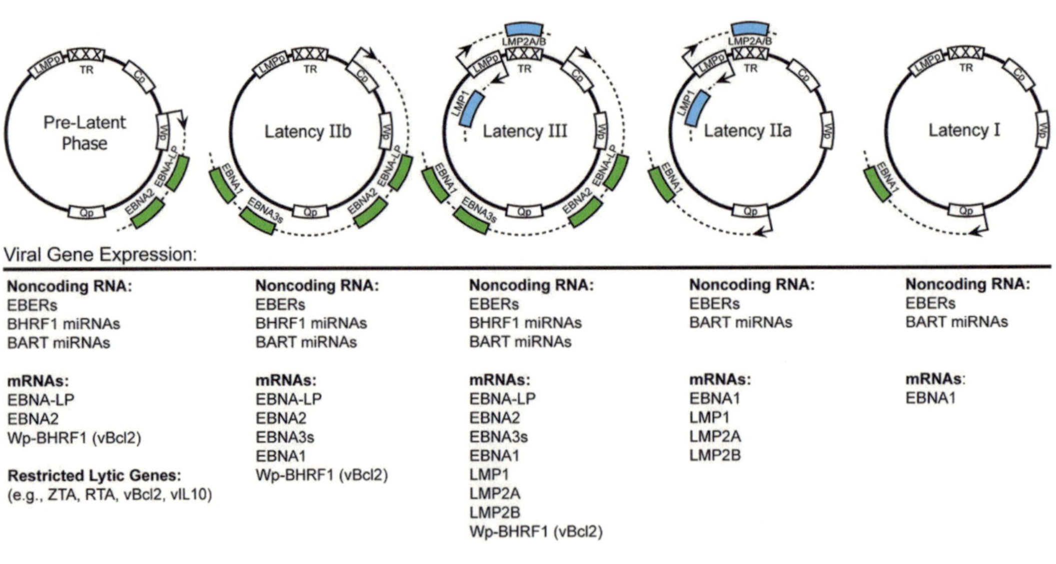

Figure 1. Gene expression patterns at different stages of EBV latency states. The theoretical progression of EBV latency gene expression from initial infection to true latency is described from left to right. The EBV genome is shown in episomal form closed at the terminal repeats (TR). Promoters are shown as white boxes and include the EBNA promoters Cp, Wp and Qp as well as the bidirectional LMPp. Primary mRNA transcripts are shown as dotted lines, while coding regions have been simplified as colored boxes. An expanded list of viral genes expressed in each latency state is listed directly underneath the representative schematic. Taken from [2] with permission.

functions [9, 10] (for review, see [3, 11]). The LMP-1 and -2 encode for transmembrane proteins with a plethora of oncogenic functions with conflicted results in gastric carcinoma (for review, see [12]). It has been proposed that variations in its sequences might be related to phylogeographic diversity of EBV-associated gastric carcinoma (EBVaGC) strains worldwide [13]. Taken together, EBV latent genes not only define the type of latency but also are associated with oncogenic transformation, immune evasion and the genetic diversity of EBVaGC.

2. Gastric cancer: novel molecular classifications

The molecular bases of gastric cancer have begun to be unraveled by a comprehensive molecular evaluation of primary tumors [14–20]. As shown in **Figure 2**, the Cancer Genome Atlas (TCGA) network has proposed a novel molecular classification of gastric carcinoma that recognized for the first time a subtype of tumor positive for Epstein-Barr virus, the EBV-associated gastric carcinoma (EBVaGC). This novel subtype of gastric cancer is characterized by frequent PIK3CA gene mutations, amplification of JAK2, CD274 (PD-L1) and PDCD1LG2 (PD-L2), and a unique CpG island methylator phenotype (CIMP) [14, 21].

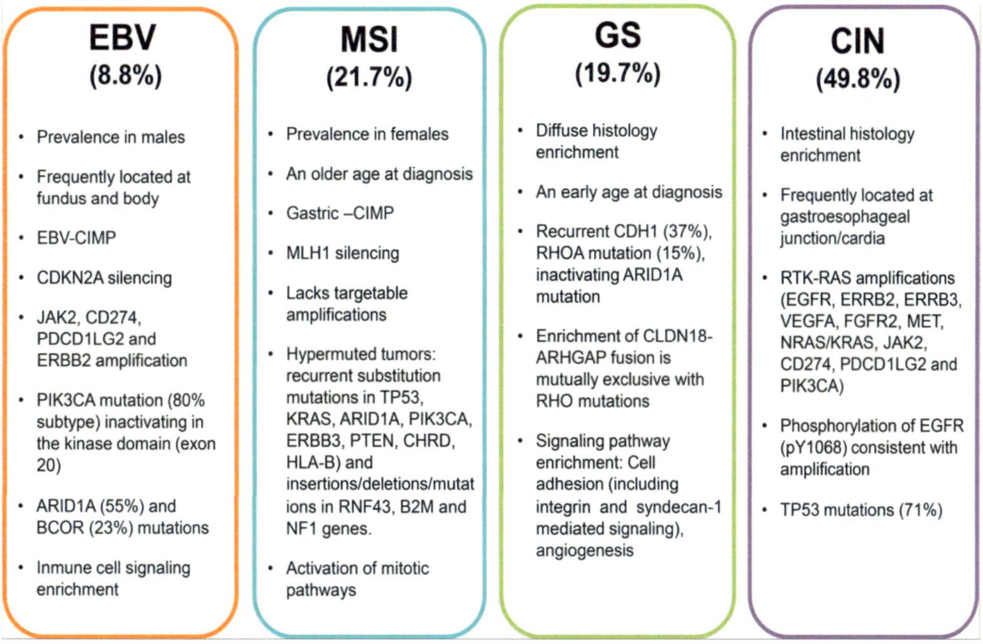

Figure 2. Major features of molecular classification of gastric cancer as proposed by the tumor cancer genome atlas (TCGA) are CIMP: CpG island methylator phenotype, EBV: Epstein-Barr virus, MSI: microsatellite instability, GS: genomically stable and CIN: chromosomal instability. Taken from [20] with permission.

3. EBV-associated gastric carcinoma: the Americas' perspective

Worldwide studies show higher EBVaGC prevalence in the Americas than in Asia [22]. These observations suggest a phylogeographic diversity of Epstein-Barr virus strains along with host and environmental associations [13]. In the Americas, the first report of gastric tumors positive for Epstein-Barr virus comes from Shibata and coworkers [23] (**Figure 3**). These authors, based on the histological resemblance between rare variant of undifferentiated gastric carcinomas with intense lymphoid infiltration (so-called lymphoepithelioma-like carcinoma [LELC]) and nasopharyngeal lymphoepithelioma, a well-established EBV-associated disease, detected EBV sequences in seven of eight LELC cases. EBV genomes were uniformly present only in carcinoma cells but not in reactive lymphoid infiltrate or normal gastric mucosa. Furthermore, the presence of a single genotype in each LELC cell was consistent with a clonal process, suggesting that EBV infection occurs before malignant transformation. Later, the same group expanded these findings to conventional gastric cancer, detecting EBV sequences in 22 of 138 (16%) cases [24]. In all these cases, the EBV genome was expressed, exclusively in gastric tumor cells. No EBV sequences were detected in surrounding lymphocytes, or precancerous lesions such as intestinal metaplasia and chronic gastritis. In addition, EBVaGC cases were most often detected in males than in females (p = 0.007). To define the clinicopathological characteristics of this novel molecular

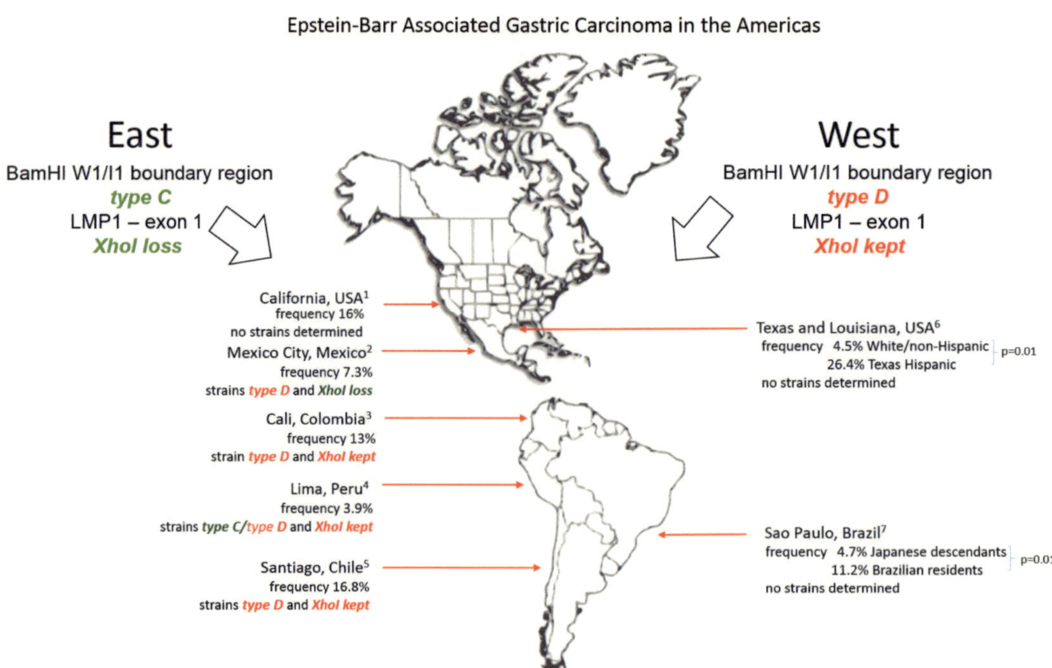

Figure 3. A consolidated overview of EBVaGC in the Americas. Phylogeographic diversity of EBV strains along with host and environmental associations might explain the high incidence of EBVaGC in the Americas [24–31].

subtype of gastric cancer, a long-term, well-characterized cohort of Japanese-Americans living in Hawaii [32, 33] was evaluated. Unfortunately, beyond male predominance, no other clinicopathological characteristic, including survival, was found [32]. A high incidence of EBVaGC has been reported in Santiago, Chile, with 31 (16.8%) EBV-positive cases identified among 185 consecutive gastric cancer patients [25]. In this series, associations with the diffuse-type histology ($p < 0.001$) and nonantrum location ($p = 0.01$) were the most significant findings. Among Mexican descendants living in the USA, Gulley and coworkers and Vo and coworkers have reported 20 out of 138 (14.5%) EBVaGC cases [26, 27]. Interestingly, prevalence of EBV was 26.4% among Mexican descendants in comparison with 4.5% among white/non-Hispanic cases. In addition, male predominance was found exclusively in those with Hispanic ancestry ($p = 0.01$) [27]. Koriyama et al. [28] examined 151 non–Japanese-Brazilian and 149 Japanese-Brazilian gastric carcinoma cases to identify an 11.2% prevalence among non–Japanese-Brazilian but only 4.7% among Japanese-Brazilian residents ($p = 0.01$). EBV-associated gastric carcinoma was predominant in males only in the non–Japanese-Brazilian cases ($p = 0.047$). Taken together, these findings suggest human phylogeographic diversity in the prevalence of EBVaGC.

Among other countries in Latin America, Carrascal et al. [29], in Cali, Colombia, examined 178 consecutive gastric carcinoma cases identifying 23 (13%) cases of EBVaGCs. In this series, EBVaGC also revealed a male ($p = 0.004$) and nonantrum ($p = 0.009$) predominance. Herrera-Goepfert et al. [30] identified 24 of 330 (7.3%) cases in Mexico City. In this series, no male predominance was confirmed, although all cases were of diffuse-type histology. The lowest frequency reported in Latin America was in Peru, where 254 gastric cancer cases from Japanese descendants were evaluated by Yoshiwara et al. [31]. In this analysis, only 3.9% (10 cases) of EBV infection was found, with no male or histological subtype predominance detected. A consolidated overview of EBVaGC in the Americas is shown in **Figure 3**.

A recent meta-analysis estimated a prevalence of 11.49% (95% CI = 8.46–15.43), with high heterogeneity among the aforementioned studies ($I2 = 73.3\%$; $p < 0.001$). Although heterogeneity for predominant sex, location and histology was low ($I2 = 16.5\%$ [$p = 0.35$], 0% [$p = 0.68$] and 33.7% [$p = 0.16$], respectively), these authors showed male predominance ($p < 0.001$) and diffuse-type histology ($p < 0.001$) as the most significant features of EBVaGC in the Americas (**Figures 4** and **5**) [13].

In Asia, low prevalence of EBV-associated gastric carcinoma has been described. The reported prevalence ranges from 6.1% in Northern China [34] to 9.1% in Southern China [35]. In Japan and Korea, the reported prevalence is 6.6 and 6.9%, respectively [35, 36]. Among European countries, Russia and the Republics of the former Soviet Union, 8.7% prevalence has been reported [37]. Interestingly, distribution of EBV-positive GCs by sex, site and histological type was similar to that in Japan. In a study carried out in Holland, EBV was detected in 7.2% of the gastric carcinomas from the Dutch D1D2 trial (N = 566; mean follow-up, 9 years) [38]. In France, only 5.8% of 85 cases of gastric adenocarcinomas were EBV-associated adenocarcinomas, from which 4 cases were of the intestinal histological type [39].

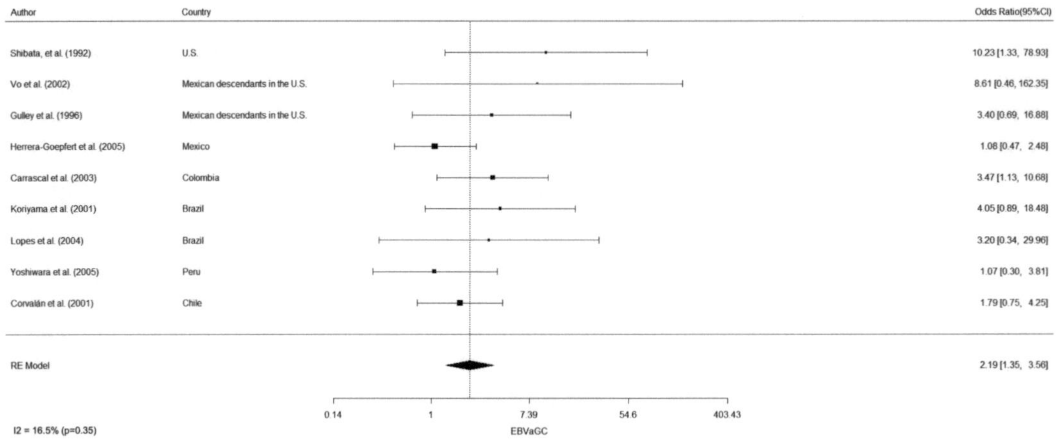

Figure 4. An estimated odds ratio (95% CI) for male predominance of EBV-associated gastric cancer in the Americas. Meta-analyses were performed by a random effects model with the inverse variance method, using the DerSimonian-Laird estimator, a logit transformation and the Clopper-Pearson confidence interval for individual studies. The results are shown in a log-scale. Taken from [4] with permission.

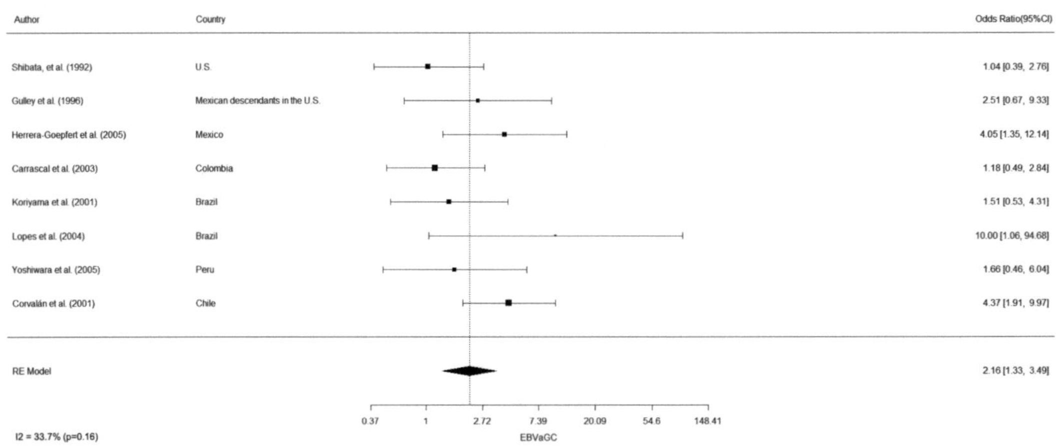

Figure 5. An estimated odds ratio (95% CI) for diffuse-type histology of EBV-associated gastric carcinoma in the Americas. Meta-analyses were performed by a random effects model with the inverse variance method, using the DerSimonian-Laird estimator, a logit transformation and the Clopper-Pearson confidence interval for individual studies. The results are shown in a log-scale. Taken from [13] with permission.

4. EBV strains and EBV-associated gastric carcinoma

Previous restriction fragment length polymorphism (RFLP) studies and the recently completed genome sequencing of 31 viruses head to the first global approach of the diversity of EBV. Seven of these sequences were obtained from healthy donors or benign lesions and twenty-five from strains present in tumors including nine EBVaGC [40–44]. By this approach, the genome diversity of EBV can be classified into five types (A–F). A substitution of 1.8 kb in the C-terminal part of the EBNA-2 gene defines types A and B [45]. Subtype A is the most common strain in the West and in Asia, while subtype B is the most common one in Africa [45, 46]. Polymorphisms at

BamHI W1/I1 boundary region identify C and D subtypes. The lack of the BamHI site defines subtype C that predominates in Asia among healthy people and EBV-associated diseases [47–50]. On the other hand, the presence of the BamHI restriction site defines subtype D that prevails in the West [47, 51]. Lastly, polymorphism at BamHI site identifies subtype F with worldwide distribution. However, the presence of an extra site defines the "f" variant and is found only in cases of nasopharyngeal carcinomas (NPC) [52]. Two more variants of EBV associated with the LMP-1 gene have been described. Polymorphisms at XhoI restriction site in position 169,425 of the LMP-1 gene define Western and Asian strains. Healthy people and EBV-associated diseases in Asia lack the XhoI restriction site [47], while in Western countries, the presence of the XhoI site is frequent [53]. The second variant in the LMP-1 gene is the deletion of 30-base pair at C-terminal (position 168,287–168,256) [54]. This variant confers an aggressive clinical behavior in Hodgkin's disease [55].

In the Americas, both polymorphisms at BamHI W1/I1 boundary region (C and D types) and XhoI RFLPs at exon 1 of the LMP-1 gene are present in healthy donors at similar proportions [56]. These authors also identified two unique novel recombinant strains (C type/kept XhoI site and D type/lack of XhoI site) [56]. As shown in **Figure 3**, these findings might reflect the mixing of different ethnic populations in this continent as has been reported in Texas and Louisiana, USA [26, 27] and Brazil [28]. Conversely of what has been found in Asian and Western countries, this mixing did not reflect in the case of EBVaGC, since almost all EBV strains studied in tumors harbored exclusively the western genotype (D type and kept XhoI site) (OR 16.3 [95% CI 2.5–685]) [56]. **Figure 3** shows a consolidated overview of phylogeographic diversity of Epstein-Barr virus strains in the Americas.

5. Epigenetic abnormalities of EBV-associated gastric carcinoma: DNA methylation

EBV-associated gastric cancer has been reported as the most extensive CpG island methylation at both human and viral genomes, being more extensive than any other tumor type from the TCGA network [14, 21, 57, 58]. CpG island methylation is an epigenetic mechanism of gene expression regulation, affecting all cellular pathways [59]. It consists of methyl groups attached to the 5′ position of cytosines, which are followed by a guanine nucleotide (CpG site) [60] (**Figure 6**). More than 50% of human genes contain CpG site in the promoter region and are known as CpG islands [62]. Methylation of CpG sites within a promoter region may inhibit the binding of transcription factors in their consensus sequence of tumor suppressor genes, thus precluding the transcription of the gene, and resulting in gene silencing [63]. Methylation of tumor suppressor genes is usually seen at early stages of gastric cancer and increases during the stomach carcinogenesis [64]. These observations suggest that the silencing of these genes by DNA methylation mechanisms plays an important role in the gastric carcinogenesis. In addition, aberrant methylation is unusually detected in EBVaGC nonneoplastic surrounding mucosa, which might indicate a critical role of EBV in tumorigenesis mechanisms [65]. Although the extensive CpG island methylation is present in EBVaGC, a distinctive pattern of methylation has been suggested, as promoter methylation of tumor suppressor gene CDKN2A, but not promoter methylation of MLH1,

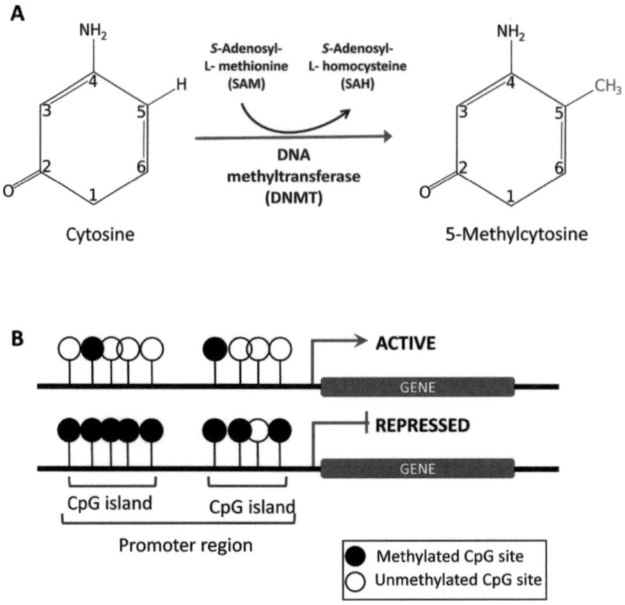

Figure 6. DNA methylation. (A) CpG methylation mechanism is mediated by DNA methyltransferases and consists in the addition of a methyl group to the carbon in the 5th position of cytosines that precedes guanine nucleotides. (B) CpG islands are DNA sequences rich in CpG sites (>50% CpG sites within a 200bp sequence). Methylation of CpG islands inside a promoter region may control gene expression.

characteristic of the microsatellite instability (MSI) GC subtype [21, 27, 66–71]. Individual methylation of p14ARF and p16INK4a, alternative reading frames of CDKN2A locus, has also been described, and many studies have proved a significant association between their methylation and EBV positivity [72, 73]. Ushiku et al. [74] observed a uniform methylation of all CpG sites on promoter regions of both genes in EBVaGC, whereas it was variable in EBV-negative tumors. In addition, methylation frequency of p16INK4a appears to be about three times higher in EBVaGC than in EBV-negative tumors [65, 75]. CDH1, p15 and p73 tumor suppressor genes are also frequently methylated in EBVaGC, representing one of the most common abnormalities described in this tumor [65, 74].

Despite EBV-induced host gene methylation in EBVaGC is well established, the exact underlying mechanisms are not entirely understood. It has been proposed that when the host cell detects the viral genome, it defends itself by starting a host-driven extensive methylation of the foreign genome, which may trigger the subsequent host genome methylation [75–77]. However, based on the specific methylation patterns observed, a possible participation of EBV in maintenance and de novo methylation has been proposed [72, 74]. Several studies have shown that EBV can modulate the expression of DNA methyltransferases (DNMT), which catalyze the transfer of methyl groups to DNA. Specifically, LMP-2A, EBV latent gene, has been shown to upregulate DNMT1 and DNMT3b expression in gastric cancer cell lines, which further induced methylation of several tumor suppressor genes, such as PTEN [78, 79]. Therefore, LMP-2A may play an essential role in the epigenetic abnormalities in host cells and in the development and maintenance of EBV-associated cancer.

http://dx.doi.org/10.5772/intechopen.70201

6. Epigenetic abnormalities of EBV-associated gastric carcinoma: microRNAs

MicroRNAs (miRNAs) are small (~22 nt) noncoding RNAs and fundamental in posttranscriptional regulation of a broad range of biological processes of different organisms. This fundamental regulation is achieved through specific complementary binding to the 3′ untranslated region (3′UTR) of one or more target mRNAs, allowing regulation of multiple genes simultaneously [80] (**Figure 7**). Increasing evidence has shown that dysregulation of specific miRNAs has a crucial role in tumorigenesis. In fact, microRNAs involved in this process are usually called oncomiRs and anti-oncomiRs, acting similar to onco- and tumor-suppressor genes [11]. Particularly, in gastric cancer, cellular miRNAs have gained special interest because they have shown differential expression between distinct cancer subtypes and have been related to progression and prognosis of the disease (for a review, see [80]). Viral microRNAs were first described in EBV [81]. It is now known that diverse virus families

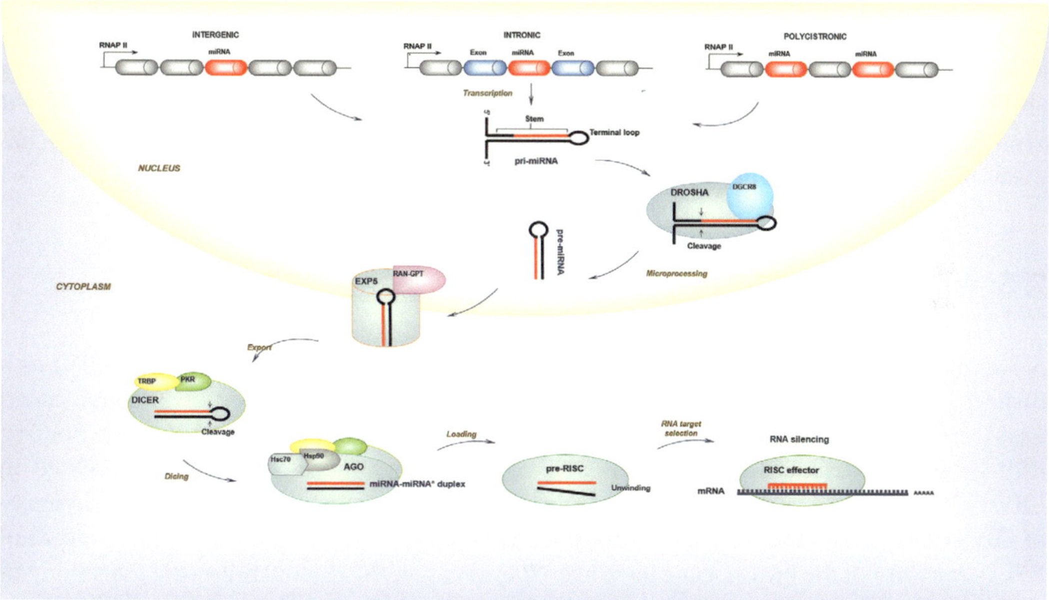

Figure 7. Canonical pathway of miRNA biogenesis in human. miRNAs are transcribed by RNA polymerase II (RNAP II) from intergenic, intronic or polycistronic loci to long primary transcript, called primary miRNA (pri-miRNA), which consists in a stem, a terminal loop and single-stranded RNA segments at both the 5′- and 3′-UTR sides. Microprocessor complex (Drosha and DGCR8 cofactor) cleaves the stem-loop and releases a small hairpin-shaped RNA, called precursor miRNA (pre-miRNA). Following, pre-miRNA is exported into the cytoplasm by the transport complex formed by protein exportin 5 (EXP5) and GTP-binding nuclear protein RAN•GTP. Subsequently, pre-miRNAs are cleaved by a ternary complex formed by dicer, TAR RNA-binding protein (TRBP) and protein activator of PKR (PACT), producing a small RNA duplexes (miRNA-miRNA*). Next, these are loaded onto an Argonaute protein (AGO) to form an immature RNA-induced silencing complex (RISC) or pre-RISC, in a process mediated for heat shock cognate 70 (Hsc70)-heat shock protein (Hsp90) chaperone complex. AGO protein separates the two strands to generate a mature RISC effector. Finally, RISC binds the target mRNA through complementary binding of six to eight base pairs of the miRNA, with a specific sequence of the target resulting in the gene silencing. Taken from [80] with permission.

encode miRNAs and that they are capable of targeting both cellular and viral genes [82]. EBV-miRNA expression is dependent on the host cellular miRNA processing machinery for its biogenesis. EBV miRNAs are encoded in two clusters within the EBV genome. As shown in **Figure 1**, the first cluster is localized in the Bam HI fragment H rightward open reading frame 1 (BHRF1) gene and originates four mature miRNAs, which express only during lytic infection and in latency type IIb/III [83]. The second cluster is localized among the Bam HI-A region rightward transcript (BART) gene, encoding 40 mature miRNAs [84], which are expressed in all EBV latency types [83]. However, variable expression patterns of BART miRNAs have been reported in different EBV-associated malignancies or cell types [83, 85]. Additionally, discrepant reports exist concerning specific BART miRNAs' relative expression within the same cellular context, which could be in part a result of different EBV strains studied [86–89]. Most BART miRNAs host targets, identified so far, are involved in proapoptotic and immune response pathways, suggesting a crucial role in promoting host cell survival [90]. For instance, EBVaGC highly expressed miRBART4-5p and miRBART5-5p that have been shown to target and downregulate the BH3-interacting domain death agonist (BID) protein [91] and the p53-upregulated modulator of apoptosis (PUMA) [92], respectively. Furthermore, EBV not only expresses its own miRNAs but also alters miRNAs' expression of the host cells. Particularly, miR-200 family has been shown to be consistently downregulated both in GC cell lines and in EBVaGC tumor samples compared to normal adjacent mucosa and other GC subtypes [93, 94]. Aberrant DNA methylation following EBV infection and viral proteins such as BRAF0, EBER, and LMP-2A have been proposed as the main mechanisms of downregulation of these miRNAs [93, 95].

7. Summary and conclusions

Novel molecular classifications and meta-analyses identified Epstein-Barr virus (EBV) as a distinct etiological agent for gastric cancer. An important characteristic of EBV-associated gastric carcinoma (EBVaGC) is the difference in incidence in Asia and the Americas. Specific EBV genes such as EBERs, EBNAs, BARTs and LMP are the most actively expressed in EBVaGC, and variations in its sequences might be associated with phylogeographic diversity of EBV strains across the world. Polymorphisms at BamHI W1/I1 boundary region and XhoI RFLPs at exon 1 of the LMP-1 gene have been found in healthy donors reflecting the mixing of different ethnic populations in the Americas. However, this is not the case for gastric cancer, since almost all types of EBVaGC studied harbor exclusively the western genotypes (subtype D and kept XhoI site). These findings propose that a disrupted coevolution between a pathogen and its healthy population might contribute to a phylogeographic origin of disease. DNA methylation and cellular and viral microRNAs play an emerging role in the pathogenesis of EBVaGC.

Disclaimer

The funders had no role in study design, data collection and analysis, decision to publish or preparation of the paper.

http://dx.doi.org/10.5772/intechopen.70201

Authors' contribution

Alejandra Alarcón: Conception or design of the work, data collection, data analysis and interpretation, drafting the article, critical revision of the article, final approval of the version to be published; Ursula Figueroa: Conception or design of the work, data collection, data analysis and interpretation, drafting the article, critical revision of the article, final approval of the version to be published; Bastian Espinoza: Conception or design of the work, data collection, data analysis and interpretation, drafting the article, critical revision of the article, final approval of the version to be published; Gonzalo Carrasco-Aviño: Conception or design of the work, data collection, data analysis and interpretation, drafting the article, critical revision of the article, final approval of the version to be published; Francisco R. Aguayo: Drafting the article, critical revision of the article, final approval of the version to be published; Alejandro H. Corvalan: Conception or design of the work, data collection, data analysis and interpretation, drafting the article, critical revision of the article, final approval of the version to be published.

Acknowledgements

This study was funded by Fondecyt grant nos. 1151411 and 1161219 from the Government of Chile.

Conflict of interest

The authors declare that there is no conflict of interest regarding the publication of this paper.

Author details

Alejandra Alarcón[1], Ursula Figueroa[1], Bastian Espinoza[1], Alejandra Sandoval[1], Gonzalo Carrasco-Aviño[1,2], Francisco R. Aguayo[1,3] and Alejandro H. Corvalan[1,4,5]*

*Address all correspondence to: corvalan@med.puc.cl

1 Advanced Center for Chronic Diseases (ACCDIS), Pontificia Universidad Catolica de Chile, Santiago, Chile

2 Department of Pathology, Faculty of Medicine, Universidad de Chile, Santiago, Chile

3 Department of Basic and Clinical Oncology, Faculty of Medicine, Universidad de Chile, Santiago, Chile

4 UC-Center for Investigational Oncology (CITO), Pontificia Universidad Catolica de Chile, Santiago, Chile

5 Department of Hematology and Oncology, School of Medicine, Pontificia Universidad Catolica de Chile, Santiago, Chile

References

[1] Stanfield BA, Luftig MA. Recent advances in understanding Epstein-Barr virus. F1000Research. 2017;6:386. DOI: 10.12688/f1000research.10591.1

[2] Price AM, Luftig MA. To be or not IIb: a multi-step process for Epstein-Barr virus latency establishment and consequences for B cell tumorigenesis. PLoS Pathogens. 2015;11:e1004656. DOI: 10.1371/journal.ppat.1004656

[3] Tsao SW, Tsang CM, To KF, Lo KW. The role of Epstein-Barr virus in epithelial malignancies. The Journal of Pathology. 2015;235:323-333. DOI: 10.1002/path.4448

[4] Weiss LM, Chen YY. EBER in situ hybridization for Epstein-Barr virus. Methods in Molecular Biology. 2013;999:223-230. DOI: 10.1007/978-1-62703-357-2_16

[5] Sivachandran N, Wang X, Frappier L. Functions of the Epstein-Barr virus EBNA1 protein in viral reactivation and lytic infection. Journal of Virology. 2012;86:6146-6158. DOI: JVI.00013-12 [pii]

[6] Malik-Soni N, Frappier L. Proteomic profiling of EBNA1-host protein interactions in latent and lytic Epstein-Barr virus infections. Journal of Virology. 2012;86:6999-7002. DOI: 10.1128/jvi.00194-12

[7] Shire K, Wong AI, Tatham MH, Anderson OF, Ripsman D, Gulstene S, Moffat J, Hay RT, Frappier L. Identification of RNF168 as a PML nuclear body regulator. Journal of Cell Science. 2016;129:580-591. DOI: 10.1242/jcs.176446

[8] Skalsky RL, Cullen BR. EBV noncoding RNAs. Current Topics in Microbiology and Immunology. 2015;391:181-217. DOI: 10.1007/978-3-319-22834-1_6

[9] Marquitz AR, Mathur A, Nam CS, Raab-Traub N. The Epstein-Barr virus BART microRNAs target the pro-apoptotic protein Bim. Virology. 2011;412:392-400. DOI: S0042-6822(11)00042-0 [pii]

[10] Marquitz AR, Mathur A, Edwards RH, Raab-Traub N. Host gene expression is regulated by two types of noncoding RNAs transcribed from the Epstein-Barr virus BamHI a rightward transcript region. Journal of Virology. 2015;89:11256-11268 DOI: JVI.01492-15 [pii]

[11] Shinozaki-Ushiku A, Kunita A, Fukayama M. Update on Epstein-Barr virus and gastric cancer (review). International Journal of Oncology. 2015;46:1421-1434. DOI: 10.3892/ijo.2015.2856

[12] Kang MS, Kieff E. Epstein-Barr virus latent genes. Experimental & Molecular Medicine. 2015;47:e131. DOI: 10.1038/emm.2014.84

[13] Carrasco-Avino G, Riquelme I, Padilla O, Villaseca M, Aguayo FR, Corvalan AH. The conundrum of the Epstein-Barr virus-associated gastric carcinoma in the Americas. Oncotarget. 2017.DOI: 10.18632/oncotarget.18497

[14] Bass AJ. Comprehensive molecular characterization of gastric adenocarcinoma. Nature. 2014;513:202-209 DOI: nature13480 [pii]10.1038/nature13480

[15] Cristescu R, Lee J, Nebozhyn M, Kim KM, Ting JC, Wong SS, Liu J, Yue YG, Wang J, Yu K, Ye XS, Do IG, Liu S, et al. Molecular analysis of gastric cancer identifies subtypes associated with distinct clinical outcomes. Natural Medicine. 2015;21:449-456. DOI: nm.3850 [pii]10.1038/nm.3850

[16] Liu N, Liu X, Zhou N, Wu Q, Zhou L, Li Q. Gene expression profiling and bioinformatics analysis of gastric carcinoma. Experimental and Molecular Pathology. 2014;96:361-366. DOI: S0014-4800(14)00022-7 [pii]10.1016/j.yexmp.2014.02.007

[17] Shah MA, Khanin R, Tang L, Janjigian YY, Klimstra DS, Gerdes H, Kelsen DP. Molecular classification of gastric cancer: A new paradigm. Clinical Cancer Research. 2011;17:2693-2701. DOI: 1078-0432.CCR-10-2203 [pii]10.1158/1078-0432.CCR-10-2203

[18] Lei Z, Tan IB, Das K, Deng N, Zouridis H, Pattison S, Chua C, Feng Z, Guan YK, Ooi CH, Ivanova T, Zhang S, Lee M, et al. Identification of molecular subtypes of gastric cancer with different responses to PI3-kinase inhibitors and 5-fluorouracil. Gastroenterology. 2013;145:554-565. DOI: S0016-5085(13)00722-1 [pii]10.1053/j.gastro.2013.05.010

[19] Tan IB, Ivanova T, Lim KH, Ong CW, Deng N, Lee J, Tan SH, Wu J, Lee MH, Ooi CH, Rha SY, Wong WK, Boussioutas A, et al. Intrinsic subtypes of gastric cancer, based on gene expression pattern, predict survival and respond differently to chemotherapy. Gastroenterology. 2011;141:476-485, 85 e1-11. DOI: S0016-5085(11)00597-X [pii]

[20] Riquelme I, Saavedra K, Espinoza JA, Weber H, Garcia P, Nervi B, Garrido M, Corvalan AH, Roa JC, Bizama C. Molecular classification of gastric cancer: Towards a pathway-driven targeted therapy. Oncotarget. 2015;6((28)):24750-24779. DOI: 10.18632/oncotarget.4990

[21] Gulley ML. Genomic assays for Epstein-Barr virus-positive gastric adenocarcinoma. Experimental & Molecular Medicine. 2015;47:e134. DOI: emm201493 [pii]

[22] Camargo MC, Anderson WF, King JB, Correa P, Thomas CC, Rosenberg PS, Eheman CR, Rabkin CS. Divergent trends for gastric cancer incidence by anatomical subsite in US adults. Gut. 2011;60:1644-1649. DOI: gut.2010.236737 [pii]10.1136/gut.2010.236737

[23] Shibata D, Tokunaga M, Uemura Y, Sato E, Tanaka S, Weiss LM. Association of Epstein-Barr virus with undifferentiated gastric carcinomas with intense lymphoid infiltration: Lymphoepithelioma-like carcinoma. The American Journal of Pathology. 1991;139:469-474

[24] Shibata D, Weiss LM. Epstein-Barr virus-associated gastric adenocarcinoma. The American Journal of Pathology. 1992;140:769-774

[25] Corvalán AH, Koriyama C, Akiba S, Eizuru Y, Backhouse C, Palma M, Argandona J, Tokunaga M. Epstein-Barr virus in gastric carcinoma is associated with location in the cardia and with a diffuse histology: A study in one area of Chile. International Journal of Cancer. 2001;94:527-530. DOI: 10.1002/ijc.1510

[26] Gulley ML, Pulitzer DR, Eagan PA, Schneider BG. Epstein-Barr virus infection is an early event in gastric carcinogenesis and is independent of bcl-2 expression and p53 accumulation. Human Pathology. 1996;27:20-27

[27] Vo QN, Geradts J, Gulley ML, Boudreau DA, Bravo JC, Schneider BG. Epstein-Barr virus in gastric adenocarcinomas: Association with ethnicity and CDKN2A promoter methylation. Journal of Clinical Pathology. 2002;55:669-675

[28] Koriyama C, Akiba S, Iriya K, Yamaguti T, Hamada GS, Itoh T, Eizuru Y, Aikou T, Watanabe S, Tsugane S, Tokunaga M. Epstein-Barr virus-associated gastric carcinoma in Japanese Brazilians and non-Japanese Brazilians in Sao Paulo. Japanese Journal of Cancer Research. 2001;92:911-917

[29] Carrascal E, Koriyama C, Akiba S, Tamayo O, Itoh T, Eizuru Y, Garcia F, Sera M, Carrasquilla G, Piazuelo MB, Florez L, Bravo JC. Epstein-Barr virus-associated gastric carcinoma in Cali, Colombia. Oncology Reports. 2003;10:1059-1062

[30] Herrera-Goepfert R, Akiba S, Koriyama C, Ding S, Reyes E, Itoh T, Minakami Y, Eizuru Y. Epstein-Barr virus-associated gastric carcinoma: Evidence of age-dependence among a Mexican population. World Journal of Gastroenterology. 2005;11:6096-6103

[31] Yoshiwara E, Koriyama C, Akiba S, Itoh T, Minakami Y, Chirinos JL, Watanabe J, Takano J, Miyagui J, Hidalgo H, Chacon P, Linares V, Eizuru Y. Epstein-Barr virus-associated gastric carcinoma in Lima, Peru. Journal of Experimental and Clinical Cancer Research. 2005;24:49-54

[32] Shibata D, Hawes D, Stemmermann GN, Weiss LM. Epstein-Barr virus-associated gastric adenocarcinoma among Japanese Americans in Hawaii. Cancer Epidemiology, Biomarkers & Prevention. 1993;2:213-217

[33] Nomura AM, Stemmermann GN, Chyou PH. Gastric cancer among the Japanese in Hawaii. Japanese Journal of Cancer Research. 1995;86:916-923 DOI: 0910505095967854 [pii]

[34] Hao Z, Koriyama C, Akiba S, Li J, Luo X, Itoh T, Eizuru Y, Zou J. The Epstein-Barr virus-associated gastric carcinoma in southern and northern China. Oncology Reports. 2002;9:1293-1298

[35] Lee HS, Chang MS, Yang HK, Lee BL, Kim WH. Epstein-barr virus-positive gastric carcinoma has a distinct protein expression profile in comparison with Epstein-Barr virus-negative carcinoma. Clinical Cancer Research. 2004;10:1698-1705

[36] Koriyama C, Akiba S, Corvalán AH, Carrascal E, Itoh T, Herrera-Goepfert R, Eizuru Y, Tokunaga M. Histology-specific gender, age and tumor-location distributions of Epstein-Barr virus-associated gastric carcinoma in Japan. Oncology Reports. 2004;12:543-547

[37] Galetsky SA, Tsvetnov VV, Land CE, Afanasieva TA, Petrovichev NN, Gurtsevitch VE, Tokunaga M. Epstein-Barr-virus-associated gastric cancer in Russia. International Journal of Cancer. 1997;73:786-789. DOI: 10.1002/(SICI)1097-0215(19971210)73:6<786::AID-IJC2>3.0.CO;2-Z [pii]

[38] van Beek J, zur Hausen A, Klein Kranenbarg E, van de Velde CJ, Middeldorp JM, van den Brule AJ, Meijer CJ, Bloemena E. EBV-positive gastric adenocarcinomas: A distinct clinicopathologic entity with a low frequency of lymph node involvement. Journal of Clinical Oncology. 2004;22:664-670. DOI: 10.1200/jco.2004.08.061

[39] Kerroucha R, Hervieu V, Chambonniere ML, Mege-Lechevallier F, Poncet G, Boulez J, Taniere P, Scoazec JY. Adenocarcinomas of the stomach and distal esophagus. Incidence and phenotypic characteristics of EBV-associated cases in the Lyons area, France. Annales de Pathologie. 2004;24:228-235

[40] Liu Y, Yang W, Pan Y, Ji J, Lu Z, Ke Y. Genome-wide analysis of Epstein-Barr virus (EBV) isolated from EBV-associated gastric carcinoma (EBVaGC). Oncotarget. 2016;7:4903-4914. DOI: 6751 [pii]

[41] Baer R, Bankier AT, Biggin MD, Deininger PL, Farrell PJ, Gibson TJ, Hatfull G, Hudson GS, Satchwell SC, Seguin C, et al. DNA sequence and expression of the B95-8 Epstein-Barr virus genome. Nature. 1984;310:207-211

[42] de Jesus O, Smith PR, Spender LC, Elgueta Karstegl C, Niller HH, Huang D, Farrell PJ. Updated Epstein-Barr virus (EBV) DNA sequence and analysis of a promoter for the BART (CST, BARF0) RNAs of EBV. The Journal of General Virology. 2003;84:1443-1450. DOI: 10.1099/vir.0.19054-0

[43] Lei H, Li T, Hung GC, Li B, Tsai S, Lo SC. Identification and characterization of EBV genomes in spontaneously immortalized human peripheral blood B lymphocytes by NGS technology. BMC Genomics. 2013;14:804. DOI: 10.1186/1471-2164-14-8041471-2164-14-804 [pii]

[44] Santpere G, Darre F, Blanco S, Alcami A, Villoslada P, Mar Alba M, Navarro A. Genome-wide analysis of wild-type Epstein-Barr virus genomes derived from healthy individuals of the 1000 genomes project. Genome Biology and Evolution. 2014;6:846-860 DOI: evu054 [pii]

[45] Zimber U, Adldinger HK, Lenoir GM, Vuillaume M, Knebel-Doeberitz MV, Laux G, Desgranges C, Wittmann P, Freese UK, Schneider U, et al. Geographical prevalence of two types of Epstein-Barr virus. Virology. 1986;154:56-66

[46] Young LS, Yao QY, Rooney CM, Sculley TB, Moss DJ, Rupani H, Laux G, Bornkamm GW, Rickinson AB. New type B isolates of Epstein-Barr virus from Burkitt's lymphoma and from normal individuals in endemic areas. The Journal of General Virology. 1987;68(Pt 11):2853-2862. DOI: 10.1099/0022-1317-68-11-2853

[47] Lung ML, Chang RS, Jones JH. Genetic polymorphism of natural Epstein-Barr virus isolates from infectious mononucleosis patients and healthy carriers. Journal of Virology. 1988;62:3862-3866

[48] Lung ML, Chang GC. Detection of distinct Epstein-Barr virus genotypes in NPC biopsies from southern Chinese and Caucasians. International Journal of Cancer. 1992;52:34-37

[49] Sidagis J, Ueno K, Tokunaga M, Ohyama M, Eizuru Y. Molecular epidemiology of Epstein-Barr virus (EBV) in EBV-related malignancies. International Journal of Cancer. 1997;72:72-76. DOI: 10.1002/(SICI)1097-0215(19970703)72:1<72::AID-IJC11>3.0.CO;2-C [pii]

[50] Lung ML, Chang RS, Huang ML, Guo HY, Choy D, Sham J, Tsao SY, Cheng P, Ng MH. Epstein-Barr virus genotypes associated with nasopharyngeal carcinoma in southern China. Virology. 1990;177:44-53

[51] Abdel-Hamid M, Chen JJ, Constantine N, Massoud M, Raab-Traub N. EBV strain variation: Geographical distribution and relation to disease state. Virology. 1992;190:168-175 DOI: 0042-6822(92)91202-6 [pii]

[52] Lung ML, Lam WP, Sham J, Choy D, Yong-Sheng Z, Guo HY, Ng MH. Detection and prevalence of the "f" variant of Epstein-Barr virus in southern China. Virology. 1991;185:67-71 DOI: 0042-6822(91)90754-Y [pii]

[53] Khanim F, Yao QY, Niedobitek G, Sihota S, Rickinson AB, Young LS. Analysis of Epstein-Barr virus gene polymorphisms in normal donors and in virus-associated tumors from different geographic locations. Blood. 1996;88:3491-3501

[54] Wohlford EM, Asito AS, Chelimo K, Sumba PO, Baresel PC, Oot RA, Moormann AM, Rochford R. Identification of a novel variant of LMP-1 of EBV in patients with endemic Burkitt lymphoma in western Kenya. Infectious Agents and Cancer. 2013;8:34. DOI: 10.1186/1750-9378-8-34

[55] Santon A, Manzanal AI, Campo E, Bellas C. Deletions in the Epstein-Barr virus latent membrane protein-1 oncogene in Hodgkin's disease. Clinical Molecular Pathology. 1995;48:M184-M187

[56] Corvalán AH, Ding S, Koriyama C, Carrascal E, Carrasquilla G, Backhouse C, Urzua L, Argandona J, Palma M, Eizuru Y, Akiba S. Association of a distinctive strain of Epstein-Barr virus with gastric cancer. International Journal of Cancer. 2006;118:1736-1742. DOI: 10.1002/ijc.21530

[57] Zouridis H, Deng N, Ivanova T, Zhu Y, Wong B, Huang D, Wu YH, Wu Y, Tan IB, Liem N, Gopalakrishnan V, Luo Q, Wu J, et al. Methylation subtypes and large-scale epigenetic alterations in gastric cancer. Science Translational Medicine. 2012;4:156ra140. DOI: 4/156/156ra140 [pii]

[58] Loh M, Liem N, Vaithilingam A, Lim PL, Sapari NS, Elahi E, Mok ZY, Cheng CL, Yan B, Pang B, Salto-Tellez M, Yong WP, Iacopetta B, et al. DNA methylation subgroups and the CpG island methylator phenotype in gastric cancer: A comprehensive profiling approach. BMC Gastroenterology. 2014;14:55. DOI: 1471-230X-14-55 [pii]

[59] Cech TR, Steitz JA. The noncoding RNA revolution-trashing old rules to forge new ones. Cell. 2014;157:77-94. DOI: 10.1016/j.cell.2014.03.008

[60] Chen ZX, Riggs AD. DNA methylation and demethylation in mammals. The Journal of Biological Chemistry. 2011;286:18347-18353. DOI: 10.1074/jbc.R110.205286

[61] Collas P, Noer A, Timoskainen S. Programming the genome in embryonic and somatic stem cells. Journal of Cellular and Molecular Medicine. 2007;11:602-620. DOI: 10.1111/j.1582-4934.2007.00079.x

[62] Vavouri T, Lehner B. Human genes with CpG island promoters have a distinct transcription-associated chromatin organization. Genome Biology. 2012;13:R110. DOI: 10.1186/gb-2012-13-11-r110

[63] Padmanabhan N, Ushijima T, Tan P. How to stomach an epigenetic insult: The gastric cancer epigenome. Nature Reviews. Gastroenterology & Hepatology. 2017;14:467-478. DOI: 10.1038/nrgastro.2017.53

[64] Oue N, Mitani Y, Motoshita J, Matsumura S, Yoshida K, Kuniyasu H, Nakayama H, Yasui W. Accumulation of DNA methylation is associated with tumor stage in gastric cancer. Cancer. 2006;106:1250-1259. DOI: 10.1002/cncr.21754

[65] Akiba S, Koriyama C, Herrera-Goepfert R, Eizuru Y. Epstein-Barr virus associated gastric carcinoma: Epidemiological and clinicopathological features. Cancer Science. 2008;99:195-201 DOI: CAS674 [pii]

[66] Ryan JL, Jones RJ, Kenney SC, Rivenbark AG, Tang W, Knight ER, Coleman WB, Gulley ML. Epstein-Barr virus-specific methylation of human genes in gastric cancer cells. Infectious Agents and Cancer. 2010;5:27. DOI: 1750-9378-5-27 [pii]

[67] Ferrasi AC, Pinheiro NA, Rabenhorst SH, Caballero OL, Rodrigues MA, de Carvalho F, Leite CV, Ferreira MV, Barros MA, Pardini MI. Helicobacter pylori and EBV in gastric carcinomas: Methylation status and microsatellite instability. World Journal of Gastroenterology. 2010;16:312-319

[68] Bernal C, Vargas M, Ossandon F, Santibanez E, Urrutia J, Luengo V, Zavala LF, Backhouse C, Palma M, Argandona J, Aguayo F, Corvalán AH. DNA methylation profile in diffuse type gastric cancer: Evidence for hypermethylation of the BRCA1 promoter region in early-onset gastric carcinogenesis. Biological Research. 2008;41:303-315

[69] McCormick TM, Canedo NH, Furtado YL, Silveira FA, de Lima RJ, Rosman AD, Almeida Filho GL, Carvalho MG. Association between human papillomavirus and Epstein-Barr virus DNA and gene promoter methylation of RB1 and CDH1 in the cervical lesions: A transversal study. Diagnostic Pathology. 2015;10:59. DOI: 10.1186/s13000-015-0283-3

[70] He D, Zhang YW, Zhang NN, Zhou L, Chen JN, Jiang Y, Shao CK. Aberrant gene promoter methylation of p16, FHIT, CRBP1, WWOX, and DLC-1 in Epstein-Barr virus-associated gastric carcinomas. Medical Oncology 2015;32:92. DOI: 10.1007/s12032-015-0525-y

[71] Qu Y, Dang S, Hou P. Gene methylation in gastric cancer. Clinica Chimica Acta. 2013;424:53-65. DOI: 10.1016/j.cca.2013.05.002

[72] Chong JM, Sakuma K, Sudo M, Ushiku T, Uozaki H, Shibahara J, Nagai H, Funata N, Taniguchi H, Aburatani H, Fukayama M. Global and non-random CpG-island methylation in gastric carcinoma associated with Epstein-Barr Virus. Cancer Science. 2003;94:76-80

[73] Geddert H, Zur Hausen A, Gabbert HE, Sarbia M. EBV-infection in cardiac and non-cardiac gastric adenocarcinomas is associated with promoter methylation of p16, p14 and APC, but not hMLH1. Analytical cellular pathology (Amsterdam). 2010;33:143-149. DOI: 10.3233/acp-clo-2010-0540

[74] Ushiku T, Chong JM, Uozaki H, Hino R, Chang MS, Sudo M, Rani BR, Sakuma K, Nagai H, Fukayama M. p73 gene promoter methylation in Epstein-Barr virus-associated gastric carcinoma. International Journal of Cancer. 2007;120:60-66. DOI: 10.1002/ijc.22275

[75] Kang GH, Lee S, Kim WH, Lee HW, Kim JC, Rhyu MG, Ro JY. Epstein-barr virus-positive gastric carcinoma demonstrates frequent aberrant methylation of multiple genes and constitutes CpG island methylator phenotype-positive gastric carcinoma. The American Journal of Pathology. 2002;160:787-794. DOI: S0002-9440(10)64901-2 [pii]10.1016/S0002-9440(10)64901-2

[76] Zong L, Seto Y. CpG island methylator phenotype, helicobacter pylori, Epstein-Barr virus, and microsatellite instability and prognosis in gastric cancer: A systematic review and meta-analysis. PLoS One 2014;9:e86097. DOI: 10.1371/journal.pone.0086097

[77] Kaneda A, Matsusaka K, Aburatani H, Fukayama M. Epstein-Barr virus infection as an epigenetic driver of tumorigenesis. Cancer Research. 2012;72:3445-3450. DOI: 0008-5472.CAN-11-3919 [pii]10.1158/0008-5472.CAN-11-3919

[78] Hino R, Uozaki H, Murakami N, Ushiku T, Shinozaki A, Ishikawa S, Morikawa T, Nakaya T, Sakatani T, Takada K, Fukayama M. Activation of DNA methyltransferase 1 by EBV latent membrane protein 2A leads to promoter hypermethylation of PTEN gene in gastric carcinoma. Cancer Research. 2009;69:2766-2774. DOI: 0008-5472.CAN-08-3070 [pii]10.1158/0008-5472.CAN-08-3070

[79] Zhao J, Liang Q, Cheung KF, Kang W, Lung RW, Tong JH, To KF, Sung JJ, Yu J. Genome-wide identification of Epstein-Barr virus-driven promoter methylation profiles of human genes in gastric cancer cells. Cancer. 2013;119:304-312. DOI: 10.1002/cncr.27724

[80] Sandoval-Borquez A, Saavedra K, Carrasco-Aviño G, Garcia-Bloj B, Fry J, Wichmann I, Corvalan AH. Noncoding genomics in gastric cancer and the gastric precancerous cascade: Pathogenesis and biomarkers. Disease Markers. 2015;2015:14. DOI: 10.1155/2015/503762

[81] Pfeffer S, Zavolan M, Grasser FA, Chien M, Russo JJ, Ju J, John B, Enright AJ, Marks D, Sander C, Tuschl T. Identification of virus-encoded microRNAs. Science. 2004;304:734-736. DOI: 10.1126/science.1096781

[82] Grundhoff A, Sullivan CS. Virus-encoded microRNAs. Virology. 2011;411:325-343. DOI: 10.1016/j.virol.2011.01.002

[83] Klinke O, Feederle R, Delecluse HJ. Genetics of Epstein-Barr virus microRNAs. Seminars in Cancer Biology. 2014;26:52-59. DOI: 10.1016/j.semcancer.2014.02.002

[84] Kozomara A, Griffiths-Jones S. miRBase: Annotating high confidence microRNAs using deep sequencing data. Nucleic Acids Research. 2014;42:D68-D73. DOI: 10.1093/nar/gkt1181

[85] Lung RW, Tong JH, To KF. Emerging roles of small Epstein-Barr virus derived non-coding RNAs in epithelial malignancy. International Journal of Molecular Sciences. 2013;14:17378-17409 DOI: ijms140917378 [pii]

[86] Edwards RH, Marquitz AR, Raab-Traub N. Epstein-Barr virus BART microRNAs are produced from a large intron prior to splicing. Journal of Virology. 2008;82:9094-9106. DOI: 10.1128/jvi.00785-08

[87] Kim do N, Chae HS, Oh ST, Kang JH, Park CH, Park WS, Takada K, Lee JM, Lee WK, Lee SK. Expression of viral microRNAs in Epstein-Barr virus-associated gastric carcinoma. Journal of Virology. 2007;81:1033-1036. DOI: JVI.02271-06 [pii]10.1128/JVI.02271-06

[88] Marquitz AR, Mathur A, Chugh PE, Dittmer DP, Raab-Traub N. Expression profile of microRNAs in Epstein-Barr virus-infected AGS gastric carcinoma cells. Journal of Virology. 2014;88:1389-1393 DOI: JVI.02662-13 [pii]

[89] Treece AL, Duncan DL, Tang W, Elmore S, Morgan DR, Dominguez RL, Speck O, Meyers MO, Gulley ML. Gastric adenocarcinoma microRNA profiles in fixed tissue and in plasma reveal cancer-associated and Epstein-Barr virus-related expression patterns. Laboratory Investigation. 2016;96:661-671. DOI: 10.1038/labinvest.2016.33

[90] Kang D, Skalsky RL, Cullen BR. EBV BART MicroRNAs target multiple pro-apoptotic cellular genes to promote epithelial cell survival. PLoS Pathogens. 2015;11:e1004979. DOI: 10.1371/journal.ppat.1004979

[91] Shinozaki-Ushiku A, Kunita A, Isogai M, Hibiya T, Ushiku T, Takada K, Fukayama M. Profiling of virus-encoded MicroRNAs in Epstein-Barr virus-associated gastric carcinoma and their roles in gastric carcinogenesis. Journal of Virology. 2015;89:5581-5591 JVI.03639-14 [pii]

[92] Choy EY, Siu KL, Kok KH, Lung RW, Tsang CM, To KF, Kwong DL, Tsao SW, Jin DY. An Epstein-Barr virus-encoded microRNA targets PUMA to promote host cell survival. The Journal of Experimental Medicine. 2008;205:2551-2560. DOI: 10.1084/jem.20072581

[93] Shinozaki A, Sakatani T, Ushiku T, Hino R, Isogai M, Ishikawa S, Uozaki H, Takada K, Fukayama M. Downregulation of microRNA-200 in EBV-associated gastric carcinoma. Cancer Research. 2010;70:4719-4727. DOI: 10.1158/0008-5472.can-09-4620

[94] Du Y, Xu Y, Ding L, Yao H, Yu H, Zhou T, Si J. Down-regulation of miR-141 in gastric cancer and its involvement in cell growth. Journal of Gastroenterology. 2009;44:556-561. DOI: 10.1007/s00535-009-0037-7

[95] Yau TO, Tang CM, Yu J. Epigenetic dysregulation in Epstein-Barr virus-associated gastric carcinoma: Disease and treatments. World Journal of Gastroenterology. 2014;20:6448-6456. DOI: 10.3748/wjg.v20.i21.6448

Chapter 3

Neuroendocrine Tumors of the Stomach: Gastric Apudomas

Alfredo José Afonso Barbosa

Additional information is available at the end of the chapter

http://dx.doi.org/10.5772/intechopen.69722

Abstract

Anatomo-clinical studies of the neuroendocrine tumors of the stomach only can be well completed with a view of the basic characteristics of the elements of the so-called neuroendocrine system or gastrointestinal APUD system. Therefore, these gastric neoplasias cannot be studied in isolation because they are derived from a special line of endocrine cells that have many common biochemical bonds which are often involved in the clinical behavior of the tumor. These cells are called "APUD" for their biochemical and morphological characteristics, and their tumors as "apudomas." APUD cells store amines and regulatory peptides and are dispersed throughout the body and concentrated mainly in the digestive tract. Other names used for tumors of the same cell line, namely, "carcinoids," "endocrine tumors," and "neuroendocrine tumors," are not yet very well defined, although they are ostensibly used. The gastric apudomas do not escape of the basic rules of behavior of their counterparts of other sites of the digestive tract. Nevertheless, most of them present peculiar pathogenetic and pathophysiological characteristics whose knowledge is important to better understand the patient with this type of lesion.

Keywords: neuroendocrine tumors, gastric apudomas, gastric carcinoids, atrophic body gastritis, APUD cells

1. Introduction

Gastrointestinal neuroendocrine tumors make up a group of heterogeneous neoplasms of somewhat unpredictable biological and clinical behavior. These tumors arise mainly in the digestive tract but can occur in other organs that harbor neuroendocrine cells. They are considered complex tumors and of unpredictable clinical evolution due to the variety of attributes that they possess as the potential capacity of secretion of a large variety of peptides.

Although they may appear benign tumors for a certain period of time, they can originate tissue infiltration and give metastasis. All these pathophysiological attributes of neuroendocrine tumors, which may occur in varying degrees of intensity in different patients, arouse general interest, and so they are studied by professionals from different expertise. In this chapter, we will turn to the study of some relevant aspects of these tumors that originate in the stomach. However, since these neoplasias are part of a large family of gastrointestinal tumors, we will carry out a summary review of the main attributes of this family which should be useful to better understand some nuances of these tumors which originate in the stomach.

2. General aspects of neuroendocrine gastrointestinal system

The terms "neuroendocrine tumors," "carcinoid tumors," and "endocrine tumors" are widely used when referring to tumors of the digestive tract. These designations can be found simultaneously even as part of the same classification. Neuroendocrine tumors were firstly called as "carcinoid tumors" by the German pathologist Oberndorfer, in 1907 [1]. And until now, the term carcinoid has been used ostensibly, colloquially, and even in almost all current classifications [2, 3].

The term "apudoma" may also be considered as being a synonym of carcinoid tumor. The denomination of "APUD cells" was proposed by Pearse in the late 1960s as an acronym of *amine precursor uptake and decarboxylation* [4]. The term APUD summarizes some of the most important characteristics of these cells, which are (a) a high amine content and/or amine precursor uptake, (b) amino acid decarboxylase activity, and (c) characteristic ultrastructural pattern. Initially, the term "apudoma" was used mainly from the clinical point of view to designate those tumors of symptomatic patients due to the pathological secretion of bioactive products and afterward also for clinically asymptomatic tumors originating from APUD cells [5–7]. As we can see, unlike the roots of the other designations for these tumors, the term "apudoma" has been derived from consistent morphologic and biochemical basis.

Apudomas are derived from the APUD cell line and so they have characteristic ultrastructural pattern recognized due the presence in the tumor cells of secretory granules where the regulatory peptides are located as well as the biogenic amines that they produce [8, 9]. Normally, the APUD cells are rich in amino acid decarboxylase, which gives them the ability to capture 5-hydroxytryptophan and dihydroxyphenylalanine and produce, respectively, serotonin and dopamine. Although this property has not been demonstrated in all the cells morphologically characteristic of this system, this biochemical link may occur in all of them whatever their specific function is. This gives these cells a familial, morphological, and biochemical bond, which extends to a greater or lesser degree to the apudomas. In addition, these morphological and biochemical characteristics give to the term "APUD" a biologically more specific designation compared to the other denominations. Thus, the term "apudoma" is less vulnerable to temporal changes than those currently used, namely, "carcinoid," "endocrine tumor," and "neuroendocrine tumor." The latter denomination is being adopted in this article because of its extensive use in modern classifications and also throughout the medical literature indexing.

2.1. Tumor sites and staining

One of the first steps, both in pathology and clinics, when we are faced with the possibility to do the diagnosis of a gastrointestinal apudoma, is the knowledge of its possible primary location (**Table 1**). It may seem like an unimportant detail, but this can be very valuable as a first step to better understand the biology of the tumor [10, 11].

Sometimes, we deal with an unknown primary site metastasis. But knowing which segment of the digestive tract derives the tumor may be helpful because this information gives an idea on the possible evolution of the apudoma. Regarding the gastric apudomas, this is a crucial knowledge as we will see later on. In addition, the pathologist gains confidence in the study of the diagnostic possibilities, including for the evaluation which stain techniques or which neuroendocrine marker should be used [12]. Most of the gastric apudomas do not produce serotonin and are negative for argentaffin staining; on the other hand, they usually are positive for argyrophilic and chromogranin staining (**Figure 1**). These properties of apudoma, in relation to certain staining techniques, often depend on their place of origin (**Table 2**) [13–15].

Currently, immunohistochemistry techniques have been used as tools of choice for the specific histologic diagnosis of apudomas. Through this methodology, it is sought to mark the presence of antigenic products typical of APUD cells and also frequently present in apudomas (**Figures 2** and **3**). Neuron-specific enolase (NSE) was the first immunohistochemical marker for histological diagnosis of apudomas [16]. Before the discovery of this marker, the most commonly available methods were silver staining. Synaptophysin is also a neuroendocrine marker, located on the membrane of the synaptic vesicles, and present in neurons, neuroendocrine cells and in many neuroendocrine tumors [17, 18]. Chromogranins comprise a group of acidic polypeptides that make up about 40–50% of the soluble protein content of the suprarenal medullar granules. The chromogranin A is the most widespread; it is present in varying amounts in the secretion granules of neuroendocrine cells and in neuroendocrine tumors [15, 18]. If the tumor is less differentiated and with fewer secretory granules in the cytoplasm, the staining can give doubtful results or even a false-negative reaction. Chromogranin is one of the main markers used for the histological diagnosis of gastric apudomas presenting high index of sensitivity and specificity. It is also tentatively used as a serologic marker of apudoma evolution [19]. It is always appropriate to remember that the antibodies used against apudoma antigens are derived from different clones and are provided by different companies. This may result in differences in sensitivity and specificity of each set of reagents, and these different properties must be under the control of each laboratory.

Foregut	Midgut	Hindgut
Esophagus	Jejunum/ileum	Distal colon
Stomach	Appendix	Rectosigmoid
Duodenum	Cecum	

Apudomas can arise in any region of the gastrointestinal tract. These regions are known as foregut, midgut, and hindgut. Apudomas from these different sites frequently present different clinical behaviors.

Table 1. Primary sites of the gastrointestinal apudomas.

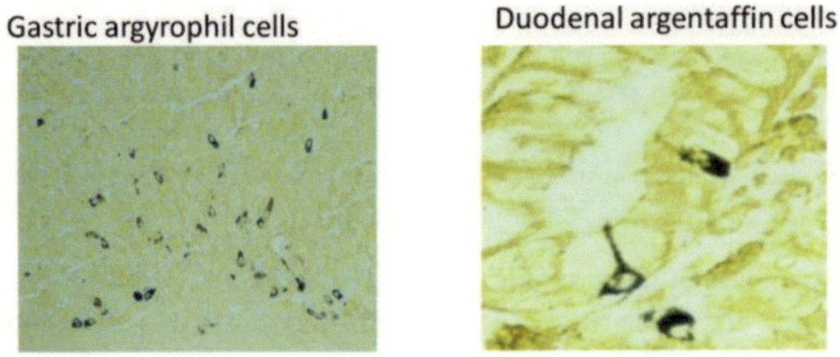

Figure 1. Although it is nonspecific staining for APUD cells and apudomas, the argentaffin and argyrophilic stains may be useful for the demonstration of these elements [13].

Gastrointestinal apudomas and silver staining properties			
	Foregut	**Midgut**	**Hindgut**
Argyrophilic tumors	+++	+++	++
Argentaffin tumors	+	+++	+

+, seldomly positive; ++, sometimes negative; +++, much frequently positive

Table 2. Almost all the gastric apudomas are demonstrated by argyrophilic staining and/or by argentaffin methods.

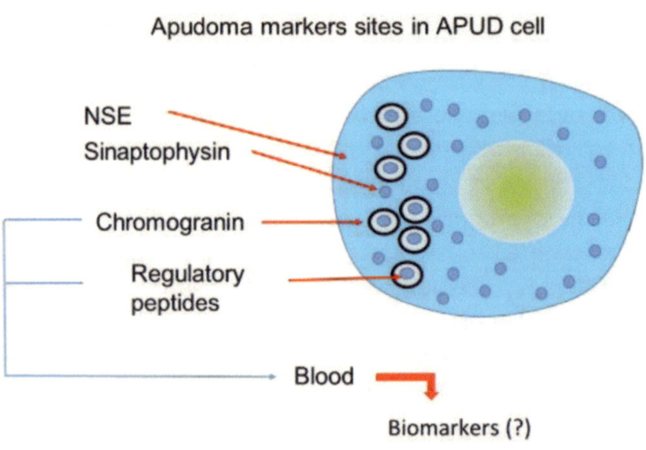

Figure 2. Some of the neuroendocrine markers are scattered in the cytoplasm of apudoma cells such as PGP 9.5, synaptophysin, and neuron specific enolase. Chromogranin and the regulatory peptides are stored in secretory granules. The amount of these granules in the neoplastic cells will determine weaker or stronger staining of the tumor.

2.2. General view on pathology of gastrointestinal apudomas

We have now reached a point which concerns more directly the attending physician. Since the apudomas frequently present unpredictable clinical evolution, how could the histopathology help on this matter? In fact, all the factors shown in **Table 3** are important to evaluate the possible clinical behavior of a given gastrointestinal apudoma. However, the two first, i.e., degree

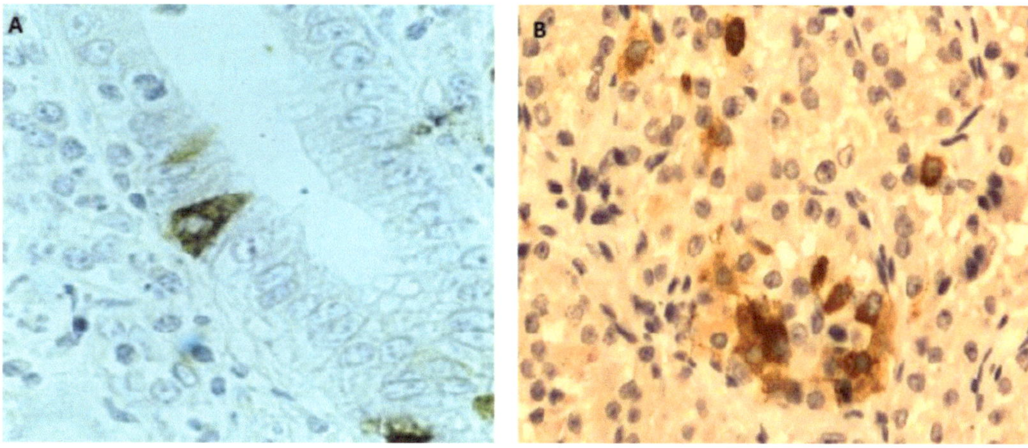

Figure 3. (A) G cell of the gastric mucosa stained specifically with antibody against gastrin. The staining is very specific by observing that the background elements, i.e., other cells and surrounding tissues, are completely negative. The very strong contrast between the positive and negative elements of tissue confers confidence of the final result in relation to the specificity of the staining reaction. (B) The staining contrast is not always very clear in regard to apudomas which may exhibit cells with various degrees of differentiation. A variable number of neoplastic cells with low secretory granule density could present a dubious or completely negative reaction. As a result, a given gastrinoma may exhibit cells strongly reactive to the gastrin antibody alongside others completely negative.

of histologic tumor differentiation and the proliferative activity of the neoplastic cells, depend exclusively on the pathologist interpretation. And unlikely, the last four parameters shown in **Table 3** depend on the opinion of different expert professionals to reach more reliable conclusions about the clinical course of the tumor.

In general pathology, the degree of differentiation of a given epithelial tumor, evaluated by histology, has always been, and still is, a criterion that together with other ones, gives an idea about the grade of malignancy that a particular carcinoma must have: a less aggressive evolution, more common among the well-differentiated ones, or a more aggressive evolution more common in those poorly differentiated (**Figure 4**). This histopathological criterion continues to be applied

PATHOLOGY (Histopathology)	Tumor histopathology Well differenciated Pourly differenciated
	Proliferative activity
IMAGE METHODS ENDOSCOPY SURGERY PATHOLOGY	Primary tumor site
	Tumor size
	Degree of tumor infiltration
	Metastasis (TNM Classification)

Table 3. Main criteria to determine the malignant potential of the apudoma.

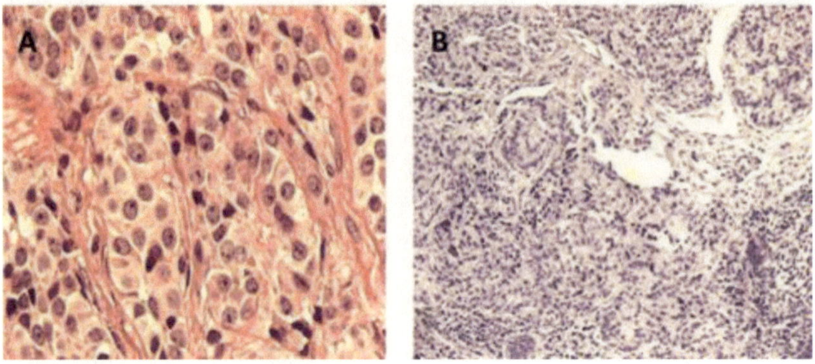

Figure 4. Well-differentiated type 1 (A) and poorly differentiated type 2 (B) gastric apudomas. Although the degree of tumor differentiated could have some importance regarding the degree of malignancy, the proliferative activity remains as a better histopathological indicator for this purpose.

mainly in relation to the nonendocrine carcinomas. Concerning the apudomas, this parameter, as an isolated element, has little value. Differently, the well-differentiated apudoma can present unpredictable clinical behavior. However, when the tumor is histologically poorly differentiated, the prognosis is often worse. In this respect, this criterion of cellular differentiation may be helpful. In addition, apudomas present varying densities of membrane receptors for different regulatory peptides, including somatostatin. And, a high density of these receptors in apudoma cells acquires current medical importance for the patient treatment. Some data indicate that the somatostatin receptor density would be dependent on the degree of tumor grade [20].

Under the view of histopathological diagnosis, the malignancy potential of a particular apudoma rests mainly on the degree of tumor cell proliferation. This criterion can be applied to all apudomas regardless of their origin. There are two histopathological tools to assess the degree of cell proliferation: (i) the number of observable mitoses in the routine preparations stained by *hematoxylin* and *eosin* and (ii) the index of cell immunoreactivity for Ki-67 antibody. The Ki-67 reactive protein is only expressed in the nucleus of cells that are in the various phases of the active cell replication cycle. This protein is not expressed in resting cells, that is, the cells that have not yet entered the active mitotic cycle. Moreover, there is not always any correspondence between the degree of differentiation of a given apudoma and the degree of cell proliferation [21, 22].

Concerning proliferative activity, the low-grade (G1) tumors present very few numbers of mitosis in routine HE preparation or otherwise less than 3% of neoplastic cells stained by Ki-67 antibody. The high-grade (G3) tumors should present more than 20 mitoses per 10 microscopic high-power field (hpf) or more than 20% of the neoplastic cells positive to Ki-67 antibody. Finally, tumors with intermediate degree of cell proliferation that lie between these two extremes are considered to be G2.

2.3. Gastric apudomas

Almost all apudomas of the stomach are derived from the endocrine cells of the body mucosa and rarely from the endocrine cells of the antral mucosa. They represent approximately 2–4% of all gastric neoplasias and 7.2% of all apudomas of the gastrointestinal tract [10].

In recent decades, there has been evidence that favors believing in an increase in the incidence of gastric apudomas. To a great extent, this increase must be occurring due to the technological evolution of the instruments connected to endoscopy of the upper digestive tract because these tumors are mostly often discovered incidentally during endoscopy. However, a real increase in the prevalence of these tumors cannot be ruled out [11, 23, 24].

The apudomas of the stomach are generally divided into three different groups based on their clinical and physiopathological characteristics: type 1, apudomas of the stomach associated with atrophic body gastritis (ABG), with or without pernicious anemia; type 2, apudomas of the stomach associated with Zollinger-Ellison syndrome, sporadic or familial; and type 3, sporadic apudoma not associated with known predisposing disease [25].

2.4. Gastric apudoma type 1

These are the most frequent gastric neuroendocrine tumors. They are characteristically associated with atrophic body gastritis (ABG) and are the most frequent of the gastric apudomas constituting about 70–80% of them. The criterion adopted for the classification of these tumors in type 1 is the recognition of the presence of established chronic autoimmune gastritis, with or without pernicious anemia, or just the presence of atrophic body gastritis confirmed by histopathology. This type of tumor appears to be more prevalent in women as well as the prevalence of the underlying disease (**Figure 5**).

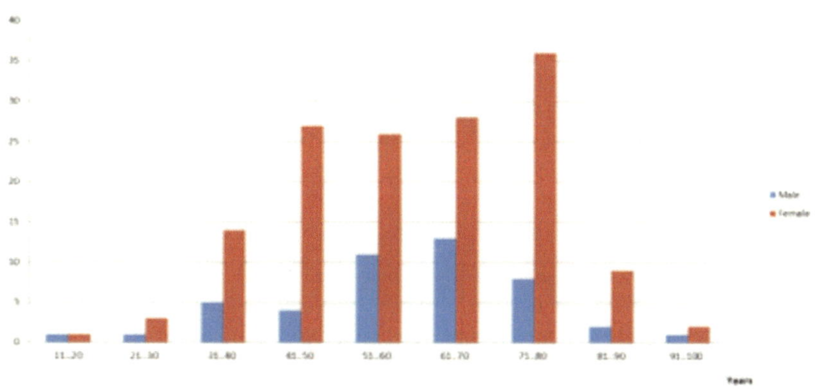

Figure 5. Distribution of 196 consecutive patients with atrophic body gastritis according to the age and gender. Patients were from a general hospital in Belo Horizonte, Brazil [26].

Therefore, it can be assumed that this type of tumor is a direct consequence of the atrophic body gastritis. According to this diagnostic criterion, we can conclude that the different types of apudomas of the stomach cannot be diagnosed based only on their endoscopic and histopathological pattern. Therefore, for the inclusion or exclusion of a gastric apudoma as type 1, it is necessary that in addition to histological samples of the tumor itself we also have samples of the gastric mucosa of the antral and body regions of the stomach to confirm or rule out the possibility of atrophic body gastritis. Recognizing an endocrine tumor as type 1 opens a range of possibilities to better understand the set of pathophysiological changes that may be occurring in the patient:

a. Gastric apudoma type 1 occurs in the mucosa of the fundus or the gastric body generally as multiple nodules, smaller than 1 cm in most cases. As they are generally multiple, they may occur according to an irregular distribution in the gastric body, the gastric fundus, or in the two regions simultaneously (**Table 4**). Usually, these nodules are projected into the lumen of the stomach and are frequently diagnosed by endoscopy as "gastric polyps." This diagnosis is not always incorrect because in ABG hyperplastic polyps are relatively frequent.

b. The neoplasia usually consists of well-differentiated neuroendocrine cells with a low Ki-67 index (G1) indicating low levels of cell proliferation. This characteristic is in agreement with the indolent evolution of these tumors; only a small number of them present metastases when diagnosed and rarely take the patient to death (**Table 4**).

c. Due to atrophy of the oxyntic mucosa these patients present hypochlorhydria or achlorhydria.

d. Since the gastric mucosa of the corpus is atrophic and the antral mucosa is preserved, the G cells are usually hyperfunctioning, and these patients frequently present hypergastrinemia (**Table 4** and **Figure 6**).

e. Even without the occurrence of high levels of serum gastrin, the constant trophic stimuli of this hormone will lead to hyperplasia of the endocrine cells of the gastric body. These hyperplastic cells are believed to be enterochromaffin-like (ECL) cells. However, other types of neuroendocrine cells may be participating in this hyperplastic process, including ghrelin-producing cells [26]. The areas of neuroendocrine cell hyperplasia can be found in almost all cases of well-established atrophic body gastritis (**Figures 7–9**). As we have already said, these areas of endocrine hyperplasia occur along the atrophic mucosa and according to their morphological aspect can be classified as (i) diffuse, (ii) linear, and (iii) nodular [27].

f. Based on these general aspects of atrophic body gastritis, it is possible to conclude that the areas of neuroendocrine hyperplasia are probably the precursor lesion of type 1 gastric apudoma. However, there are no histological signs that highlight where the hyperplasia ends and where the neoplasm begins. In this regard, the large, confluent hyperplastic nodules with a diameter about 300–500 μm associated with infiltration of mucosa tissues would already be classified as indicative of emerging neoplastic lesion (**Figure 9**). Just for comparison, 500 μm is equivalent, on average, to half thickness of normal oxyntic mucosa in formalin-fixed histologic sections.

g. The infiltration of the submucosa by the hyperplastic endocrine cells is already a sign of malignant behavior. However, for the most part, these type 1 gastric apudomas present indolent evolution, and few of them present metastasis at the time of diagnosis (**Table 4**).

2.5. Gastric apudoma type 2

Type 2 gastric apudomas are those associated with sporadic or familial Zollinger-Ellison syndrome. They account for only 5–6% of the gastric apudomas. Almost always these tumors

	Type 1	Type 2	Type 3
Frequency (%)	70–80	5–10	10–15
Endoscopic view	Multiple and small	Multiple and small	Single (>2 cm)
Site	Gastric body/fundus	Gastric body/fundus	Any region
Cellular proliferation index	G1	G1/G2	G3
Gastrinemia	Generally high	Generally high	Normal
Metastasis (%)	2–5	10–30	50–100

Table 4. Differential profiles between the three groups of gastric apudomas.

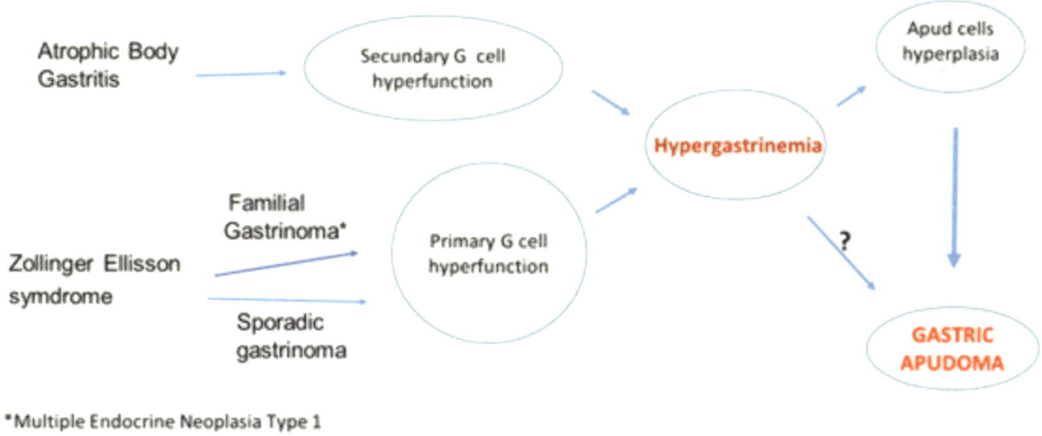

Figure 6. Drawing showing the pathogenetic mechanisms of the gastric apudomas type 1 and type 2. The pathophysiological central mechanism associated with these two types of tumors is the occurrence of hypergastrinemia or a persistent supra-basal gastrinemia.

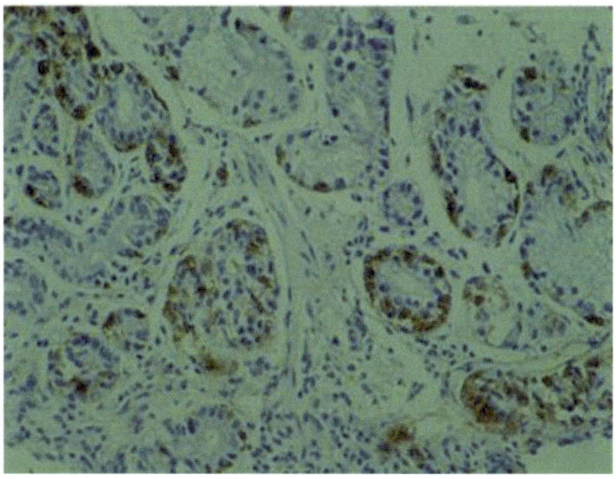

Figure 7. Diffuse and linear types of endocrine cell hyperplasia in atrophic body gastritis. The hyperplastic cells are stained for chromogranin.

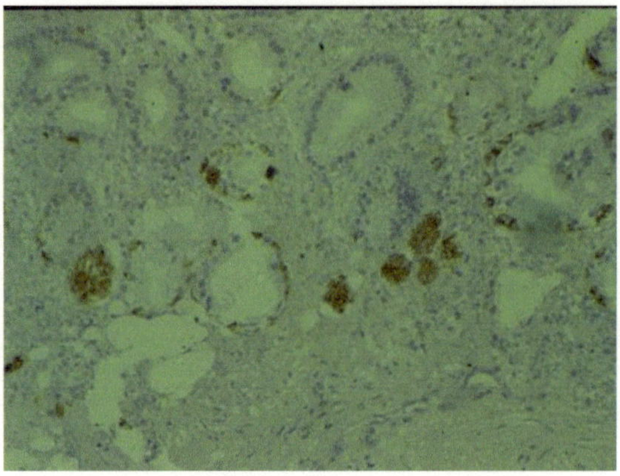

Figure 8. Nodular type of endocrine cell hyperplasia in atrophic body gastritis. The hyperplastic cells form small nodules in the lamina propria. Chromogranin staining.

occur in patients with multiple endocrine neoplasia (MEN) type 1. Rarely, there is also a Zollinger-Ellison syndrome (ZES) not associated with multiple endocrine neoplasia (MEN) which leads to gastric apudoma development. In this case the ZES may be due to the presence of a sporadic gastrinoma, the main location of which is believed to be the tail of the pancreas. Thus, most frequently, the patient presenting a type 2 gastric apudoma may be a carrier of the genetic transmission of MEN syndrome. MEN-1 is an inherited autosomal dominant syndrome caused by an inactivating mutation of the MEN-1 gene, which is a tumor suppressor gene. MEN-1 syndrome may include the development of primary hyperparathyroidism, pancreatic islet tumors, and pituitary adenomas. In addition, some patients may develop other neoplasms such as thyroid tumors, adrenal adenomas, pheochromocytomas, and neuroendocrine tumors mainly of the gastroduodenal area.

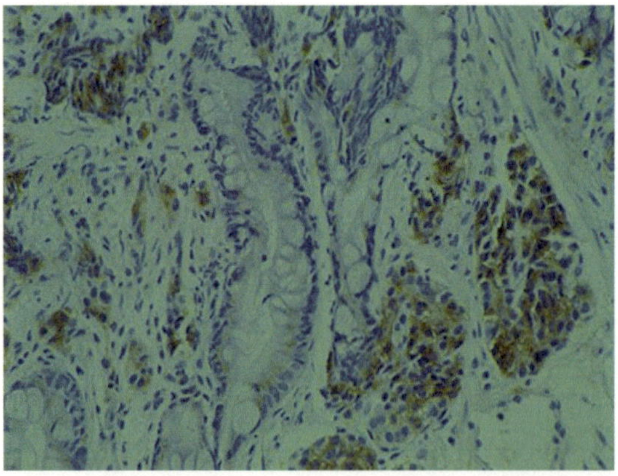

Figure 9. Endocrine cell forming large hyperplastic nodules in the lamina propria. This type of lesions may be indicative of an emerging gastric apudoma. As these tumors may be multicentric, it is possible that more strongly suspected lesions occur in other areas of the gastric mucosa. Chromogranin staining.

2.6. Gastric apudoma type 3

Type 3 gastric apudomas are known as sporadic gastric tumors, representing about 10–15% of all gastric apudomas, and develop independently hypergastrinemia as well as gastric endocrine cell hyperplasia (**Table 4**). More frequently they present as a single polypoid tumor usually greater than 2 cm in size [28]. These tumors are composed mainly by enterochromaffin-like cells, and differently from the other gastric apudoma, they have an aggressive clinical evolution. These tumors present histopathological signs corresponding to the clinical evolution of worse prognosis such as angioinvasion, rapid growth, mitotic activity, and high Ki-67 index.

Author details

Alfredo José Afonso Barbosa

Address all correspondence to: ajabarbosa@uol.com.br

Faculdade de Medicina, Universidade Federal de Minas Gerais, Belo Horizonte, Brazil

References

[1] Oberndorfer S. Karzinoide Tumoren des Dunndarms. Frankfurter Zeitschrift für Pathologie. 1907;**1**:426-429 (German)

[2] Kloppel G. Classification and pathology of gastroenteropancreatic neuroendocrine neoplasms. Endocrine-related Cancer. 2011 Oct;**18**(Suppl 1):S1-S16. PubMed PMID: 22005112

[3] Pinchot SN, Holen K, Sippel RS, Chen H. Carcinoid tumors. Oncologist. 2008 Dec;**13**(12): 1255-1269. PubMed PMID: 19091780. Pubmed Central PMCID: 2901509

[4] Pearse AG. Common cytochemical and ultrastructural characteristics of cells producing polypeptide hormones (the APUD series) and their relevance to thyroid and ultimobranchial C cells and calcitonin. Proceedings of the Royal Society of London Series B, Biological Sciences. 1968 May 14;**170**(1018):71-80. PubMed PMID: 4384885

[5] Temple WJ, Sugarbaker EV, Ketcham AS. The APUD system and its apudomas. International Advances in Surgical Oncology. 1981;4:255-276. PubMed PMID: 6114040

[6] Nakano PH, Bloom RR, Brown BC, Gray SW, Skandalakis JE, Kibbe JM. Apudomas. American Surgeon. 1987 Sep;**53**(9):505-509. PubMed PMID: 2820286

[7] Whitwam JG. APUD cells and the apudomas. A concept relevant to anaesthesia and endocrinology. Anaesthesia. 1977 Oct;**32**(9):879-888. PubMed PMID: 23705

[8] Pearse AG. The cytochemistry and ultrastructure of polypeptide hormone-producing cells of the APUD series and the embryologic, physiologic and pathologic implications of the concept. The Journal of Histochemistry and Cytochemistry : Official Journal of the Histochemistry Society. 1969 May;**17**(5):303-313. PubMed PMID: 4143745

[9] Fujita T, Kobayashi S. Structure and function of gut endocrine cells. International Review of Cytology Supplement. 1977;**6**:187-233. PubMed PMID: 25850

[10] Maggard MA, O'Connell JB, Ko CY. Updated population-based review of carcinoid tumors. Annals of Surgery. 2004 Jul;**240**(1):117-122. PubMed PMID: 15213627. Pubmed Central PMCID: 1356383

[11] Yao JC, Hassan M, Phan A, Dagohoy C, Leary C, Mares JE, et al. One hundred years after "carcinoid": epidemiology of and prognostic factors for neuroendocrine tumors in 35,825 cases in the United States. Journal of Clinical Oncology : Official Journal of the American Society of Clinical Oncology. 2008 Jun 20;**26**(18):3063-3072. PubMed PMID: 18565894

[12] Titlbach M, Chejfec G, Grimelius L, Falkmer S. Neuroendocrine background of the pathology of the islets of Langerhans. A minireview with particular reference to synaptophysin and chromogranin A as neuroendocrine markers and to the ontogeny of argyrophil insulin immunoreactive cells in the rabbit. Experimental and Clinical Endocrinology. 1987 Aug;**89**(3):242-250. PubMed PMID: 3117578

[13] Wilander E, Grimelius L, Lundqvist G, Skoog V. Polypeptide hormones in argentaffin and argyrophil gastroduodenal endocrine tumors. The American Journal of Pathology. 1979 Aug;**96**(2):519-530. PubMed PMID: 224707. Pubmed Central PMCID: 2042450

[14] Wilander E, Sundstrom C, Grimelius L. Pernicious anaemia in association with argyrophil (Sevier-Munger) gastric carcinoid. Scandinavian Journal of Haematology. 1979 Nov;**23**(5):415-420. PubMed PMID: 94457

[15] Oberg K. Gastric neuroendocrine cells and secretory products. The Yale Journal of Biology and Medicine. 1998 May-Aug;**71**(3-4):149-154. PubMed PMID: 10461347. Pubmed Central PMCID: 2578979

[16] Tapia FJ, Polak JM, Barbosa AJ, Bloom SR, Marangos PJ, Dermody C, et al. Neuron-specific enolase is produced by neuroendocrine tumours. Lancet. 1981 Apr 11;**1**(8224):808-811. PubMed PMID: 6111674

[17] Redecker P, Grube D. Synaptophysin in the nervous system and endocrine cells [Synaptophysin im Nervensystem und in endokrinen Zellen]. Acta Histochemica Supplement. 1992;**42**:33-38. PubMed PMID: 1584984

[18] Erickson LA, Lloyd RV. Practical markers used in the diagnosis of endocrine tumors. Advances in Anatomic Pathology. 2004 Jul;**11**(4):175-189. PubMed PMID: 15220821

[19] Kidd M, Bodei L, Modlin IM. Chromogranin A: Any relevance in neuroendocrine tumors? Current Opinion in Endocrinology, Diabetes, and Obesity. 2016 Feb;**23**(1):28-37. PubMed PMID: 26627724

[20] Wada H, Matsuda K, Akazawa Y, Yamaguchi Y, Miura S, Ueki N, et al. Expression of somatostatin receptor type 2A and PTEN in neuroendocrine neoplasms is associated with tumor grade but not with site of origin. Endocrine Pathology. 2016 Sep;**27**(3):179-187. PubMed PMID: 27256098

[21] Miller HC, Drymousis P, Flora R, Goldin R, Spalding D, Frilling A. Role of Ki-67 proliferation index in the assessment of patients with neuroendocrine neoplasias regarding the stage of disease. World Journal of Surgery. 2014 Jun;**38**(6):1353-1361. PubMed PMID: 24493070

[22] Lee HE, Mounajjed T, Erickson LA, Wu TT. Sporadic gastric well-differentiated neuroendocrine tumors have a higher Ki-67 proliferative index. Endocrine Pathology. 2016 Sep;**27**(3):259-267. PubMed PMID: 27306997

[23] Ellis L, Shale MJ, Coleman MP. Carcinoid tumors of the gastrointestinal tract: Trends in incidence in England since 1971. The American Journal of Gastroenterology. 2010 Dec;105(12):2563-2569. PubMed PMID: 20823835

[24] Ito T, Sasano H, Tanaka M, Osamura RY, Sasaki I, Kimura W, et al. Epidemiological study of gastroenteropancreatic neuroendocrine tumors in Japan. Journal of Gastroenterology. 2010 Feb;**45**(2):234-243. PubMed PMID: 20058030

[25] Rindi G, Luinetti O, Cornaggia M, Capella C, Solcia E. Three subtypes of gastric argyrophil carcinoid and the gastric neuroendocrine carcinoma: A clinicopathologic study. Gastroenterology. 1993 Apr;**104**(4):994-1006. PubMed PMID: 7681798

[26] Barbosa AJA, Miranda CG. Atrophic body gastritis: A challenge for the presumptive endoscopic and histologic diagnosis of autoimmune gastritis. In: Pascu O, editor. Gastrointestinal Endoscopy. Rijeka, Croatia: InTech; 2011. pp. 169-182

[27] Solcia E, Fiocca R, Villani L, Luinetti O, Capella C. Hyperplastic, dysplastic, and neoplastic enterochromaffin-like-cell proliferations of the gastric mucosa. Classification and histogenesis. American Journal of Surgical Pathology. 1995;19(Suppl 1):S1-S7. PubMed PMID: 7762735

[28] Scherubl H, Cadiot G, Jensen RT, Rosch T, Stolzel U, Kloppel G. Neuroendocrine tumors of the stomach (gastric carcinoids) are on the rise: Small tumors, small problems? Endoscopy. 2010 Aug;**42**(8):664-671. PubMed PMID: 20669078

Chapter 4

Impact of Stem Cell Genes in Gastric Cancer

Estefania Carrasco-Garcia, Mikel García-Puga,
Manuel Moreno, Nicolas Sampron,
Sara Arevalo and Ander Matheu

Additional information is available at the end of the chapter

http://dx.doi.org/10.5772/intechopen.69776

Abstract

Gastric cancer remains one of the leading causes of global cancer mortality. It has been shown that gastric cancer may originate from adult gastric stem cells and that it contains a subpopulation of cancer cells with stem cell characteristics, which are linked to *Helicobacter pylori* infection, therapy resistance and metastasis. Thus, the identification of transcription factors and related signal transduction pathways that regulate stem cell maintenance and lineage allocation is attractive from a clinical standpoint in that it may provide targets for novel cell- or drug-based therapies. This chapter summarizes the role of several important stem cell factors in gastric cancer biology.

Keywords: cancer stem cells, gastric cancer, SOX genes, *Helicobacter pylori*

1. Introduction

Gastric adenocarcinoma (GC) is the second most common cause of cancer-related mortality in the world, with developing countries being the most affected regions [1, 2]. GC is a complex disease influenced by different environmental and genetic factors. Among them, *Helicobacter pylori* (*H. pylori*) is the main etiological agent of gastrointestinal infections in children and adults and the prevalence of infection varies considerably across different geographical regions [3]. Natural acquisition of *H. pylori* infection occurs, for the most part, in childhood [4]. Infection with *Helicobacter pylori* (*H. pylori*) promotes chronic inflammation and sequential histological changes of chronic active gastritis, atrophic gastritis, intestinal metaplasia, dysplasia and ultimately invasive carcinoma [2]. Symptomatic diseases occur in approximately 10% of infected individuals, and in these cases, the risk of gastric adenocarcinoma is higher in persons carrying certain strain types as, for example, those that contain cagA or vacA alleles [1].

Gastric cancer accounts for around 10% of all new cancers (one million per year), and it is the second leading cause of cancer death globally (700,000 deaths per year). The prognosis of CG is very poor, with a survival rate below 30% at 5 years post diagnosis [1, 2]. It is usually asymptomatic or causes nonspecific symptoms at early stages. When symptoms appear, the cancer has usually reached an advanced stage and there is presence of metastasis, being this dissemination a main cause of the severe prognosis. GC-associated high mortality is the result of its silent nature and the extremely high heterogeneity exhibited between individuals and also within gastric tumors. This heterogeneity involves, at the molecular level, a broad variety of gene mutations, amplifications and/or expression alterations, diverse DNA methylation profiles and differences in the activation or inactivation of particular signaling pathways. Thus, in the last years there has been substantial progress in the elucidation of the genomic landscape of GC due to advances in high-throughput technologies and the effort of international consortiums. Consequently, gastric cancer has been recently reclassified and stratified into several distinct subtypes based on molecular and genetic/epigenetic alterations [5, 6]. In particular, GCs have been classified according to defined genetic signatures, the status of *TP53* and the presence of microsatellite instability [5, 6]. Importantly, the heterogeneity in GC involves critical consequences in terms of differential response to therapy, resistance and recurrence [6]. Nevertheless, current therapeutic strategies in GC are not adapted to GC heterogeneity and depend on the stage of the tumor. Clinically, first-line treatment consists of surgical resection (except in cases with advanced metastasis), followed by chemotherapy with cytostatic agents such as cisplatin, 5-fluorouracil (5-FU), taxanes or irinotecan, or in combinations as ECF (epirubicin, cisplatin and 5-FU) and 5-FU plus docetaxel or cisplatin (or irinotecan) [1, 7]. These treatments have been internationally and generally accepted and used since last century. In the case of metastatic dissemination, patients whose tumors exhibit high levels of HER2 receptor expression also receive Trastuzumab, a monoclonal antibody against HER2. Initially, patients respond to chemotherapy, but cancer cells eventually become resistant, facilitating the occurrence of relapses. Even with the increase in survival facilitated by the incorporation of chemotherapy, the median overall survival of patients with CG remains low, being one of the survivals associated with cancer lower.

It has been noticed that the incidence of GC has declined over time mostly in developed countries, due to improving living standards. However, and despite increasing knowledge and improvements in the standard of care, therapy resistance and metastasis remain the main causes of treatment failure and death in GC patients and GC as a disease remains a serious and significant social concern. Consequently, identifying the major GC drivers and the molecular and cellular mechanisms responsible for the GC heterogeneity and maintenance is crucial to understand the pathobiology of GC and establish optimal therapies that able to improve the prognosis of patients.

2. Cancer stem cells in gastric cancer

Several types of solid cancers, including gastric cancers, contain phenotypically and functionally heterogeneous cancer cells [8]. These cancers present a small subpopulation of cells that display characteristics similar to normal stem cells, including unlimited self-renewal, proliferation and multi-lineage differentiation. These cells are called cancer stem cells (CSCs), which are supposed to maintain long-term tumor growth, recurrence and chemotherapy resistance. The origin of gastric CSCs is not completely clear, but it has been observed that this subpopulation of cells can derive from the differentiated gastric epithelial cells, local progenitor cells in the gastric mucosa and bone marrow-derived cells (BMDCs) [9]. In line with this idea, chronic infection of C57BL/6 mice with *Helicobacter felis* results in chronic inflammation and injury in gastric mucosa, which leads to the loss of resident gastric stem cells, followed by hyperplasia, metaplasia, dysplasia and, ultimately, gastric cancer [10, 11]. *H. pylori* can attach and invade *Lgr5+* gastric stem cells and this residency results in more susceptibility to DNA damage and cancer initiation [12, 13]. This suggests that *H. pylori* infection directly affects epithelial stem cells in the stomach and plays an important role in transforming resident stem cells into tumor cells. In addition, *H. pylori cag*A virulence factor unveils CSC-like properties by induction of EMT-like changes in gastric epithelial cancer cells [14]. Increasing studies support the existence of these cancer cells exhibiting stem cell characteristics and involved in GC metastasis [14]. Among the underlying mechanisms of chemoresistance, CG cells resistant to 5-Fluoroacyl (5-FU) or cisplatin therapy have been identified as exhibiting high expression of stem cell markers such as BMI1, CD44, CD133 or SOX9. In addition, the inhibition of these regulators reverses the chemoresistance. This resistance is due in part to the acquisition or presence of quiescence and self-renewal characteristics by the small percentage of gCSCs. It is well known that conventional chemo and radiotherapy therapies have maximum efficacy in proliferative cells and when target events are present in all cancer cells. However, they do not affect the quiescent cells and do not take into account inter and intratumoral heterogeneity at the cellular and molecular level. Thus, identifying the major regulators of gastric CSCs is a prominent need in order to understand GC pathobiology and identify novel therapeutic targets. In this sense, in the last years, the identification of several stem cell-related genes or transcription factors has provided relevant information of the impact of gCSCs in GC initiation and progression, and how *H. pylori* or chronic inflammation affects gastric stem cells. This chapter summarizes the impact of some of the most relevant genes in gastric CSCs and gastric cancer pathobiology, including LGR5, CD133, CD44, SOX2 and SOX9.

2.1. Regulators of gastric cancer stem cells

2.1.1. LGR5

The human leucine-rich repeat-containing G protein-coupled receptor 5 (LGR5) is a member of the G protein-coupled transmembrane receptor (GPCR) superfamily. LGR5 is a receptor for R-spondins that belong to the WNT signalling complex at the membrane level [15] and is also a target gene of this pathway [16]. LGR5 is overexpressed in a variety of human cancers, including tumors of the digestive tract such as colorectal [17] or gastric cancer [18–20], wherein it has been postulated as a CSC marker. LGR5 is an established stem cell marker of the intestine, and several studies on mice and humans have shown that LGR5-positive stem cells are the cells-of-origin of intestinal and colorectal cancer [21–27]. In the stomach, there are also increasing evidence postulating LGR5 as a stem cell and CSC marker. Thereby, LGR5 expression in gastric mucosa is almost restricted to a subset of cells located at the base of the pyloric glands, distribution that fits well with the multiple sites of the gastric cancer in humans

[28]. Through *in vivo* lineage tracing experiments, these authors found that LGR5-positive cells were self-renewing and multipotent and were responsible for the renewal of the gastric epithelium. Interestingly, they observed that the transformation of this population of stem cells could drive gastric tumorigenesis *in vivo* [28], fact that has been strongly demonstrated more recently by Li and collaborators [29]. Consistently with the observation in mice, in human gastric tissue, LGR5 expression has also been found in the bottom of gastric glands [30]. Supporting the putative role of LGR5 as a gastric CSC regulator in humans, independent studies have reported LGR5 overexpression in human gastric cancer samples respect to normal gastric mucosa in a progressively increasing manner from well-differentiated to poorly differentiated gastric carcinomas [20, 31]. Furthermore, LGR5 expression has been strongly linked to a high degree of tumor infiltration, high TNM stage, recurrence and dismal prognosis of gastric cancer patients [18–20, 31]. More recently, Wang and collaborators have shown that sphere cells derived from a gastric cancer cell line presented increased expression of some canonical stem regulators, being LGR5 particularly elevated [32]. They also showed that ectopic LGR5 overexpression potentiated the sphere cell growth and cell migration capabilities of gastric cancer cells and also their tolerance to oxaliplatin, associating LGR5 expression with the characteristic features of CSCs [32]. These findings are in concordance with previous observations showing the impairment of the invasiveness and the reduction in the expression of metalloproteinase 2 (MMP2) and β-catenin in gastric cancer cells in response to LGR5 silencing *in vitro*; and revealing a positive correlation between the expression of LGR5 and MMP2 in gastric cancer tissue samples [20]. Regarding the implications of the carcinogenic agent *H. pylori* in the LGR5-positive cells in the stomach, it has been found that this population of cells is expanded in gastric cancer tissues affected by the bacteria, indicating that LGR5 likely represents a marker of stem cells susceptible of oncogenic transformation driven by *H. pylori* [13, 33].

2.1.2. CD133

CD133 (also Prominin 1) is a pentaspan transmembrane glycoprotein present in embryonic epithelial structures, thought to function as an organizer of plasma membrane topology, and regulating the maintenance of the appropriate lipid composition within the plasma membrane [34]. CD133 has been presented as a marker of cancer stem cells in colon, pancreas, brain or lung cancer [35], yet its role in gastric CSCs is controversial. Several findings related to different aspects of gastric CSCs have been published in support of its role as a gastric CSC marker and regulator. In gastric cancer cell lines, CD133 silencing abrogates sphere formation capacity [36] and, consistently, CD133 has been found overexpressed in gastric sphere cultures [37, 38]. Noteworthy, a large number of publications show increased CD133 expression in human gastric cancer tissue respect to non-neoplastic gastric mucosa and highlight the prognostic significance of CD133, associating its overexpression with a big plethora of adverse clinic-pathological features, such as elevated cellular proliferation rates, high T stage, venous invasion, lymph node and distant metastasis, chemoresistance, recurrence, poor 5-year disease-free and overall survival and so on [37, 39–42]. According to this, studies performed in gastric cancer cell lines demonstrate that CD133-positive gastric cancer cells present a CSC phenotype, since they are more tumorigenic, more chemoresistant and exhibit higher migration or invasion capacities than CD133-negative cells [37, 38, 43]. However, some controversial findings have been published indicating that CD133 expression is not a *sine qua non* condition for gastric cancer cells to exhibit properties of CSCs. Thus, Takaishi et al. isolated different subpopulations of cells from gastric cancer cell lines according to the expression of CD133, CD44, CD26 and other cell surface markers and showed that CD133-positive cells did not exhibit characteristics of CSCs [44]. Similar results have been obtained in other investigations using human gastric cancer specimens as source of cells, in which CD133-positive cells were not able to reproduce tumors in immunodeficient mouse models [45, 46].

2.1.3. CD44

CD44 is a transmembrane glycoprotein expressed on leukocytes, endothelial cells, hepatocytes or gastric epithelial cells, which acts as a receptor for hyaluronic acid (HA) [47] and can also interact with other ligands, such as osteopontin, collagens and MMPs. CD44 is a fetal and adult hematopoietic stem cell regulator that is involved in cell-cell interactions, cell adhesion and migration and participates in a wide variety of cellular functions, including hematopoiesis and lymphocyte activation, recirculation and homing [48]. CD44 gene contains 20 exons. Ten of these exons (exons l–5 and 16–20) are expressed together on many cell types and the product is referred to as the "standard" form of CD44. Additionally, complex alternative splicing of the transcripts affecting exons from 6 to 15 (variant exons) results in many functionally distinct isoforms or variants (CD44v) [49]. The role of CD44 as a CSC marker has been broadly studied in myeloid leukemia and also in several solid tumors such as lung, brain, liver, head and neck or gastric cancer [50]. In gastric cancer, the first temptative characterization of CSCs in terms of markers was performed by Takaishi and collaborators, who found that CD44+ cells isolated from different gastric cancer cell lines presented sphere formation ability *in vitro* and tumorigenic potential when inoculated into stomach and skin of immunodeficient mice, abilities that were abrogated by CD44 silencing. Moreover, these CD44+ gastric cancer cells showed the stem cell characteristics of self-renewal and the ability to give rise to differentiated progeny [44]. In concordance, other authors have documented CD44 enrichment in spheres derived from gastric cancer cell lines [51] or have identified that CD44-positive cells derived from gastric cancer cell lines are resistant to 5-fluorouracil and cisplatin chemotherapy and also exhibit significantly more migration, invasion and anchorage-independent growth capabilities [52]. Regarding gastric cancer clinical samples, CD44 is expressed in 80% of gastric tumor resected specimens [40] and its high expression has been associated with tumor size, lymphatic vessel and intravenous invasion, moderate grade of differentiation and low response to chemotherapy [52–54]. Furthermore, the presence of CD44+ cancer cells at the invasive front of gastric tumors entails poor survival and constitutes a prognostic factor for this malignancy [55]. In relation to this aspect, Watanabe and collaborators have found that in gastric cancer patients, the frequency of circulating CD44-positive tumor cells correlates with disease stage, depth of tumors and venous invasion [56]. Moreover, it has been suggested that the emergence of gastric CSCs induced by *H. pylori* infection of gastric mucosa may rely on CD44 upregulation [57]. Nevertheless, in contraposition to these evidences, some works have not found CSC characteristics in the subpopulations of CD44-positive cells isolated from gastric tumors [45, 58]. Besides, it is being sustained the notion that some CD44 variants are more relevant for gastric CSCs than standard CD44. An example of it is the work of Lau and collaborators, who show that CD44v8-10 is the predominant CD44 variant expressed in gastric cancer cells, whose expression levels, unlike those of standard CD44, are increased in gastric tumors respect to adjacent normal tissue. The authors also showed that ectopic expression of CD44v8-10, but not standard CD44, in gastric cancer cells potentiates their ability to initiate tumors in mice at limiting cell concentrations and that total CD44 silencing impairs tumor-initiating potential of cells, which could be rescued by restoration of CD44v8-10, but not standard CD44, expression [46].

2.1.4. CD24

CD24 encodes a cell surface sialoglycoprotein that is physiologically expressed in developing or regenerating tissues and regulates processes such as lymphocyte development [59] or neurogenesis [60]. As other stem cell genes, CD24 is expressed in hematologic malignancies and several solid tumors including gastric cancer. Suggesting a role for CD24 in gastric CSCs, some studies by using gastric cancer cell lines have shown that derived spheres are enriched in the expression of CD24 (and CD44) [51] and also that CD24 modulates positively cell migration, while its inhibition entails apoptosis [61]. However, Takaishi et al. were unable to find properties of CSCs in a CD24-positive population in terms of sphere forming capacity and tumorigenicity in mice models [44]. With regard to patients with gastric cancer, CD24 expression progressively increases in samples of normal gastric mucosa, non-atrophic chronic gastritis, chronic atrophic gastritis, intestinal metaplasia, dysplasia and gastric cancer [61]. Moreover, CD24 expression has been associated with adverse clinicopathological and prognostic aspects such as depth of tumors, lymph node status, TNM stage and reduced overall survival [62], fact that underlines its relevance in the disease.

2.1.5. SOX transcription factors

SOX factors are a family of transcription factors that are emerging as potent regulators of stem cell maintenance and cell fate decisions in multiple organ systems including the gastrointestinal tract [63]. There are at least 20 members divided into eight groups (from A to H), based on their HMG sequence identity in humans. Members within a group preserve higher than 80% identity in their HMG-domain and share other well-conserved regions. In addition, they share biochemical properties, have overlapping expression patterns and perform synergistic or redundant functions [63]. SOX proteins play critical roles during the development of several cell types and tissues in the embryo. They are also essential for stem cell types in the adult through the regulation of the cell fate determination, differentiation and proliferation [63]. SOX members fulfill their role by activating or repressing transcription and their action on target genes is context dependent, relying on other transcription factors with which they may directly interact for specificity. Dysfunction of SOX factors has been implicated in several human diseases. Such diseases are consistent with SOX function and expression pattern during embryonic development. A growing number of evidences are demonstrating that the expression and function of SOX factors are altered in a variety of cancers, and their roles in these malignancies are related to their stemness feature [64].

2.1.5.1. SOX2

SOX2 belongs to the SOXB1 subgroup along with the closely related SOX1 and SOX3. SOX2 is required for establishing embryonic stem cells and the maintenance of the early embryo [65]. It is also one of the factors necessary for reprogramming terminally differentiated cells into induced pluripotent stem cells [66]. Furthermore, SOX2 belongs to the core transcriptionally circuitry found on the regulatory regions of many genes with embryonic stem cell-specific expression [67]. This evidence demonstrates that SOX2 is a key factor in the control of embryonic stem cells fate and activity. SOX2 has additional functions during development, thus emerging as a critical regulator of stem cell maintenance and cell fate decisions. Furthermore, SOX2 also plays a relevant role during adulthood controlling tissue homeostasis and regeneration. Its expression is elevated in different populations of stem cells [68–71], and its high levels can be used to identify quiescent stem cells and distinguish them from transient amplifying progenitors [72, 73]. SOX2 is a regulator of gastric stem cells highly relevant for gastric patterning during development [74] and involved in the physiological renewal of the gastric epithelium in the adulthood [71, 75]. SOX2 displays several roles in cancer as an oncogenic driver, prognostic factor or a marker and regulator of CSCs [76–80]. In GC, its action is controversial. Several authors observed that SOX2 is frequently downregulated in gastric cancer [81–86]. Furthermore, low SOX2 expression is associated with shorter survival time [82] and also with worse prognosis [84]. In contrast, higher SOX2 levels are found among patients who have better prognosis [84]. In a large set of patients, Wang and coworkers demonstrated that SOX2 expression is progressively reduced during gastric carcinogenesis, from normal into invasive cancers including a series of premalignant states, supporting the role of SOX2 decrease as a robust predictor of disease outcome [85]. Similarly, SOX2 downregulation is linked with diffuse type of cancer with SOX2 expression becoming a good biomarker to discriminate between tumor (negative) and non-tumor (positive expression) and also high/low grades of tumor malignancy [86]. The regulation of SOX2 expression in GC has been mostly associated to epigenetic changes. Thus, aberrant DNA methylation has been shown as a key mechanism underlying SOX2 downregulation in a set of primary gastric carcinoma samples [82]. Besides promoter methylation, miR-126 overexpression also decreases SOX2 levels and therefore acts as a tumor suppressor [83]. Recently, it has been shown that SOX2 has an important role in gastric differentiation [87]. It is known that during gastric carcinogenesis, the homeobox transcription factor CDX2 is critical for intestinal differentiation driving the onset of intestinal metaplasia (IM) [88, 89]. Thereafter, Camilo and coworkers showed that SOX2 is associated with gastric differentiation in incomplete IM and is lost in the progression to dysplasia, whereas CDX2 is acquired *de novo* in IM and maintained in dysplasia [87]. Taken it into account, the authors hypothesized that balance between gastric and intestinal differentiation programs might interfere on the gastric carcinogenesis progression [87]. Since SOX2 and CDX2 expression were found in about half of the cases, the interaction of both transcription factors in gastric carcinogenesis remains to be investigated. Functional characterization performed in gastric epithelial cell lines showed that SOX2 ectopic activation inhibits cell proliferation through G1 cell-cycle arrest and induces apoptosis by decreasing cyclin D1 and phosphorylated Rb and increasing p27Kip1 protein levels [82]. Overall, the authors observed that SOX2 performs a critical part in gastric carcinogenesis, operating as a tumor suppressor.

Similarly, Wang and coworkers verified that enforced SOX2 expression inhibited proliferation, increased apoptosis and reduced invasion and motility, both in vitro and in vivo [85]. Mechanistically, SOX2 directly transactivates PTEN. Therefore, this SOX2-dependent PTEN upregulation may directly orchestrate downstream phospho-Akt dephosphorylation, affecting diverse cellular phenotypes such as survival, growth, proliferation and migration [85]. These studies show that SOX2 plays important roles in gastric epithelial cells growth inhibition through cell-cycle arrest and apoptosis [90]. Regarding its relationship with *H. pylori*, SOX2 expression is decreased by the bacteria, and this inhibition leads to an upregulation of CDX2 expression [75, 91, 92]. Additionally, *in vitro* and in a mice model infected with *Helicobacter* spp. demonstrated that CDX2 and SOX2 are downstream targets of the BMP (bone morphogenetic protein) pathway in gastric carcinogenesis. The authors showed that *H. pylori* upregulates BMP pathway, through an increase in BMP2, SMAD4 and pSMAD1/5/8 expression. Thus, SOX2 expression was downregulated by *H. pylori* and the BMP pathway [93]. From a mechanistic perspective, it was postulated that the activation of an intestinal differentiation program may occur concomitantly with the silencing of a gastric differentiation, induced or controlled by SOX2 [93]. Another recent study identified that the bacteria might trigger its pro-carcinogenic activity through a blockage of SOX2 [85]. However, other authors verified that overexpression of SOX2 is associated with tumor invasion, lymph node metastasis and chemoresistance [94–97]. Tian and coworkers were able to show that SOX2 enhances the tumorigenicity and chemoresistance of cancer stem-like cells derived from gastric cancer, suggesting an oncogenic effect of SOX2 in the stomach [94]. In addition, it has been demonstrated that SOX2 overexpression was significantly correlated with lymph node metastasis and the stage of tumor invasion in gastric cancer indicating that SOX2 might be a predictive prognostic factor [95]. Hutz and coworkers proved that high levels of SOX2 are involved in gastric carcinogenesis by regulating the expression of genes associated with proliferation, apoptosis and cell cycle regulation, *in vitro* and *in vivo* [96]. Functionally, the SOX2 suppression induced a decrease in cell proliferation, which coincided with an increase of apoptosis in AZ-521 cells. Similarly, blocking of SOX2 in a xenograft mouse model resulted in reduced tumor growth [96]. Moreover, the expression of SOX2 in human gastric tumor samples was observed at high proliferation rate sites [96]. Likewise, SOX2 overexpression in gastric cancer has been recently observed in other study, where the surge in the expression is attributed to SOX2 locus copy number variation, being related as well with the presence of regional lymph node metastases [98].

2.1.5.2. SOX9

SOX9 is overexpressed in a variety of human cancers, being its high levels correlated with malignant character and progression in prostate, lung, breast and brain tumors [80, 99, 100]. SOX9 expression is also elevated in tumors of the digestive system such as esophageal, colorectal and pancreatic cancers [101, 102]. In esophageal and pancreatic tumors, SOX9 stimulate self-renewal properties [102, 103]. However, in colorectal cancer, there are contradictory results between functional studies and clinical samples, suggesting a context-dependent activity of SOX9 [100, 104]. Remarkably, several studies have reported clinical implications of SOX9 in GC. Thereby, in GC patients, high tumoral SOX9 expression has been observed and associated with advanced TNM stages and lower overall patient survival [105]. Interestingly, in clinical samples, high levels of SOX9 correlate with elevated expression of the carcinoembryonic antigen-related cell adhesion molecule 1 (CEACAM1) [106], which facilitates GC metastasis, and are positively associated with lymph nodes metastasis and advanced TNM stage [107]. In samples from patients, there is also an inverse relation between SOX9 and the tumor suppressor gastrokine 1 (GKN1), relationship also observed in GC cell lines, wherein GKN1 negatively regulates SOX9 expression [106, 108]. Furthermore, elevated SOX9 expression in gastric tumors is associated with the activation of the WNT canonical oncogenic pathway, with whom it establishes a feedback regulatory loop [105].

Noteworthy, SOX9 is a critical executor of the carcinogenic action of *H. pylori*. According to this notion, the bacterium induces SOX9 expression in pre-tumorigenic gastric mouse cells [109] and also in GC cells [105], being the induction more pronounced in response to specimens of *H. pylori* containing the pathogenically significant *CagA* virulence factor. Notably, SOX9 is required for bacteria-induced GC cell proliferation, induction of β-catenin and acquisition of stem cell-like properties. Mechanistically, it has been found that TNFα and IL-1β cytokines, involved in the inflammatory response to *H. pylori*, induce the expression of SOX9 in mouse models and GC cells [105, 109], being probably the action of TNFα in human GC cells stronger and more extensive. In fact, TNFα high levels correlated with SOX9 upregulation in *H. pylori*-positive GC samples, and there was a positive association between them in two independent large cohorts of GC samples [TCGA and ACRG] [105]. Overall, these results identified a novel association between SOX9 and *IL1-β* and *TNFα* cytokines, which links *H. pylori* infection with SOX9 and GC outcome in patients, evidence supported by other studies [110–114]. SOX9 represents a key driver of GC and given the importance of its strong clinical implications, elucidating the molecular mechanism of its action in GC has constituted an important challenge to identify novel and suitable therapeutic targets. With respect to that, it is known that SOX9 establishes a feedback regulatory loop with WNT/β-catenin signaling pathway. Consistently, SOX9 abrogation in GC cells diminishes *CYCLIN D1* and *c-MYC* expression, and there is a positive correlation between these genes and SOX9 in patient samples [105]. Functionally, SOX9 silencing in GC cells promotes apoptosis and senescence through BMI1 decline and the consequent upregulation of $p21^{CIP}$ [105]. SOX9 silencing also supposes detrimental effects on the subpopulation of gCSCs, reflected by a reduction in tumorsphere self-renewal and decreased tumor initiating capability [105]. Paralleling these effects, and likely due to its functions in gCSCs, SOX9 mediates cisplatin chemoresistance [105, 114], fact that might explain the reduced disease-free survival of patients presenting tumors with high *SOX9* expression levels [105]. Additionally, there are other SOX members associated to GC. Thus, SOX4 has been shown to display pro-oncogenic activities and become upregulated with gastric cancer progression, in the population of gCSCs and in response to *H. pylori* infection [115–117]. Finally, SOX18 mRNA levels are increased in gastric cancer tissues compared to normal tissue, and the frequencies of both lymphovascular invasion and lymph node metastases are higher in SOX18 positive than in the negative group. Furthermore, both the 5-year survival and the recurrence-free survival were shorter for SOX18-positive cancers suggesting that SOX18 expression might be a prognostic tumor marker and a potential therapeutic target in gastric cancer [118].

Author details

Estefania Carrasco-Garcia[1], Mikel García-Puga[1], Manuel Moreno[1,2], Nicolas Sampron[1,2], Sara Arevalo[1,2] and Ander Matheu[1,3*]

*Address all correspondence to: ander.matheu@biodonostia.org

1 Cellular Oncology Group, Biodonostia Health Research Institute, San Sebastian, Spain

2 Donostia Hospital, San Sebastian, Spain

3 Ikerbasque, Basque Foundation, Bilbao, Spain

References

[1] Wadhwa R, Song S, Lee JS, Yao Y, Wei Q, Ajani JA: Gastric cancer-molecular and clinical dimensions. Nature Reviews Clinical Oncology. 2013;**10**:643-655. DOI: 10.1038/nrclinonc.2013.170

[2] Correa P, Piazuelo MB. The gastric precancerous cascade. Journal of Digestive Diseases. 2012;**13**:2-9. DOI: 10.1111/j.1751-2980.2011.00550.x

[3] Wang F, Meng W, Wang B, Qiao L: Helicobacter pylori-induced gastric inflammation and gastric cancer. Cancer Letters. 2014;**345**:196-202. DOI: 10.1016/j.canlet.2013.08.016.

[4] Drumm B, Day AS, Gold B, Gottrand F, Kato S, Kawakami E, et al. *Helicobacter pylori* and peptic ulcer: Working Group Report of the second World Congress of Pediatric Gastroenterology, Hepatology, and Nutrition. Journal of Pediatric Gastroenterology and Nutrition. 2004;**39**(Suppl 2):S626-S631.

[5] Cristescu R, Lee J, Nebozhyn M, Kim KM, Ting JC, Wong SS, et al. Molecular analysis of gastric cancer identifies subtypes associated with distinct clinical outcomes. Nature Medicine. 2015;**21**:449-456. DOI: 10.1038/nature13480

[6] Cancer Genome Atlas Research Network. Comprehensive molecular characterization of gastric adenocarcinoma. Nature. 2014;**513**: 202-209. DOI: 10.1002/ijc.29352

[7] Cunningham D, Allum WH, Stenning SP, Thompson JN, Van de Velde CJ, Nicolson M, et al. Perioperative chemotherapy versus surgery alone for resectable gastroesophageal cancer. The New England Journal of Medicine. 2006;**355**:11-20. DOI: 10.1056/NEJMoa055531

[8] Clevers H. The cancer stem cell: Premises, promises and challenges. Nature Medicine. 2011;**17**:313-319. DOI: 10.1038/nm.2304

[9] Xu G, Shen J, Ou Yang X, Sasahara M, Su X. Cancer stem cells: The 'heartbeat' of gastric cancer. Journal of Gastroenterology. 2013;**48**:781-797. DOI: 10.1007/s00535-012-0712-y

[10] Varon C, Dubus P, Mazurier F, Asencio C, Chambonnier L, Ferrand J, et al. *Helicobacter pylori* infection recruits bone marrow-derived cells that participate in gastric preneoplasia in mice. Gastroenterology. 2012;**142**:281-291. DOI: 10.1053/j.gastro.2011.10.036

[11] Houghton J, Stoicov C, Nomura S, Rogers AB, Carlson J, Li H, et al. Gastric cancer originating from bone marrow-derived cells. Science (New York, NY). 2004;**306**:1568-1571. DOI: 10.1126/science.1099513

[12] Giannakis M, Chen SL, Karam SM, Engstrand L, Gordon JI. *Helicobacter pylori* evolution during progression from chronic atrophic gastritis to gastric cancer and its impact on gastric stem cells. Proceedings of the National Academy of Sciences of the United States of America. 2008;**105**:4358-4363. DOI: 10.1073/pnas.0800668105

[13] Uehara T, Ma D, Yao Y, Lynch JP, Morales K, Ziober A, et al. *H. pylori* infection is associated with DNA damage of Lgr5-positive epithelial stem cells in the stomach of patients with gastric cancer. Digestive Diseases and Sciences. 2013;**58**:140-149. DOI: 10.1007/s10620-012-2360-8

[14] Bessede E, Staedel C, Acuna Amador LA, Nguyen PH, Chambonnier L, Hatakeyama M, et al. *Helicobacter pylori* generates cells with cancer stem cell properties via epithelial-mesenchymal transition-like changes. Oncogene. 2014;**33**:4123-4131. DOI: 10.1038/onc.2013.380

[15] de Lau W, Barker N, Low TY, Koo BK, Li VS, Teunissen H, et al. Lgr5 homologues associate with Wnt receptors and mediate R-spondin signalling. Nature. 2011;**476**:293-297. DOI:10.1038/nature103337

[16] Van der Flier LG, Sabates-Bellver J, Oving I, Haegebarth A, De Palo M, Anti M, et al. The intestinal Wnt/TCF signature. Gastroenterology. 2007;**132**:628-632. DOI: 10.1053/j.gastro.2006.08.039

[17] Uchida H, Yamazaki K, Fukuma M, Yamada T, Hayashida T, Hasegawa H, et al. Overexpression of leucine-rich repeat-containing G protein-coupled receptor 5 in colorectal cancer. Cancer Science. 2010;**101**:1731-1737. DOI: 10.1111/j.1349-7006.2010.01571.x

[18] Simon E, Petke D, Boger C, Behrens HM, Warneke V, Ebert M, et al. The spatial distribution of LGR5+ cells correlates with gastric cancer progression. PLoS One. 2012;**7**:e35486

[19] Yamanoi K, Fukuma M, Uchida H, Kushima R, Yamazaki K, Katai H, et al. Overexpression of leucine-rich repeat-containing G protein-coupled receptor 5 in gastric cancer. Pathology International. 2013;**63**:13-19. DOI: 10.1111/pin.12013

[20] Xi HQ, Cai AZ, Wu XS, Cui JX, Shen WS, Bian SB, et al. Leucine-rich repeat-containing G-protein-coupled receptor 5 is associated with invasion, metastasis, and could be a potential therapeutic target in human gastric cancer. British Journal of Cancer. 2014;**110**:2011-2020. DOI: 10.1038/bjc.2014.112

[21] Barker N, van Es JH, Kuipers J, Kujala P, van den Born M, Cozijnsen M, et al. Identification of stem cells in small intestine and colon by marker gene Lgr5. Nature. 2007;**449**:1003-1007. DOI: 10.1038/nature06196

[22] Barker N, van Es JH, Jaks V, Kasper M, Snippert H, Toftgard R, et al. Very long-term self-renewal of small intestine, colon, and hair follicles from cycling Lgr5+ve stem cells. Cold Spring Harbor Symposia on Quantitative Biology. 2008;**73**:351-356. DOI: 10.1101/sqb.2008.72.003

[23] Barker N, Ridgway RA, van Es JH, van de Wetering M, Begthel H, van den Born M, et al. Crypt stem cells as the cells-of-origin of intestinal cancer. Nature. 2009;**457**:608-611. DOI: 10.1038/nature07602

[24] Schepers AG, Snippert HJ, Stange DE, van den Born M, van Es JH, van de Wetering M, et al. Lineage tracing reveals Lgr5+ stem cell activity in mouse intestinal adenomas. Science (New York, NY). 2012;**337**:730-735. DOI: 10.1126/science.1224676

[25] Vermeulen L, Todaro M, de Sousa Mello F, Sprick MR, Kemper K, Perez Alea M, et al. Single-cell cloning of colon cancer stem cells reveals a multi-lineage differentiation capacity. Proceedings of the National Academy of Sciences of the United States of America. 2008;**105**:13427-13432. DOI: 10.1073/pnas.0805706105

[26] Takahashi H, Ishii H, Nishida N, Takemasa I, Mizushima T, Ikeda M, et al. Significance of Lgr5(+ve) cancer stem cells in the colon and rectum. Annals of Surgical Oncology. 2011;**18**:1166-1174. DOI: 10.1245/s10434-010-1373-9

[27] Takeda K, Kinoshita I, Shimizu Y, Matsuno Y, Shichinohe T, Dosaka-Akita H. Expression of LGR5, an intestinal stem cell marker, during each stage of colorectal tumorigenesis. Anticancer Research. 2011;**31**:263-270.

[28] Barker N, Huch M, Kujala P, van de Wetering M, Snippert HJ, van Es JH, et al. Lgr5(+ve) stem cells drive self-renewal in the stomach and build long-lived gastric units in vitro. Cell Stem Cell. 2010;**6**:25-36. DOI: 10.1016/j.stem.2009.11.013

[29] Li XB, Yang G, Zhu L, Tang YL, Zhang C, Ju Z, et al. Gastric Lgr5(+) stem cells are the cellular origin of invasive intestinal-type gastric cancer in mice. Cell Research. 2016;**26**:838-849. DOI: 10.1038/cr.2016.47

[30] Wu C, Xie Y, Gao F, Wang Y, Guo Y, Tian H, et al. Lgr5 expression as stem cell marker in human gastric gland and its relatedness with other putative cancer stem cell markers. Gene. 2013;**525**:18-25. DOI: 10.1016/j.gene.2013.04.067

[31] Zheng ZX, Sun Y, Bu ZD, Zhang LH, Li ZY, Wu AW, et al. Intestinal stem cell marker LGR5 expression during gastric carcinogenesis. World Journal of Gastroenterology. 2013;**19**:8714-8721. DOI: 10.3748/wjg.v19.i46.8714

[32] Wang B, Chen Q, Cao Y, Ma X, Yin C, Jia Y, et al. LGR5 is a gastric cancer stem cell marker associated with stemness and the EMT signature genes NANOG, NANOGP8, PRRX1, TWIST1, and BMI1. PLoS One. 2016;**11**:e0168904. DOI: 10.1371/journal.pone.0168904

[33] Sigal M, Rothenberg ME, Logan CY, Lee JY, Honaker RW, Cooper RL, et al. *Helicobacter pylori* activates and expands Lgr5(+) stem cells through direct colonization of the gastric glands. Gastroenterology. 2015;**148**:1392-1404.e21. DOI: 10.1053/j.gastro.2015.02.049

[34] Mizrak D, Brittan M, Alison M. CD133: Molecule of the moment. The Journal of Pathology. 2008;**214**:3-9. DOI: 10.1002/path.2283

[35] Brungs D, Aghmesheh M, Vine KL, Becker TM, Carolan MG, Ranson M. Gastric cancer stem cells: Evidence, potential markers, and clinical implications. Journal of Gastroenterology. 2016;**51**:313-326. DOI: 10.1007/s00535-015-1125-5

[36] Yu JW, Wang SL, Wu JG, Lu RQ, Ni XC, Cai C, et al. Study on the biological characteristics of CD133 (+) cells interfered by RNA interference in gastric cancer. ISRN Gastroenterology. 2014;**2014**:329519. DOI: 10.1155/2014/329519

[37] Zhang X, Hua R, Wang X, Huang M, Gan L, Wu Z, et al. Identification of stem-like cells and clinical significance of candidate stem cell markers in gastric cancer. Oncotarget. 2016;**7**:9815-9831. DOI: 10.18632/oncotarget.6890

[38] Song Z, Yue W, Wei B, Wang N, Li T, Guan L, et al. Sonic hedgehog pathway is essential for maintenance of cancer stem-like cells in human gastric cancer. PLoS One. 2011;**6**:e17687. DOI: 10.1371/journal.pone.0017687

[39] Zhao P, Li Y, Lu Y. Aberrant expression of CD133 protein correlates with Ki-67 expression and is a prognostic marker in gastric adenocarcinoma. BMC Cancer. 2010;**10**:218. DOI: 10.1186/1471-2407-10-218

[40] Wang T, Ong CW, Shi J, Srivastava S, Yan B, Cheng CL, et al. Sequential expression of putative stem cell markers in gastric carcinogenesis. British Journal of Cancer. 2011;**105**:658-665. DOI: 10.1038/bjc.2011.287

[41] Lee HH, Seo KJ, An CH, Kim JS, Jeon HM. CD133 expression is correlated with chemoresistance and early recurrence of gastric cancer. Journal of Surgical Oncology. 2012;**106**:999-1004. DOI: 10.1002/jso.23178

[42] Yiming L, Yunshan G, Bo M, Yu Z, Tao W, Gengfang L, et al. CD133 overexpression correlates with clinicopathological features of gastric cancer patients and its impact on survival: A systematic review and meta-analysis. Oncotarget. 2015;**6**:42019-42027. DOI: 10.18632/oncotarget.5714

[43] Zhu Y, Yu J, Wang S, Lu R, Wu J, Jiang B. Overexpression of CD133 enhances chemoresistance to 5-fluorouracil by activating the PI3K/Akt/p70S6K pathway in gastric cancer cells. Oncology Reports. 2014;**32**:2437-2444. DOI: 10.3892/or.2014.3488

[44] Takaishi S, Okumura T, Tu S, Wang SS, Shibata W, Vigneshwaran R, et al. Identification of gastric cancer stem cells using the cell surface marker CD44. Stem Cells. 2009;**27**:1006-1020. DOI: 10.1002/stem.30

[45] Rocco A, Liguori E, Pirozzi G, Tirino V, Compare D, Franco R, et al. CD133 and CD44 cell surface markers do not identify cancer stem cells in primary human gastric tumors. Journal of Cellular Physiology. 2012;**227**:2686-2693. DOI: 10.1002/jcp.23013

[46] Lau WM, Teng E, Chong HS, Lopez KA, Tay AY, Salto-Tellez M, et al. CD44v8-10 is a cancer-specific marker for gastric cancer stem cells. Cancer Research. 2014;**74**:2630-2641. DOI: 10.1158/0008-5472.can-13-2309

[47] Lesley J, Hascall VC, Tammi M, Hyman R. Hyaluronan binding by cell surface CD44. The Journal of Biological Chemistry. 2000;**275**:26967-26975. DOI: 10.1074/jbc.M002527200

[48] Thorne RF, Legg JW, Isacke CM. The role of the CD44 transmembrane and cytoplasmic domains in co-ordinating adhesive and signalling events. Journal of Cell Science. 2004;**117**:373-380. DOI: 10.1242/jcs.00954

[49] Tolg C, Hofmann M, Herrlich P, Ponta H. Splicing choice from ten variant exons establishes CD44 variability. Nucleic Acids Research. 1993;**21**:1225-1229.

[50] Morath I, Hartmann TN, Orian-Rousseau V. CD44: More than a mere stem cell marker. The International Journal of Biochemistry & Cell Biology. 2016;**81**:166-173. DOI: 10.1016/j.biocel.2016.09.009

[51] Wang X, Zou F, Deng H, Fu Z, Li Y, Wu L, et al. Characterization of sphereforming cells with stemlike properties from the gastric cancer cell lines MKN45 and SGC7901. Molecular Medicine Reports. 2014;**10**:2937-2941. DOI: 10.3892/mmr.2014.2601

[52] Yoon C, Park DJ, Schmidt B, Thomas NJ, Lee HJ, Kim TS, et al. CD44 expression denotes a subpopulation of gastric cancer cells in which Hedgehog signaling promotes chemotherapy resistance. Clinical Cancer Research: An Official Journal of the American Association for Cancer Research. 2014;**20**:3974-3988. DOI: 10.1158/1078-0432.ccr-14-0011

[53] Lu L, Wu M, Sun L, Li W, Fu W, Zhang X, et al. Clinicopathological and prognostic significance of cancer stem cell markers CD44 and CD133 in patients with gastric cancer: A comprehensive meta-analysis with 4729 patients involved. Medicine. 2016;**95**:e5163. DOI: 10.1097/md.0000000000005163

[54] Nosrati A, Naghshvar F, Khanari S. Cancer stem cell markers CD44, CD133 in primary gastric adenocarcinoma. International Journal of Molecular and Cellular Medicine. 2014;**3**:279-286.

[55] Kodama H, Murata S, Ishida M, Yamamoto H, Yamaguchi T, Kaida S, et al. Prognostic impact of CD44-positive cancer stem-like cells at the invasive front of gastric cancer. British Journal of Cancer. 2017;**116**:186-194. DOI: 10.1038/bjc.2016.401

[56] Watanabe T, Okumura T, Hirano K, Yamaguchi T, Sekine S, Nagata T, et al. Circulating tumor cells expressing cancer stem cell marker CD44 as a diagnostic biomarker in patients with gastric cancer. Oncology Letters. 2017;**13**:281-288. DOI: 10.3892/ol.2016.5432

[57] Choi YJ, Kim N, Chang H, Lee HS, Park SM, Park JH, et al. *Helicobacter pylori*-induced epithelial-mesenchymal transition, a potential role of gastric cancer initiation and an emergence of stem cells. Carcinogenesis. 2015;**36**:553-563. DOI: 10.1093/carcin/bgv022

[58] Fukamachi H, Seol HS, Shimada S, Funasaka C, Baba K, Kim JH, et al. CD49f(high) cells retain sphere-forming and tumor-initiating activities in human gastric tumors. PLoS One. 2013;**8**:e72438. DOI: 10.1371/journal.pone.0072438

[59] Allman DM, Ferguson SE, Lentz VM, Cancro MP. Peripheral B cell maturation. II. Heat-stable antigen(hi) splenic B cells are an immature developmental intermediate in the

production of long-lived marrow-derived B cells. Journal of Immunology (Baltimore, Md: 1950). 1993;**151**:4431-4444.

[60] Gilliam DT, Menon V, Bretz NP, Pruszak J. The CD24 surface antigen in neural development and disease. Neurobiology of Disease. 2016;**99**:133-144. DOI: 10.1016/j.nbd.2016.12.011

[61] Wang YC, Wang JL, Kong X, Sun TT, Chen HY, Hong J, et al. CD24 mediates gastric carcinogenesis and promotes gastric cancer progression via STAT3 activation. Apoptosis: An International Journal on Programmed Cell Death. 2014;**19**:643-656. DOI: 10.1007/s10495-013-0949-9

[62] Wu JX, Zhao YY, Wu X, An HX. Clinicopathological and prognostic significance of CD24 overexpression in patients with gastric cancer: A meta-analysis. PLoS One. 2014;**9**:e114746. DOI: 10.1371/journal.pone.0114746

[63] Sarkar A, Hochedlinger K. The sox family of transcription factors: Versatile regulators of stem and progenitor cell fate. Cell Stem Cell. 2013;**12**:15-30. DOI: 10.1016/j.stem.2012.12.007

[64] Castillo SD, Sanchez-Cespedes M. The SOX family of genes in cancer development: Biological relevance and opportunities for therapy. Expert Opinion on Therapeutic Targets. 2012;**16**:903-919. DOI: 10.1517/14728222.2012.709239

[65] Avilion AA, Nicolis SK, Pevny LH, Perez L, Vivian N, Lovell-Badge R. Multipotent cell lineages in early mouse development depend on SOX2 function. Genes & Development. 2003;**17**:126-140. DOI: 10.1101/gad.224503

[66] Takahashi K, Yamanaka S. Induction of pluripotent stem cells from mouse embryonic and adult fibroblast cultures by defined factors. Cell. 2006;**126**:663-676. DOI: 10.1016/j.cell.2006.07.024

[67] Chen X, Xu H, Yuan P, Fang F, Huss M, Vega VB, et al. Integration of external signaling pathways with the core transcriptional network in embryonic stem cells. Cell. 2008;**133**:1106-1117. DOI: 10.1016/j.cell.2008.04.043

[68] Ellis P, Fagan BM, Magness ST, Hutton S, Taranova O, Hayashi S, et al. SOX2, a persistent marker for multipotential neural stem cells derived from embryonic stem cells, the embryo or the adult. Developmental Neuroscience. 2004;**26**:148-165. DOI: 10.1159/000082134

[69] Taranova OV, Magness ST, Fagan BM, Wu Y, Surzenko N, Hutton SR, et al. SOX2 is a dose-dependent regulator of retinal neural progenitor competence. Genes & Development. 2006;**20**:1187-1202. DOI: 10.1101/gad.1407906

[70] Fauquier T, Rizzoti K, Dattani M, Lovell-Badge R, Robinson IC. SOX2-expressing progenitor cells generate all of the major cell types in the adult mouse pituitary gland. Proceedings of the National Academy of Sciences of the United States of America. 2008;**105**:2907-2912. DOI: 10.1073/pnas.0707886105

[71] Arnold K, Sarkar A, Yram MA, Polo JM, Bronson R, Sengupta S, et al. Sox2(+) adult stem and progenitor cells are important for tissue regeneration and survival of mice. Cell Stem Cell. 2011;**9**:317-329. DOI: 10.1016/j.stem.2011.09.001

[72] Hutton SR, Pevny LH. SOX2 expression levels distinguish between neural progenitor populations of the developing dorsal telencephalon. Developmental Biology. 2011;**352**:40-47. DOI: 10.1016/j.ydbio.2011.01.015

[73] Urban S, Kobi D, Ennen M, Langer D, Le Gras S, Ye T, et al. A Brn2-Zic1 axis specifies the neuronal fate of retinoic-acid-treated embryonic stem cells. Journal of Cell Science. 2015;**128**:2303-2318. DOI: 10.1242/jcs.168849

[74] Que J, Okubo T, Goldenring JR, Nam KT, Kurotani R, Morrisey EE, et al. Multiple dose-dependent roles for Sox2 in the patterning and differentiation of anterior foregut endoderm. Development (Cambridge, England). 2007;**134**:2521-2531. DOI: 10.1242/dev.003855

[75] Asonuma S, Imatani A, Asano N, Oikawa T, Konishi H, Iijima K, et al. *Helicobacter pylori* induces gastric mucosal intestinal metaplasia through the inhibition of interleukin-4-mediated HMG box protein Sox2 expression. American Journal of Physiology Gastrointestinal and Liver Physiology. 2009;**297**:G312-G322. DOI: 10.1152/ajpgi.00518.2007

[76] Bass AJ, Watanabe H, Mermel CH, Yu S, Perner S, Verhaak RG, et al. SOX2 is an amplified lineage-survival oncogene in lung and esophageal squamous cell carcinomas. Nature Genetics. 2009;**41**:1238-1242. DOI: 10.1038/ng.465

[77] Liu K, Jiang M, Lu Y, Chen H, Sun J, Wu S, et al. Sox2 cooperates with inflammation-mediated Stat3 activation in the malignant transformation of foregut basal progenitor cells. Cell Stem Cell. 2013;**12**:304-315. DOI: 10.1016/j.stem.2013.01.007

[78] Boumahdi S, Driessens G, Lapouge G, Rorive S, Nassar D, Le Mercier M, et al. SOX2 controls tumour initiation and cancer stem-cell functions in squamous-cell carcinoma. Nature. 2014;**511**:246-250. DOI: 10.1038/nature13305

[79] Siegle JM, Basin A, Sastre-Perona A, Yonekubo Y, Brown J, Sennett R, et al. SOX2 is a cancer-specific regulator of tumour initiating potential in cutaneous squamous cell carcinoma. Nature Communications. 2014;**5**:4511. DOI: 10.1038/ncomms5511

[80] Garros-Regulez L, Aldaz P, Arrizabalaga O, Moncho-Amor V, Carrasco-Garcia E, Manterola L, et al. mTOR inhibition decreases SOX2-SOX9 mediated glioma stem cell activity and temozolomide resistance. Expert Opinion on Therapeutic Targets. 2016;**20**:393-405. DOI: 10.1517/14728222.2016.1151002

[81] Li XL, Eishi Y, Bai YQ, Sakai H, Akiyama Y, Tani M, et al. Expression of the SRY-related HMG box protein SOX2 in human gastric carcinoma. International Journal of Oncology. 2004;**24**:257-263

[82] Otsubo T, Akiyama Y, Yanagihara K, Yuasa Y. SOX2 is frequently downregulated in gastric cancers and inhibits cell growth through cell-cycle arrest and apoptosis. British Journal of Cancer. 2008;**98**:824-831. DOI: 10.1038/sj.bjc.6604193

[83] Otsubo T, Akiyama Y, Hashimoto Y, Shimada S, Goto K, Yuasa Y. MicroRNA-126 inhibits SOX2 expression and contributes to gastric carcinogenesis. PLoS One. 2011;**6**:e16617. DOI: 10.1371/journal.pone.0016617

[84] Zhang X, Yu H, Yang Y, Zhu R, Bai J, Peng Z, et al. SOX2 in gastric carcinoma, but not Hath1, is related to patients' clinicopathological features and prognosis. Journal of Gastrointestinal Surgery: Official Journal of the Society for Surgery of the Alimentary Tract. 2010;**14**:1220-1226. DOI: 10.1007/s11605-010-1246-3

[85] Wang S, Tie J, Wang R, Hu F, Gao L, Wang W, et al. SOX2, a predictor of survival in gastric cancer, inhibits cell proliferation and metastasis by regulating PTEN. Cancer Letters. 2015;**358**:210-219. DOI: 10.1016/j.canlet.2014.12.045

[86] Khalili M, Vasei M, Khalili D, Alimoghaddam K, Sadeghizadeh M, Mowla SJ. Downregulation of the genes involved in reprogramming (SOX2, c-MYC, miR-302, miR-145, and P21) in gastric adenocarcinoma. Journal of Gastrointestinal Cancer. 2015;**46**:251-258. DOI: 10.1007/s12029-015-9695-2

[87] Camilo V, Garrido M, Valente P, Ricardo S, Amaral AL, Barros R, et al. Differentiation reprogramming in gastric intestinal metaplasia and dysplasia: Role of SOX2 and CDX2. Histopathology. 2015;**66**:343-350. DOI: 10.1111/his.12544

[88] Chawengsaksophak K, James R, Hammond VE, Kontgen F, Beck F. Homeosis and intestinal tumours in Cdx2 mutant mice. Nature. 1997;**386**:84-87. DOI: 10.1038/386084a0

[89] Beck F, Chawengsaksophak K, Waring P, Playford RJ, Furness JB. Reprogramming of intestinal differentiation and intercalary regeneration in Cdx2 mutant mice. Proceedings of the National Academy of Sciences of the United States of America. 1999;**96**:7318-7323.

[90] Sarkar A, Huebner AJ, Sulahian R, Anselmo A, Xu X, Flattery K, et al. Sox2 suppresses gastric tumorigenesis in mice. Cell Reports. 2016;**16**:1929-1941. DOI: 10.1016/j.celrep.2016.07.034

[91] Matsuda K, Yamauchi K, Matsumoto T, Sano K, Yamaoka Y, Ota H. Quantitative analysis of the effect of *Helicobacter pylori* on the expressions of SOX2, CDX2, MUC2, MUC5AC, MUC6, TFF1, TFF2, and TFF3 mRNAs in human gastric carcinoma cells. Scandinavian Journal of Gastroenterology. 2008;**43**:25-33

[92] Niu H, Jia Y, Li T, Su B. SOX2 inhibition promotes promoter demethylation of CDX2 to facilitate gastric intestinal metaplasia. Digestive Diseases and Sciences. 2017;**62**:124-132. DOI: 10.1007/s10620-016-4361-5

[93] Camilo V, Barros R, Sousa S, Magalhaes AM, Lopes T, Mario Santos A, et al. *Helicobacter pylori* and the BMP pathway regulate CDX2 and SOX2 expression in gastric cells. Carcinogenesis. 2012;**33**:1985-1992. DOI: 10.1093/carcin/bgs233

[94] Tian T, Zhang Y, Wang S, Zhou J, Xu S. Sox2 enhances the tumorigenicity and chemoresistance of cancer stem-like cells derived from gastric cancer. Journal of Biomedical Research. 2012;**26**:336-345. DOI: 10.7555/jbr.26.20120045

[95] Matsuoka J, Yashiro M, Sakurai K, Kubo N, Tanaka H, Muguruma K, et al. Role of the stemness factors sox2, oct3/4, and nanog in gastric carcinoma. The Journal of Surgical Research. 2012;**174**:130-135. DOI: 10.1016/j.jss.2010.11.903

[96] Hutz K, Mejias-Luque R, Farsakova K, Ogris M, Krebs S, Anton M, et al. The stem cell factor SOX2 regulates the tumorigenic potential in human gastric cancer cells. Carcinogenesis. 2014;**35**:942-950. DOI: 10.1093/carcin/bgt410

[97] Camilo V, Barros R, Celestino R, Castro P, Vieira J, Teixeira MR, et al. Immunohistochemical molecular phenotypes of gastric cancer based on SOX2 and CDX2 predict patient outcome. BMC Cancer. 2014;**14**:753. DOI: 10.1186/1471-2407-14-753

[98] Yang L, Xu JF, Kang Q, Li AQ, Jin P, Wang X, et al. Predictive value of stemness factor Sox2 in gastric cancer is associated with tumor location and stage. PLoS One. 2017;**12**:e0169124. DOI: 10.1371/journal.pone.0169124

[99] Riemenschnitter C, Teleki I, Tischler V, Guo W, Varga Z. Stability and prognostic value of Slug, Sox9 and Sox10 expression in breast cancers treated with neoadjuvant chemotherapy. SpringerPlus. 2013;**2**:695. DOI: 10.1186/2193-1801-2-695

[100] Matheu A, Collado M, Wise C, Manterola L, Cekaite L, Tye AJ, et al. Oncogenicity of the developmental transcription factor Sox9. Cancer Research. 2012;**72**:1301-1315. DOI: 10.1158/0008-5472.can-11-3660

[101] Kopp JL, von Figura G, Mayes E, Liu FF, Dubois CL, Morris JPt, et al. Identification of Sox9-dependent acinar-to-ductal reprogramming as the principal mechanism for initiation of pancreatic ductal adenocarcinoma. Cancer Cell. 2012;**22**:737-750. DOI: 10.1016/j.ccr.2012.10.025

[102] Song S, Ajani JA, Honjo S, Maru DM, Chen Q, Scott AW, et al. Hippo coactivator YAP1 upregulates SOX9 and endows esophageal cancer cells with stem-like properties. Cancer Research. 2014;**74**:4170-4182. DOI: 10.1158/0008-5472.can-13-3569

[103] Sun L, Mathews LA, Cabarcas SM, Zhang X, Yang A, Zhang Y, et al. Epigenetic regulation of SOX9 by the NF-kappaB signaling pathway in pancreatic cancer stem cells. Stem Cells. 2013;**31**:1454-1466. DOI: 10.1002/stem.1394

[104] Shi Z, Chiang CI, Labhart P, Zhao Y, Yang J, Mistretta TA, et al. Context-specific role of SOX9 in NF-Y mediated gene regulation in colorectal cancer cells. Nucleic Acids Research. 2015;**43**:6257-6269. DOI: 10.1093/nar/gkv568

[105] Santos JC, Carrasco-Garcia E, Garcia-Puga M, Aldaz P, Montes M, Fernandez-Reyes M, et al. SOX9 elevation acts with canonical WNT signaling to drive gastric cancer progression. Cancer Research. 2016;**76**:6735-6746. DOI: 10.1158/0008-5472.can-16-1120

[106] Liu JN, Shang Guan YM, Qi YZ, Wang HB, Zhang TG, Zhou CJ. The evaluation of SOX9 expression and its relationship with carcinoembryonic antigen-related cell adhesion molecule 1 in gastric neoplastic and nonneoplastic lesions. Annals of Diagnostic Pathology. 2012;**16**:235-244. DOI: 10.1016/j.anndiagpath.2011.10.003

[107] Shi JF, Xu SX, He P, Xi ZH. Expression of carcinoembryonic antigen-related cell adhesion molecule 1(CEACAM1) and its correlation with angiogenesis in gastric cancer. Pathology, Research and Practice. 2014;**210**:473-476. DOI: 10.1016/j.prp.2014.03.014

[108] Choi YJ, Song JH, Yoon JH, Choi WS, Nam SW, Lee JY, et al. Aberrant expression of SOX9 is associated with gastrokine 1 inactivation in gastric cancers. Gastric Cancer: Official Journal of the International Gastric Cancer Association and the Japanese Gastric Cancer Association. 2014;**17**:247-254. DOI: 10.1007/s10120-013-0277-3

[109] Serizawa T, Hirata Y, Hayakawa Y, Suzuki N, Sakitani K, Hikiba Y, et al. Gastric metaplasia induced by *Helicobacter pylori* is associated with enhanced SOX9 expression via interleukin-1 signaling. Infection and Immunity. 2015;**84**:562-572. DOI: 10.1128/iai.01437-15

[110] Oshima H, Oshima M. The role of PGE2-associated inflammatory responses in gastric cancer development. Seminars in Immunopathology. 2013;**35**:139-150. DOI: 10.1007/s00281-012-0353-5

[111] Echizen K, Hirose O, Maeda Y, Oshima M. Inflammation in gastric cancer: Interplay of the COX-2/prostaglandin E2 and Toll-like receptor/MyD88 pathways. Cancer Science. 2016;**107**:391-397. DOI: 10.1111/cas.12901

[112] Nardone G, Rippa E, Martin G, Rocco A, Siciliano RA, Fiengo A, et al. Gastrokine 1 expression in patients with and without *Helicobacter pylori* infection. Digestive and Liver Disease: Official Journal of the Italian Society of Gastroenterology and the Italian Association for the Study of the Liver. 2007;**39**:122-129. DOI: 10.1016/j.dld.2006.09.017

[113] Yoon JH, Seo HS, Choi SS, Chae HS, Choi WS, Kim O, et al. Gastrokine 1 inhibits the carcinogenic potentials of *Helicobacter pylori* CagA. Carcinogenesis. 2014;**35**:2619-2629. DOI: 10.1093/carcin/bgu199

[114] Wang J, Xue X, Hong H, Qin M, Zhou J, Sun Q, et al. Upregulation of microRNA-524-5p enhances the cisplatin sensitivity of gastric cancer cells by modulating proliferation and metastasis via targeting SOX9. Oncotarget. 2017;**8**:574-582. DOI: 10.18632/oncotarget.13479

[115] Fang CL, Hseu YC, Lin YF, Hung ST, Tai C, Uen YH, et al. Clinical and prognostic association of transcription factor SOX4 in gastric cancer. PLoS One. 2012;**7**:e52804. DOI: 10.1371/journal.pone.0052804

[116] Zhou X, Li L, Su J, Zhang G. Decreased miR-204 in *H. pylori*-associated gastric cancer promotes cancer cell proliferation and invasion by targeting SOX4. PLoS One. 2014;**9**:e101457. DOI: 10.1371/journal.pone.0101457

[117] Wang CY, Hua L, Sun J, Yao KH, Chen JT, Zhang JJ, et al. MiR-211 inhibits cell proliferation and invasion of gastric cancer by down-regulating SOX4. International Journal of Clinical and Experimental Pathology. 2015;**8**:14013-14020

[118] Eom BW, Jo MJ, Kook MC, Ryu KW, Choi IJ, Nam BH, et al. The lymphangiogenic factor SOX 18: A key indicator to stage gastric tumor progression. International Journal of Cancer. 2012;**131**:41-48. DOI: 10.1002/ijc.26325

Chapter 5

Gastric Cancer: A Stem Cell Disease?

Julie Giraud, Emilie Bessède, Francis Mégraud and
Christine Varon

Additional information is available at the end of the chapter

http://dx.doi.org/10.5772/intechopen.69947

Abstract

Gastric stem cells have been recently identified and are not yet fully characterized. Each gastric gland or unit is composed of different specialized cells and a small number of discrete stem cells. These gastric stem cells play key roles. They have self-renewal and multipotent properties and are the origin of specialized gastric epithelial cells. These properties are the basis for the stem cells' role in tissue homeostasis, tissue repair, and cancer. In tumors, growing evidence indicates that a cell subpopulation with stem cell features, the so-called cancer stem cells (CSCs), represents the "fuel" for the tumor: they are at the origin of tumor initiation, growth, and dissemination, and they also display resistance to conventional chemotherapy treatments. The recent identification of CSCs in gastric carcinoma opens the door to the development of new therapeutic strategies targeting more specifically the CSCs at the origin of the disease, which is the third leading cause of cancer-related deaths worldwide.

Keywords: stem cells, gastric cancer stem cells, CD44, stomach cancer, *Helicobacter pylori*, chemoresistance, ALDH, markers

1. Introduction

Gastric cancer is the third leading cause of cancer-related deaths and the fifth most frequent cancer worldwide. The cancer in its nonmetastatic form is essentially treated by surgery associated with conventional chemotherapy or by chemotherapy alone when metastatic. Its poor prognosis, with less than 10% survival, is due to frequent relapses in metastatic forms even after multimodal therapy. This relapse is associated with the persistence of a cell subpopulation that has acquired or possesses intrinsic mechanisms to resist chemotherapeutic drugs. Indeed, gastric carcinoma, as other solid tumors, is heterogeneous and, a part of their cell population, the gastric cancer stem cells (GCSCs) are responsible for tumor initiation, progression, recurrence, and metastasis. Herein, we first review the major markers of stem/progenitor cells in the stomach, then we describe the cells at the origin of gastric tumors, and finally, we focus on the characterization of the GCSC subpopulation.

2. Existence of stem cells in the stomach

In the stomach, the gastric epithelium is a physiologically self-renewing tissue with a cycle of 2–7 days. Anatomically, the stomach is divided into three main parts: the cardiac region (in humans) or the forestomach (in mice), the main body (corpus), and the distal part (antrum/pylorus). The mucosa of the stomach is composed of a glandular epithelium with millions of gastric units. Each gland is considered to be monoclonal [1] and is subdivided into the foveolus, isthmus, neck, and bottom regions (**Figure 1**). In the gastric corpus, the glands are long and, from the bottom to the top of the gland, contain zymogenic/chief cells implicated in digestion, parietal cells that are essential for acid production, enterochromaffin-like cells that control acid production, mucous neck cells, and superficial pit cells. In the antrum, the glands are shorter and are composed mainly of mucus-producing cells and enteroendocrine hormone-secreting cells that regulate acid and digestive enzyme production in the corpus. In both regions, some discrete gastric stem cells exist and are instrumental in stomach epithelium renewal under pathophysiological conditions.

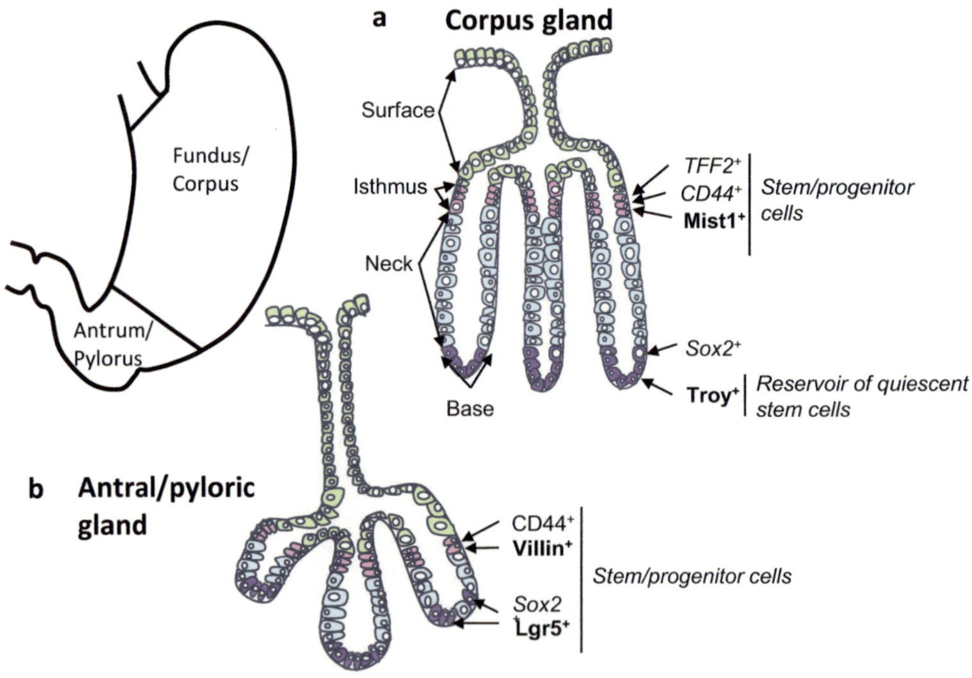

Figure 1. Architecture of the gastric glands and localization of stem/progenitor cells in the main parts of the stomach. (a) Fundic/corpus gastric gland. (b) Antral/pyloric gastric gland. Stem/progenitor markers identified by lineage tracing are indicated in bold.

In adult organs, tissue stem cells are characterized by self-renewal and asymmetrical division properties, giving rise after mitosis to another stem cell and to a progenitor cell that will undergo expansion and then differentiation into mature cells. These stem cells reside in a physiologically limited and specialized microenvironment, called the niche, which is comprised of cells and extracellular matrices forming the surrounding stroma (including mesenchymal cells, vessels, nerves) and which plays a key role in the maintenance of the stem cell number and functions and in preventing tumorigenesis. The localization of the niche of stem/progenitor cells varies according to the part of the stomach considered: in the corpus, they are located in the isthmus just below the glandular narrowing, and in the antropyloric region, there are located at the bottom of the glands. Moreover, as is the case in other organs [2], the coexistence of two stem cell populations has been described in the stomach: (1) a population of dividing gastric stem cells recruited under "homeostatic conditions", expressing CD44 or Lgr5 markers and (2) a rare population of quiescent cells recruited mainly upon tissue damage, expressing Villin, Troy, and Mist1 markers (**Figure 1**).

2.1. Discovery of gastric stem cells and their markers

Using radiolabeling experiments and analyses of the cells by electron microscopy, Leblond et al. first identified a group of small undifferentiated and granule-free cells with the highest labeling index as the putative stem/progenitor cells. These cells are localized in the isthmus region from where they migrate toward both the pit and the bottom [3, 4]. However, the first evidence of the existence of multipotent stem cells in adult mouse gastric glands was found later using chemical mutagenesis of single cells and long-term gastric epithelial cell analyses where many clones spanned entire glands containing all specialized gastric cell lineages [5]. The use of inducible Cre recombinase activity to indelibly label putative stem/progenitor cells and their progeny in the stomach has been widely practiced and is considered as the gold standard method for lineage tracing studies. The first marker of gastric stem/progenitor cells revealed by lineage tracing in the gastric mucosa was **Villin**. *Villin-lacZ* transgenic mice revealed a rare population of quiescent β-galactosidase-positive cells located at the bottom of antropyloric glands or at the isthmus in the corpus [6]. These quiescent Villin$^+$ cells can be activated after stimulation by interferon-γ and moved from the isthmus toward the base of the gland to generate all of the specialized cells of the gastric glands. Villin$^+$ cells may act as a stem cell reservoir with a high proliferative potential to regenerate the gastric mucosa after injury. The presence of such a cell population that highly responds to inflammation is very interesting, especially in the context of gastric cancer which is initiated by a chronic inflammation of the gastric mucosa.

Leucine-rich G protein-coupled receptor 5 (**Lgr5**), a well-recognized stem cell maker in the intestine, is expressed at the bottom of prospective corpus and pyloric glands in the stomach of neonates, whereas its expression in adults is predominantly restricted to the bottom of pyloric glands in mice and in humans [7]. Lineage tracing experiments revealed that Lgr5$^+$ cells are multipotent stem cells responsible for the long-term renewal of the gastric epithelium. In vitro, single Lgr5$^+$ cells generated long-lived organoids resembling the pyloric epithelium in three-dimensional culture. Lgr5$^+$ cells divide symmetrically to generate clonal gland units via neutral competition and lateral expansion of stem cell clones via gland fission under non-damaging conditions [8].

These two markers identified stem cells in the gastric antrum/pyloric region, where most of distal gastric carcinoma arises in humans. In the corpus, some studies suggested that **Sox2$^+$** cells may represent long-lived stem cells scattered throughout the isthmus and in the lower part of the gastric unit [9]. Trefoil factor family 2 (**Tff2$^+$**) cells were also described as short-lived progenitors in the isthmus region of the corpus [10]. More recently, lineage tracing experiments have shown that differentiated mature chief cells expressing the **Troy** marker at the base of the corpus gastric glands can generate entirely labeled gastric units over a period of several months in vivo and long-lived organoids in vitro [11]. This phenomenon is accelerated upon depletion of the proliferating isthmus compartment mediated by 5-fluorouracile treatment, suggesting that the gastric corpus also seems to contain two stem cell populations: (1) an actively dividing population located in the isthmus region and (2) a smaller reserve population of *Troy*$^+$ stem-like chief cells located at the base of the gland [11]. This property of a differentiated cell to reenter the cell cycle and to act as a multipotent stem cell highlights the plasticity of gastric epithelial cells. Surprisingly, Stange et al. detected Lgr5$^+$ cells at the base of the corpus glands using another Lgr5 reporter construction in transgenic mice, and transcriptomic analyses demonstrated that Troy$^+$ cells expresses several Wnt target genes including Lgr5 and CD44 [11].

Likewise, **Mist1** is a marker of stem-like quiescent chief cells located in the lower third of the glands and in rare single cells of the isthmus in the gastric corpus [12, 13]. The vast majority of Mist1$^+$ chief cells at the base of the glands are Lgr5$^+$, whereas Mist1$^+$ cells in the isthmus are Lgr5$^-$, and only 1.1% of them are proliferative. Ablation of Lgr5$^+$/Mist1$^+$ chief cells by expression of the diphtheria toxin in *Lgr5*-DTR-GFP transgenic mice results in an increase of Mist1$^+$ cells in the isthmus which reconstitute the entire glands, suggesting that Mist1$^+$ isthmus cells are multipotent stem cells [13]. Finally, Mist1$^+$ isthmus cells can form organoids in an Lgr5-independent manner in the corpus.

In addition, the Runx1 enhancer element, **eR1**, is expressed in the isthmus and marks a small number of terminally differentiated chief cells at the base in the stomach corpus as well as near the bottom of the pyloric gland. eR1$^+$ cells generated entirely labeled gastric units after a year and formed organoids in vitro, suggesting that they are composed of gastric stem cells [14]. Nevertheless, it appears that some Runx1-expressing cells are stem cells, whereas others are differentiated cells, such as pit cells. Moreover, 80% of eR1$^+$ cells expressed Ki67, whereas only 1.1% of Mist1$^+$ cells in the isthmus expressed it, suggesting that Mist1$^+$ cells are quiescent cells and that eR1$^+$ cells are rapidly dividing cells [13, 14].

Additional markers have been proposed for gastric stem cells (e.g., DCKL1/DCAMKL1, CD133/PROM1, and CD44), but the multipotency of these cells has not yet been analyzed by lineage tracing [15, 16]. Khurana et al. found that **CD44** (cluster of differentiation 44) is mainly expressed at the base of antral/pyloric glands, in a region overlapping Lgr5, and in the isthmus region of the corpus glands [17, 18]. When parietal cell loss and atrophy were induced chemically or by *Helicobacter* infection, the CD44$^+$ cells expanded from the isthmus and replenished the base of the gastric units (**Figure 2**). CD44 expression is enriched in the Mist1$^+$ isthmus stem cell population in the corpus, suggesting again that they could represent stem/progenitor cells.

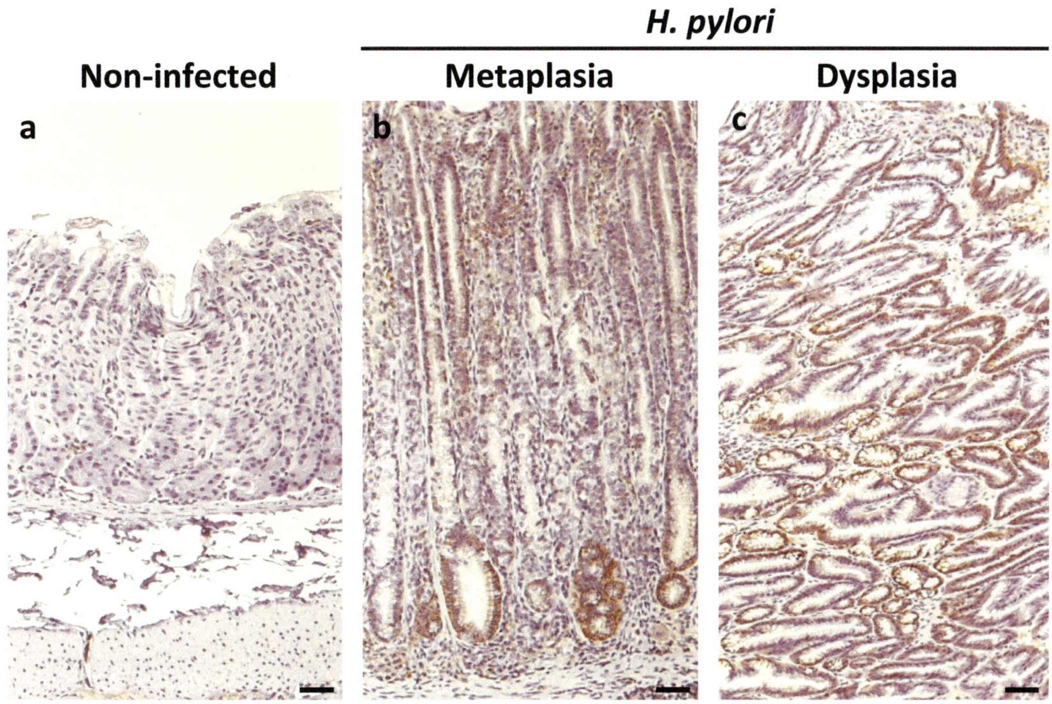

Figure 2. CD44 expression in *H. pylori*-induced metaplasia and dysplasia. Representative pictures of CD44 detection by immunohistochemistry in mouse stomachs: (a) normal gastric mucosa of a noninfected mouse; (b) metaplasia; and (c) intraepithelial dysplasia in *H. pylori SS1*-infected stomachs. Scale bars, 50 μm.

2.2. Factors sustaining gastric stem cell self-renewal and multipotency

Until very recently, suitable models to study gastric stem cells in vitro were lacking. Cell lines from cell banks are all derived from carcinomas, and primary culture of gastric epithelial cells from biopsies is not successful under conventional adherent culture conditions. Culture of antrum and fundus cells has been rendered possible very recently by the development of mouse and human protocols allowing the development of organoids, named gastroids, under three-dimensional culture conditions, in media containing epithelial growth factor (EGF) and Noggin, with either Wnt3A and R-spondin, a molecule binding Lgr4/5 and potentiating Wnt/β-catenin activity [19], or supplemented with the Notch ligand Jagged-1 [7, 13]. In vitro studies of organoid formation by gastric stem cells or gastric glands have allowed insight in the necessary growth factors and signaling molecules of the niche implicated in stem cell properties and gland formation and can offer new therapeutic applications in patient that suffer malignant diseases, for example, for ulcer treatment. Engevik et al. have shown that gastric stem cells/organoid isolated from young mice can be transplanted into sites of acetic acid-induced ulcer within the stomachs of older mice and that this results in accelerated repair injury [20].

Wnt5a, a noncanonical Wnt ligand, is highly expressed by $Cxcr4^{+}$ cells in the isthmus part of the corpus. Histological analyses show that Wnt5A is secreted by $Cxcr4^{+}$ resident hematopoietic cells recruited to the isthmus and stimulated by Cxcl12 endothelial cell production. The efficiency of organoid formation is enhanced by Wnt5a or coculture with $Cxcr4^+$ intraepithelial gastric innate lymphoid cells [13], suggesting that cells in the niche regulate stem/progenitor proliferation.

The enteric nervous system also has the ability to regulate gastric homeostasis via direct innervation of the glands. In three independent mouse models of gastric cancer, Zhao et al. elegantly demonstrated that surgical or pharmacological denervation suppresses gastric tumorigenesis, even if performed at an early preneoplastic step [21]. Further analyses revealed that cholinergic nerves surround the base of glands and modulate epithelial stem cells through activation of the Wnt signaling pathway via the muscarinic acetylcholine receptor 3 (M_3R) expressed by $Lgr5^+$ cells. In stomach organoid models, coculture with neurons or treatment with pilocarpine, a cholinomimetic drug, increased organoid formation and the expression of *Lgr5* and *Cd44* stem cell markers, whereas the effects were reversed by botox treatment [21]. Another publication reported that $Dclk1^+$ tuft cells and nerves, the main sources of acetylcholine in the gastric mucosa, induced nerve growth factor (NGF) secretion from epithelial cells that expand enteric nerves and promote carcinogenesis [22]. Remarkably, *Tff2*-Cre;*R29*-NGF mice developed metaplasia and dysplasia by 8 months of age with $CD44^+$ dysplastic cell expansion and intramucosal adenocarcinomas by 18 months. Ablation of $Dclk1^+$ cells in this context led to the inhibition of epithelial proliferation and tumorigenesis in a M_3R-dependent manner [22].

The Notch signaling pathway is also inhibited in vagotomized mice [21]. The Notch inhibitor dibenzazepine (DBZ) reduced the proliferation in the isthmus region, decreased the Mist1-lineage tracing, and blocked the growth of corpus organoids in vitro, suggesting that Notch activity is important for corpus gastric stem cell maintenance and activity [13].

3. Is gastric cancer a stem cell disease?

Gastric carcinoma is a multifactorial disease, involving a chronic *Helicobacter pylori* infection as the main cause as well as the Epstein-Barr Virus to a small extent, diet (low vitamins, nitrosamines, chemicals, etc.), smoking, and genetic susceptibility of the host [23, 24]. At the histological level, the WHO described more than five different histological subtypes, divided into two main groups in the Lauren classification of gastric tumors, i.e., the intestinal type and the diffuse type [25]. At the molecular level, gastric carcinomas are classified in four main groups based on their mutational profile [26, 27]. These classifications are not currently used in clinical practice to orientate toward a specific targeted therapy.

More than 93% of distal gastric carcinoma cases are associated with a chronic *H. pylori* infection of the gastric mucosa [28]. Most of these cases represent the intestinal histological subtype. *H. pylori* infection induces a chronic inflammation of the gastric mucosa, i.e., gastritis. In 5–10% of cases, gastritis evolves into gastric or duodenal ulcer, and in 1% of cases, gastritis leads to stomach cancers. In this last case, the loss of specialized epithelial cells results in a chronic atrophic gastritis and to the compensatory cellular hyperproliferation and aberrant differentiation at the origin of the intestinal metaplasia (firstly appearing in the pylorus) and/or spasmolytic polypeptide-expressing metaplasia (SPEM) (mainly in the corpus). These metaplastic lesions can further progress into dysplasia and ultimately into an intestinal-type carcinoma according to the Lauren classification [29, 30]. So, chronic atrophic gastritis is considered to be the first step of gastric adenocarcinomas. All of these lesions are well characterized histologically and can be reproduced experimentally in Mongolian gerbils [31] and in mice [32, 33] in response to *H. pylori* and *Helicobacter felis* infection. Gastric carcinoma of the diffuse type or signet ring cell carcinoma corresponds to poorly differentiated adenocarcinomas for which the glandular structure has disappeared. It is the second most frequent histological subtype of gastric tumors, which is frequently linked to sporadic or hereditary mutations of the *CDH1* gene encoding E-cadherin, and appears most of the time without precancerous lesions.

H. pylori is mainly present at the surface of gastric units but also as microcolonies deep in the stomach glands; the bacteria can interact directly with gastric stem/progenitor cells in the stomach of mice and humans. Regarding their long lifetime and high division ability, stem cells are more susceptible to accumulate genetic/epigenetic modifications than their progeny. Some current evidence suggests that, in the context of chronic *H. pylori* infection, gastric cancer stem cells originate from the transformation of stem cells of two different origins: local, for most of the cases, and to a lesser extent from bone marrow-derived stem cells that home into the gastric mucosa in response to the chronic injury mediated by *Helicobacter*, contributing to metaplasia and dysplasia [34–36]. It is important, however, to distinguish between the origin of cancer cells which initiate and drive the primary tumor development and those which accumulate and contribute to tumor growth once the process is initiated. These two main mechanisms leading to the emergence of gastric cancer cells will be discussed below.

3.1. Tumors can originate from epithelial stem cell transformation

Interestingly, the parietal cell atrophy induced after *H. pylori* infection causes an increase in the proliferation of stem/progenitor cells in the isthmus [37] that is associated with an induction of CD44 expression in this region, which then expands toward the bottom of the gastric unit [17, 35, 36] (**Figure 2**). Sigal et al. also reported an increase of the number of antral $Lgr5^+$ cells in *H. pylori*-associated gastritis and carcinoma in humans. As these cells are susceptible to DNA damage, it suggests that $Lgr5^+$ stem cells could be at the origin of cancer [38, 39]. An $Lgr5^+$ gene signature in pyloric gastric units identified Wnt target genes, including *Sox9* and *Cd44*, suggesting canonical Wnt signaling activity at the base of the pyloric glands. Gastric cancer patients exhibit a dysregulation of Wnt signaling [21]. Spontaneous Wnt activation in the mouse model APC^{min} leads to the development of gastric adenomas in the pyloric region; *Apc* depletion specifically in $Lgr5^+$ via a single tamoxifen injection in *Lgr5-EGFP-CreERT2;*$APC^{flox/flox}$ mice leads to adenoma formation in the gastric antrum, but not in the corpus [7].

KRAS is one of the most commonly mutated oncogenes in gastric cancer. The *Kras* mutation in the $Mist1^+$ isthmus cells, and not in the $Mist1^+$ chief cells, results in the formation of metaplastic/dysplastic foci from the isthmus to the bottom of glands. $Mist1^+$ stem cells give rise to intramucosal intestinal-type gastric cancer induced by *Apc* loss of function but only in the context of KRAS-induced metaplasia [13].

E-cadherin expression is lost in most diffuse-type gastric carcinomas, but E-cadherin loss alone is not sufficient to initiate diffuse-type gastric cancer in mice [40]. Loss of the tight junction protein IQGAP1 is also insufficient to induce diffuse-type gastric carcinoma in transgenic mice after challenge with *Helicobacter* infection, as it indeed promotes intestinal-type carcinogenesis [41]. To try to reproduce the diffuse-type gastric cancer, some authors infected *Mist1*;CreERT2;*Cdh1*$^{flox/flox}$ mice with *H. felis* to induce chronic inflammation. In this context, E-cadherin loss in Mist1^{+} cells resulted in the development of diffuse-type gastric carcinomas [13]. The double inactivation of E-cadherin and p53 in a conditional mouse model also successfully led to metastatic diffuse-type gastric cancer [42].

3.2. Tumors originating from bone marrow-derived cells

Some data have shown that bone marrow-derived cells (BMDCs) can migrate to peripheral tissues in case of injury or inflammation where they are engrafted and participate in tissue repair, giving rise to all cell lineages. Houghton et al. showed that BMDCs are recruited into the gastric mucosa of C57BL/6 mice chronically infected by *H. felis* and contribute overtime to metaplasia, dysplasia, and finally cancer [34]. In fact, to the contrary, they found that it was a rare event in the context of a normal homeostasis, without injury. Results from this study did not exclude the possibility that BMDCs participate in the development of lesions via fusion with epithelial cells. Our group confirmed these observations in the same mouse genetic background but with different strains of the human pathogen *H. pylori* and found that nearly a quarter of high-grade dysplastic lesions are composed of BMDCs [35]. BMDC epithelial gland repopulation was significantly associated with pseudointestinal metaplasia, suggesting that BMDC recruitment may play a role in preneoplastic lesion progression. These BMDCs are recruited only in response to chronic *H. felis* and *H. pylori* infection but not in response to acute injury [34]. BMDC recruitment occurs in response to the secretion of several chemokines such as SDF1 and TNFα by infected epithelial cells in a NF-κB-dependent manner [34, 43]. Once recruited, the BMDCs can differentiate into local gastric epithelial cells via transdifferentiation or cell/cell fusion with local gastric epithelial cells [35, 44]. Interestingly, BMDC recruitment into the gastric mucosa was a late event in the cascade of gastric carcinogenesis, occurring only in infected animals of more than 1 year of age. In these chimera mice, metaplastic lesions were comprised, inside the same gland, of a mosaic of tagged-BMDCs and native gastric epithelial cells, revealing a multiclonal composition [35]. These metaplastic lesions are now considered as a "point of no return," after which, most of the time, eradication of *H. pylori* cannot lead to a regression of the metaplastic and associated dysplastic lesions, because mutations deregulating stem cell properties and proliferation are already present. A monoclonal conversion will occur during the evolution of intestinal metaplasia toward dysplasia and finally carcinoma. As the mice never develop real metastatic gastric adenocarcinoma in contrast to the human situation, there is no evidence in the literature to date of the role of BMDCs composing metaplastic/dysplastic lesions as the tumor-initiating cells in invasive gastric adenocarcinoma. However, it is very interesting to note that BMDCs were also detected in gastric carcinoma of the esophagus in mice models and in humans, which also develop on a background of chronic inflammation and intestinal metaplasia cascade [45, 46]. Very few studies have been described in humans to strengthen the results obtained in animal models, because there is a limited possibility to trace BMDCs in an individual developing a carcinoma of the GI tract. The only technical approach tested was to detect the Y chromosome of BM cells of a male donor in female transplanted patients by fluorescence in situ hybridization (FISH). In such transplanted cases having developed carcinoma of the GI tract, BMDCs were detected in some rare cases of carcinoma and dysplasia of the esophagus [45, 46]. Concerning the stomach, the study of Whortley et al., performed on only four cases of sex-mismatch transplanted cases having developed gastric carcinoma, failed to report a carcinoma composed of cells of BM origin. However, one of the cases showed aneuploidy, so a contribution of the BMDCs cannot be totally excluded [47].

Unfortunately, in those models, full proof of the concept that gastric stem cells or other populations of differentiated cells or BMDCs are the cells of origin of cancer has not been found, because the tumorigenic effect mediated, for instance, by *Apc* and *Cdh1* inactivation or by *Kras* oncogenic activation in non-stem cell populations, i.e., in progenitor or differentiated cells, has not been followed. Moreover, in contrast to squamous skin tumors [48] or intestinal adenomas [49], the in vivo contribution of GCSCs to tumorigenesis has not yet been fully elucidated. Nevertheless, regardless of their origin, dysplastic lesions and gastric adenocarcinomas are composed of CD44$^+$ cells (**Figure 2**) [17, 36] that have been recently described to possess cancer stem cell properties [50, 51].

3.3. Tumor originates from dedifferentiation of epithelial cells

In an inflammatory setting, differentiated cells can reacquire the ability to divide and to give rise to all cell lineages. In vitro, *H. pylori* infection induces a destabilization of cell/cell junctions and an elongated phenotype associated with motility [52]. We reported that *H. pylori* infection leads to the generation of a CD44$^+$ cancer stem-like cell population with mesenchymal phenotype and tumorigenic properties, through complex signaling pathways involving activation of the mitogen-activated protein kinase ERK, c-Jun N-terminal kinase, miR200, and NF-κB signaling pathways, leading to the activation of ZEB1 and Snail1 transcription factors, the main drivers of the epithelial-mesenchymal transition (EMT) [36]. We showed that this effect was associated with the bacterial oncoprotein CagA produced by *H. pylori* and with secreted factors such as hepatocyte growth factor (HGF) as described by others [36, 53]. In vivo, the expansion of the compartment of CD44$^+$ stem cells at the isthmus in the corpus and at the base of the glands in the antro-pyloric region is associated with the expression of mesenchymal markers in the context of *H. pylori*-associated gastritis, metaplasia, and dysplasia, in humans and in wild-type mice [23, 36, 41]. We recently showed that invalidation of *iqgap1*, a partner of E-cadherin at the cell/cell junctions, increased EMT both in vitro and in vivo, promoted *H. felis*- and *H. pylori*-induced regenerative hyperplasia expressing CD44 and mesenchymal markers, and accelerated and worsened metaplasia and dysplasia development, reinforcing the causal link between EMT and emergence of CSC-like cells [41].

4. Properties of gastric cancer stem cells

Tumor cells are heterogeneous in terms of mutations carried, susceptibility to drugs, markers expressed or morphology, and not all are tumorigenic. This genetic heterogeneity would come not only from intrinsic factors such as genetic mutations acquired progressively and amplified within new clones but also from extrinsic factors related to the variation of the tumor microenvironment [54, 55]. To explain these observations, two concepts have been proposed: the cancer stem cell (CSC) theory, also named the hierarchical model, and the stochastic model. In the stochastic model, all cancer cells have similar tumorigenic properties, with cancer arising after a series of genetic and epigenetic events leading to successive waves of clonal selections depending on the proliferative and survival benefits acquired. In the hierarchical model, there is a cellular hierarchy between cancer cells inside the tumor, with CSCs being at the origin of the more or less differentiated cells, not all proliferative and tumorigenic, composing the tumor mass. CSCs represent a small percentage of tumor cells and possess particular properties compared to non-CSCs (**Figure 3**): (1) the first and most important is their capacity to self-renew and divide asymmetrically and to generate a new CSC and a non-CSC progenitor cell, a property that maintains a constant CSC pool; (2) CSCs are able to initiate tumor growth when injected in low cell numbers in immunocompromised mice; (3) CSCs display differentiation properties giving rise to the more or less differentiated cells composing the tumor mass, reconstructing the tumor heterogeneity observed within the primary tumor; (4) CSCs have increased resistance to current chemo- and radiotherapies; and (5) CSCs express

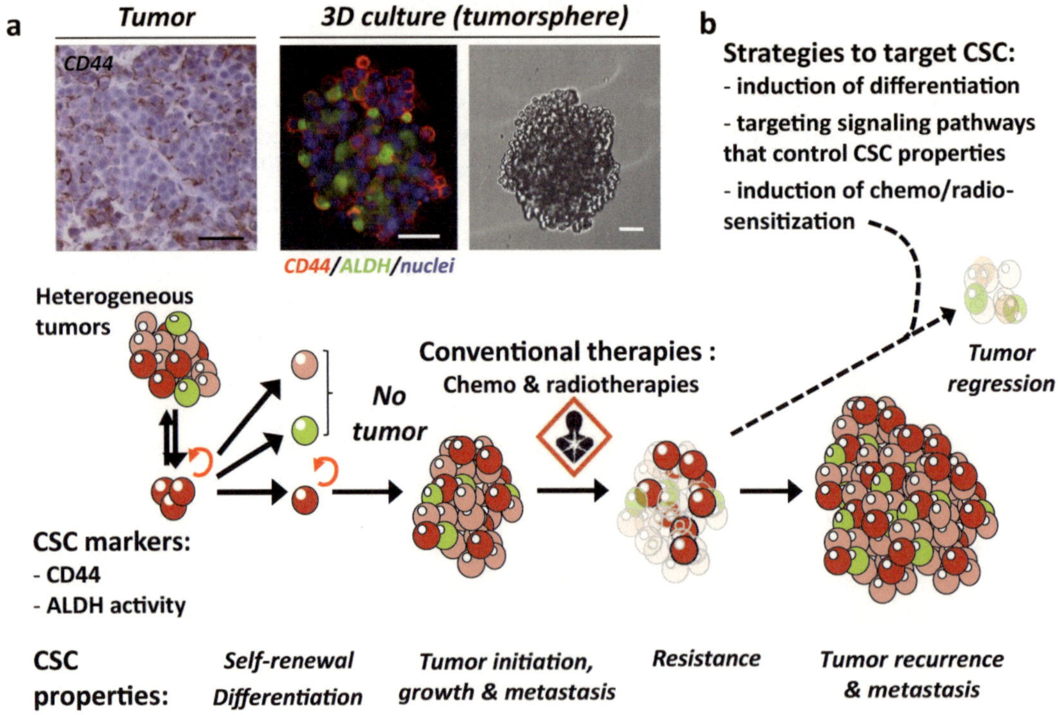

Figure 3. Hierarchical model illustrating the heterogeneity of the tumors. (a) Representative images of CD44 detection by immunohistochemistry on tumor tissue section (left panel) and of the detection of CD44 by immunofluorescence and ALDH activity (Aldefluor™ reagent) with Hoescht 33342 dye (middle panel) on tumor spheres of MKN45 gastric cancer cells (right panel, phase contrast microscopy). Scale bars, 50 μm. (b) Hypothetical strategies to target CSC to cure gastric cancer. The main gastric CSC markers are CD44 and ALDH activity. Cancer stem cells represent a subpopulation of cells implicated in tumor initiation, growth, metastasis, and chemo-/radio-resistance.

specific markers [55]. This hierarchical model is not exclusive but is now the most accepted model with the recent identification of CSCs in most cancers since their first discovery in acute myeloid leukemia in 1995, then in solid tumors in 2003, and more recently in gastric carcinoma. However, we must keep in mind that this hierarchical model is also subjected to clonal evolution even if it has not been clearly demonstrated for gastric carcinoma [56].

4.1. Functional characterization of gastric cancer stem cells

By taking advantage of the capacity of stem cells to self-renew, differentiate, and initiate tumors, functional assays have been developed to evaluate the amount of GCSCs or to isolate them from a global population of tumor cells. In vitro, under conditions in which cells are seeded at low-density in low-adherent plates, without serum and in the presence of some growth factors such as EGF, bFGF, and insulin, only GCSCs can survive, self-renew, and form tumorspheres [36, 50, 51, 57]. Long self-renewal ability is evaluated after tumorsphere dissociation into single cells and several passages; indeed only GCSCs can generate tumorspheres after several passages [51, 58]. In vivo, frequency of GCSCs in a given population is determined after subcutaneous xenograft in immunocompromised mice using different cell doses and an analysis of their ability to initiate a new heterogenous tumor after several weeks. Immunocompromised mouse phenotypes, nonobese diabetic/severe combined immunodeficiency (NOD/SCID) and NOD/SCID/IL2Rg− (NSG), can influence the CSC frequency as reported in the case of melanoma by Morrison's group [59]. In both methods, cells were seeded for an extreme limiting dilution assay, and a mathematical method was applied to calculate the CSC frequency in a given cell population [51, 60].

4.2. Phenotypic characterization of gastric cancer stem cells

Several phenotypic characteristics have been proposed to isolate GCSCs using fluorescence-activated cell sorting (FACS), including (1) the expression of cell membrane markers (or combinations of markers), and among them CD44; (2) the exclusion of Hoechst 33342 dye by the "side population" of cells (SP cells); and (3) the enzymatic activity of aldehyde dehydrogenases (ALDH).

CD44 was among the first markers of CSCs described in solid tumors and initially in breast carcinoma [61]. CD44 is a type I transmembrane glycoprotein expressed in many normal and tumoral cells. It plays a role in adhesion/homing, supporting cell migration and transmitting survival signals, thereby being pro-oncogenic by nature. The principal ligand of the CD44 receptor coordinating signalization is hyaluronic acid, but it can also interact with additional molecules of the extracellular matrix, such as collagen, fibronectin, fibrinogen, laminin, or osteopontin [62]. Cytoplasmic partner molecules of CD44 are the cytoskeletal proteins Ezrin, Radixin, Moesin, and Ankyrin, which influence the signaling pathway. Loss of CD44 in mice models results in a decrease in gastric mucosa proliferation in the isthmus region. The critical role of CD44 in proliferation involves its interaction with hyaluronic acid and the downstream activation of the STAT3 signaling pathway [17], RhoGTPases, the PI3K/AKT pathway, and the MAPK signaling pathway [63]. CD44 is encoded by the 20-exon *CD44* gene, in which exons 1–5 and 16–20 are spliced together and translated into CD44s, the standard or small isoform.

In addition, the variant exons 6–15 can be alternatively spliced and assembled in different combinations with the standard exons to generate other variant (CD44v) protein isoforms [62, 64]. We and others reported that CD44 is expressed following *H. pylori* infection in patients and in mouse models in the case of regenerative hyperplasia, intestinal metaplasia, dysplasia, and gastric carcinoma (**Figure 2**) [35, 36, 50, 51, 65]. Histological and molecular analyses of tumor collections have shown that CD44 is positively and significantly associated with tumor recurrence and mortality in gastric cancer, and the expression of CD44 and CD44v has also been associated with metastasis formation [57, 65–70].

Takaishi et al. were the first to propose CD44 as a marker of GCSCs in a study performed on several gastric cancer cell lines [50]. Their $CD44^+$ cells were able to form tumorspheres and initiate tumors after subcutaneous and orthotopic engraftment in mice, and they were resistant to anticancer drugs, whereas $CD44^-$ sorted cells were not. Moreover, it seems that CD44 is not only a GCSC marker, but it also plays an oncogenic role, assessed by a decrease in tumor growth using siRNA targeting CD44. More recently, further relevant results from patient-derived xenograft models (PDXs) of gastric carcinoma have confirmed that CD44 is also a marker of GCSCs in primary gastric carcinoma. The FACS-sorted $CD44^+$ cells, but not their $CD44^-$ counterpart, displayed CSC properties such as growing as tumorspheres in vitro and lead to tumor formation in vivo that reconstitute the heterogeneity of the primary tumor of the patients and are more chemoresistant [51, 71, 72]. ESA, CD24, CD133, and CD166 are also expressed by $CD44^+$ cells, but they do not allow a better enrichment of GCSCs in combination with CD44 compared to CD44 alone [51, 73]. Although CD44 marks GCSCs, not all $CD44^+$ cells are tumorigenic [51]. CD44v8-10, also named CD44E, has been identified as the predominant CD44 variant expressed in gastric cancer cells, and its expression is low in normal tissues [57]. It plays a functional role in tumor initiation, most likely by increasing CSC resilience to adverse conditions such as hypoxia or oxidative stress. Indeed, there is evidence that CD44v8-10 stabilizes the cystine-glutamate transporter subunit xCT and promotes the synthesis of glutathione, thereby protecting cancer cells from reactive oxygen species [70]. Depletion of the expression of CD44 leads to a decrease in the tumorigenicity of cancer cell lines [50], and Yoon et al. demonstrated implication of the Hedgehog signaling in the maintenance, chemoresistance, and migration capacity of the GCSC $CD44^+$ cells [74].

ALDH activity has also been described as a GCSC marker [51, 75]. In an extensive screening of the expression of 10 putative CSC surface markers, as well as in eight PDX models, we found that CSCs expressed both CD44 and ALDH activity and that ALDH activity revealed a subpopulation within the $CD44^+$ cells that possessed CSC properties, i.e., the ability to generate a new heterogeneous tumor in vivo and a tumorsphere in vitro. Xenograft experiments using the ELDA mathematical model showed that the frequency of GCSCs expressing CD44 and ALDH was 0.1–3.5% of the cancer cells [51]. These $CD44^+/ALDH^+$ cells did not incorporate the vital DNA dye Hoechst 33342, whereas the $ALDH^-$ cells incorporated it, suggesting that $CD44^+/ALDH^+$ cells may correspond to **SP cells** with CSC properties as previously described in gastric carcinoma cell lines by others [76–78]. The ability of $CD44^+/ALDH^+$ cells to efflux the Hoechst 33342 dye and to resist conventional chemotherapy was reversed by treatment with efflux pump inhibitors [51]. Nevertheless, Takaishi et al. found that both gastric SP and non-SP cells possess a tumorigenic ability in vitro and in vivo [50]. Therefore, the detection of the SP cells does not seem to be a good marker for GCSCs; rather the best markers to detect them are CD44 and ALDH.

4.3. Missing data: implication of gastric cancer stem cells in metastasis?

Another important property of CSCs is their ability to initiate metastasis. Metastasis is a rare event [79] requiring the acquisition of invasive properties through epithelial-mesenchymal transition (1) to escape from the niche of the primary tumor in order to disseminate to distant organs after extravasation as circulating tumor cells (CTCs) and (2) to initiate secondary tumors [80]. We reported that the $CD44^+$ cells with CSC-like properties induced by *H. pylori* infection but not the $CD44^-$ cells overexpressed mesenchymal markers such as Vimentin and Zeb1 and downregulated epithelial markers and tumorigenic, migratory, and invasive properties [36, 81]. Chen et al. identified CTCs characterized by $CD44^+CD54^+$ expression in the peripheral blood from patients with gastric cancer which were able to form tumorspheres and generate heterogeneous tumors when injected into immunodeficient mice; these CTCs had a self-renewal capability both in cell culture and in mouse models [82]. This study suggested that $CD44^+CD54^+$ CTCs could represent metastatic GCSCs. Nevertheless, the characterization of the CSC subpopulation capable of initiating metastases needs to be determined.

5. Conclusion

Since 2007, researchers have increased efforts to identify real gastric stem cells, the cell population capable of replenishing an entire gastric gland containing of all cell lineages. Many of the markers involved have been reviewed here, and their stemness properties have been clearly demonstrated in mouse models. It will be of interest to understand why there are different localizations of stem cells, one in the isthmus and one at the bottom of the gland. These two stem/progenitor cell niches could play different roles, one being more proliferative than the other one which seems to behave like a reservoir, but they could also play distinct roles in response to different stimuli and damage to the gastric mucosa.

Regarding to the gastric tumor, an in-depth analysis of putative CSC markers identified CD44 as well as ALDH activity as the "gold" gastric CSC markers in cancer cell lines and in PDX models [51]. Determination of the signaling pathways controlling their properties is now instrumental to find new targeted therapies for gastric cancer, for which there is a crucial unmet need to find new efficient therapy. In this aim, we have shown by different strategies that the targeting of gastric CSCs expressing CD44 by blocking specific microRNAs or by inducing their differentiation by all-trans retinoic acid allows inhibition of tumor growth in vivo [58, 83].

Nevertheless, the characterization of gastric CSCs was limited in some publications by the cellular model used. To date, the best models to study the efficiency of new therapeutic strategies on primary gastric CSCs remain PDX models, with the restriction that almost all of those described are subcutaneous engraftments which never give rise to metastasis. Moreover, mouse models of gastric carcinogenesis induced by *Helicobacter* infection and/or carcinogens do not reproduce invasion of the deeper layers of the stomach, peritoneal carcinomatosis, and distant metastases as in humans. Consequently, there is an urgent need to develop mouse models of metastatic gastric carcinoma, in order to study the efficiency of new therapeutic strategies targeting CSCs not only on tumor initiation but also on metastasis formation.

Author details

Julie Giraud[1,2], Emilie Bessède[1,2,3], Francis Mégraud[1,2,3] and Christine Varon[1,2*]

*Address all correspondence to: christine.varon@u-bordeaux.fr

1 INSERM, U1053, Bordeaux, France

2 University of Bordeaux, Bordeaux, France

3 Hopital Pellegrin, Bordeaux, France

References

[1] McDonald SA, Greaves LC, Gutierrez-Gonzalez L, Rodriguez-Justo M, Deheragoda M, Leedham SJ, et al. Mechanisms of field cancerization in the human stomach: The expansion and spread of mutated gastric stem cells. Gastroenterology. 2008 Feb;**134**(2):500-510

[2] Li L, Clevers H. Coexistence of quiescent and active adult stem cells in mammals. Science (New York, NY). 2010 Jan 29;**327**(5965):542-545

[3] Karam SM, Leblond CP. Dynamics of epithelial cells in the corpus of the mouse stomach. I. Identification of proliferative cell types and pinpointing of the stem cell. The Anatomical Record. 1993 Jun;**236**(2):259-279

[4] Lee ER, Leblond CP. Dynamic histology of the antral epithelium in the mouse stomach: II. Ultrastructure and renewal of isthmal cells. The American Journal of Anatomy. 1985 Mar;**172**(3):205-224

[5] Bjerknes M, Cheng H. Multipotential stem cells in adult mouse gastric epithelium. American Journal of Physiology. 2002 Sep;**283**(3):G767-G777

[6] Qiao XT, Ziel JW, McKimpson W, Madison BB, Todisco A, Merchant JL, et al. Prospective identification of a multilineage progenitor in murine stomach epithelium. Gastroenterology. 2007 Dec;**133**(6):1989-1998

[7] Barker N, Huch M, Kujala P, van de Wetering M, Snippert HJ, van Es JH, et al. Lgr5(+ve) stem cells drive self-renewal in the stomach and build long-lived gastric units *in vitro*. Cell Stem Cell. 2010 Jan 8;**6**(1):25-36

[8] Leushacke M, Ng A, Galle J, Loeffler M, Barker N. Lgr5(+) gastric stem cells divide symmetrically to effect epithelial homeostasis in the pylorus. Cell Reports. 2013 Oct 31;**5**(2):349-356

[9] Arnold K, Sarkar A, Yram MA, Polo JM, Bronson R, Sengupta S, et al. Sox2(+) adult stem and progenitor cells are important for tissue regeneration and survival of mice. Cell Stem Cell. 2011 Oct 04;**9**(4):317-329

[10] Quante M, Marrache F, Goldenring JR, Wang TC. TFF2 mRNA transcript expression marks a gland progenitor cell of the gastric oxyntic mucosa. Gastroenterology. 2010 Dec;**139**(6):2018-27 e2

[11] Stange DE, Koo BK, Huch M, Sibbel G, Basak O, Lyubimova A, et al. Differentiated Troy+ chief cells act as reserve stem cells to generate all lineages of the stomach epithelium. Cell. 2013 Oct 10;**155**(2):357-368

[12] Nam KT, Lee HJ, Sousa JF, Weis VG, O'Neal RL, Finke PE, et al. Mature chief cells are cryptic progenitors for metaplasia in the stomach. Gastroenterology. 2010 Dec;**139**(6): 2028-37 e9

[13] Hayakawa Y, Ariyama H, Stancikova J, Sakitani K, Asfaha S, Renz BW, et al. Mist1 expressing gastric stem cells maintain the normal and neoplastic gastric epithelium and are supported by a perivascular stem cell niche. Cancer Cell. 2015 Dec 14;**28**(6):800-814

[14] Matsuo J, Kimura S, Yamamura A, Koh CP, Hossain MZ, Heng DL, et al. Identification of stem cells in the epithelium of the stomach corpus and antrum of mice. Gastroenterology. 2017 Jan;**152**(1):218-31 e14

[15] Mills JC, Shivdasani RA. Gastric epithelial stem cells. Gastroenterology. 2011 Feb;**140**(2): 412-424

[16] Qiao XT, Gumucio DL. Current molecular markers for gastric progenitor cells and gastric cancer stem cells. Journal of Gastroenterology. 2011 Jul;**46**(7):855-865

[17] Khurana SS, Riehl TE, Moore BD, Fassan M, Rugge M, Romero-Gallo J, et al. The hyaluronic acid receptor CD44 coordinates normal and metaplastic gastric epithelial progenitor cell proliferation. The Journal of Biological Chemistry. 2013 May 31;**288**(22):16085-16097

[18] Simon E, Petke D, Boger C, Behrens HM, Warneke V, Ebert M, et al. The spatial distribution of LGR5+ cells correlates with gastric cancer progression. PLoS One. 2012;**7**(4):e35486

[19] de Lau W, Barker N, Low TY, Koo BK, Li VS, Teunissen H, et al. Lgr5 homologues associate with Wnt receptors and mediate R-spondin signalling. Nature. 2011 Jul 04; **476**(7360):293-297

[20] Engevik AC, Feng R, Choi E, White S, Bertaux-Skeirik N, Li J, et al. The development of spasmolytic polypeptide/TFF2-expressing metaplasia (SPEM) during gastric repair is absent in the aged stomach. Cellular and Molecular Gastroenterology and Hepatology. 2016 Sep;**2**(5):605-624

[21] Zhao CM, Hayakawa Y, Kodama Y, Muthupalani S, Westphalen CB, Andersen GT, et al. Denervation suppresses gastric tumorigenesis. Science Translational Medicine. 2014 Aug 20;**6**(250):250ra115.

[22] Hayakawa Y, Sakitani K, Konishi M, Asfaha S, Niikura R, Tomita H, et al. Nerve growth factor promotes gastric tumorigenesis through aberrant cholinergic signaling. Cancer Cell. 2017 Jan 09;**31**(1):21-34

[23] Bessede E, Dubus P, Megraud F, Varon C. Helicobacter pylori infection and stem cells at the origin of gastric cancer. Oncogene. 2015 May 14;**34**(20):2547-55

[24] Megraud F, Bessede E, Varon C. *Helicobacter pylori* infection and gastric carcinoma. Clinical Microbiology and Infection. 2015 Nov;**21**(11):984-990

[25] Lauren P. The two histological main types of gastric carcinoma: Diffuse and so-called intestinal-type carcinoma. An attempt at a histo-clinical classification. Acta Pathologica et Microbiologica Scandinavica. 1965;**64**:31-49

[26] TCGARN. Comprehensive molecular characterization of gastric adenocarcinoma. Nature. 2014 Sep 11;**513**(7517):202-209

[27] Wang K, Yuen ST, Xu J, Lee SP, Yan HH, Shi ST, et al. Whole-genome sequencing and comprehensive molecular profiling identify new driver mutations in gastric cancer. Nature Genetics. 2014 Jun;**46**(6):573-582

[28] Gonzalez CA, Megraud F, Buissonniere A, Lujan Barroso L, Agudo A, Duell EJ, et al. *Helicobacter pylori* infection assessed by ELISA and by immunoblot and noncardia gastric cancer risk in a prospective study: The Eurgast-EPIC project. Annals Oncology. 2012 May;**23**(5):1320-1324

[29] Correa P, Haenszel W, Cuello C, Tannenbaum S, Archer M. A model for gastric cancer epidemiology. Lancet. 1975 Jul 12;**2**(7924):58-60

[30] Correa P, Houghton J. Carcinogenesis of *Helicobacter pylori*. Gastroenterology. 2007 Aug;**133**(2):659-672

[31] Watanabe T, Tada M, Nagai H, Sasaki S, Nakao M. *Helicobacter pylori* infection induces gastric cancer in Mongolian gerbils. Gastroenterology. 1998 Sep;**115**(3):642-648

[32] Cai X, Carlson J, Stoicov C, Li H, Wang TC, Houghton J. *Helicobacter felis* eradication restores normal architecture and inhibits gastric cancer progression in C57BL/6 mice. Gastroenterology. 2005 Jun;**128**(7):1937-1952

[33] Rogers AB, Taylor NS, Whary MT, Stefanich ED, Wang TC, Fox JG. *Helicobacter pylori* but not high salt induces gastric intraepithelial neoplasia in B6129 mice. Cancer Research. 2005 Dec 1;**65**(23):10709-10715

[34] Houghton J, Stoicov C, Nomura S, Rogers AB, Carlson J, Li H, et al. Gastric cancer originating from bone marrow-derived cells. Science (New York, NY). 2004 Nov 26;**306**(5701):1568-1571

[35] Varon C, Dubus P, Mazurier F, Asencio C, Chambonnier L, Ferrand J, et al. *Helicobacter pylori* infection recruits bone marrow-derived cells that participate in gastric preneoplasia in mice. Gastroenterology. 2012 Feb;**142**(2):281-291

[36] Bessede E, Staedel C, Acuna Amador LA, Nguyen PH, Chambonnier L, Hatakeyama M, et al. *Helicobacter pylori* generates cells with cancer stem cell properties via epithelial-mesenchymal transition-like changes. Oncogene. 2014 Aug 7;**33**(32):4123-4131

[37] Nozaki K, Ogawa M, Williams JA, Lafleur BJ, Ng V, Drapkin RI, et al. A molecular signature of gastric metaplasia arising in response to acute parietal cell loss. Gastroenterology. 2008 Feb;**134**(2):511-522

[38] Sigal M, Rothenberg ME, Logan CY, Lee JY, Honaker RW, Cooper RL, et al. *Helicobacter pylori* activates and expands Lgr5(+) stem cells through direct colonization of the gastric glands. Gastroenterology. 2015 Jun;**148**(7):1392-404 e21

[39] Uehara T, Ma D, Yao Y, Lynch JP, Morales K, Ziober A, et al. *H. pylori* infection is associated with DNA damage of Lgr5-positive epithelial stem cells in the stomach of patients with gastric cancer. Digestive Diseases and Sciences. 2013 Jan;**58**(1):140-149

[40] Humar B, Blair V, Charlton A, More H, Martin I, Guilford P. E-cadherin deficiency initiates gastric signet-ring cell carcinoma in mice and man. Cancer Research. 2009 Mar 1;**69**(5):2050-2056

[41] Bessede E, Molina S, Amador LA, Dubus P, Staedel C, Chambonnier L, et al. Deletion of IQGAP1 promotes *Helicobacter pylori*-induced gastric dysplasia in mice and acquisition of cancer stem cell properties *in vitro*. Oncotarget. 2016 Dec 06;**7**(49):80688-80699

[42] Shimada S, Mimata A, Sekine M, Mogushi K, Akiyama Y, Fukamachi H, et al. Synergistic tumour suppressor activity of E-cadherin and p53 in a conditional mouse model for metastatic diffuse-type gastric cancer. Gut. 2012 Mar;**61**(3):344-353

[43] Ferrand J, Lehours P, Schmid-Alliana A, Megraud F, Varon C. *Helicobacter pylori* infection of gastrointestinal epithelial cells *in vitro* induces mesenchymal stem cell migration through an NF-kappaB-dependent pathway. PLoS One. 2011;**6**(12):e29007

[44] Ferrand J, Noel D, Lehours P, Prochazkova-Carlotti M, Chambonnier L, Menard A, et al. Human bone marrow-derived stem cells acquire epithelial characteristics through fusion with gastrointestinal epithelial cells. PLoS One. 2011;**6**(5):e19569

[45] Janin A, Murata H, Leboeuf C, Cayuela JM, Gluckman E, Legres L, et al. Donor-derived oral squamous cell carcinoma after allogeneic bone marrow transplantation. Blood. 2009 Feb 19;**113**(8):1834-1840

[46] Hutchinson L, Stenstrom B, Chen D, Piperdi B, Levey S, Lyle S, et al. Human Barrett's adenocarcinoma of the esophagus, associated myofibroblasts, and endothelium can arise from bone marrow-derived cells after allogeneic stem cell transplant. Stem Cells and Development. 2011 Jan;**20**(1):11-17

[47] Worthley DL, Ruszkiewicz A, Davies R, Moore S, Nivison-Smith I, Bik To L, et al. Human gastrointestinal neoplasia-associated myofibroblasts can develop from bone marrow-derived cells following allogeneic stem cell transplantation. Stem Cells (Dayton, Ohio). 2009 Jun;**27**(6):1463-1468

[48] Driessens G, Beck B, Caauwe A, Simons BD, Blanpain C. Defining the mode of tumour growth by clonal analysis. Nature. 2012 Aug 23;**488**(7412):527-530

[49] Schepers AG, Snippert HJ, Stange DE, van den Born M, van Es JH, van de Wetering M, et al. Lineage tracing reveals Lgr5+ stem cell activity in mouse intestinal adenomas. Science (New York, NY). 2012 Aug 10;**337**(6095):730-735

[50] Takaishi S, Okumura T, Tu S, Wang SS, Shibata W, Vigneshwaran R, et al. Identification of gastric cancer stem cells using the cell surface marker CD44. Stem Cells (Dayton, Ohio). 2009 May;**27**(5):1006-1020

[51] Nguyen PH, Giraud J, Chambonnier L, Dubus P, Wittkop L, Belleannee G, et al. Characterization of biomarkers of tumorigenic and chemoresistant cancer stem cells in human gastric carcinoma. Clinical Cancer Research. 2017 Mar 15;**23**(6):1586-1597

[52] Bagnoli F, Buti L, Tompkins L, Covacci A, Amieva MR. *Helicobacter pylori* CagA induces a transition from polarized to invasive phenotypes in MDCK cells. Proceedings of the National Academy of Sciences of the United States of America. 2005 Nov 08;**102**(45):16339-16344

[53] Yin Y, Grabowska AM, Clarke PA, Whelband E, Robinson K, Argent RH, et al. *Helicobacter pylori* potentiates epithelial:mesenchymal transition in gastric cancer: Links to soluble HB-EGF, gastrin and matrix metalloproteinase-7. Gut. 2010 Aug;**59**(8):1037-1045

[54] Greaves M, Maley CC. Clonal evolution in cancer. Nature. 2012 Jan 18;**481**(7381):306-313

[55] Shackleton M, Quintana E, Fearon ER, Morrison SJ. Heterogeneity in cancer: Cancer stem cells versus clonal evolution. Cell. 2009 Sep 04;**138**(5):822-829

[56] Magee JA, Piskounova E, Morrison SJ. Cancer stem cells: Impact, heterogeneity, and uncertainty. Cancer Cell. 2012 Mar 20;**21**(3):283-296

[57] Lau WM, Teng E, Chong HS, Lopez KA, Tay AY, Salto-Tellez M, et al. CD44v8-10 is a cancer-specific marker for gastric cancer stem cells. Cancer Research. 2014 May 1;**74**(9): 2630-2641

[58] Nguyen PH, Giraud J, Staedel C, Chambonnier L, Dubus P, Chevret E, et al. All-trans retinoic acid targets gastric cancer stem cells and inhibits patient-derived gastric carcinoma tumor growth. Oncogene. 2016 Oct 27;**35**(43):5619-5628

[59] Quintana E, Shackleton M, Sabel MS, Fullen DR, Johnson TM, Morrison SJ. Efficient tumour formation by single human melanoma cells. Nature. 2008 Dec 04;**456**(7222):593-598

[60] Hu Y, Smyth GK. ELDA: extreme limiting dilution analysis for comparing depleted and enriched populations in stem cell and other assays. Journal of immunological methods. 2009 Aug 15;**347**(1-2):70-78

[61] Al-Hajj M, Wicha MS, Benito-Hernandez A, Morrison SJ, Clarke MF. Prospective identification of tumorigenic breast cancer cells. Proceedings of the National Academy of Sciences of the United States of America. 2003 Apr 1;**100**(7):3983-3988

[62] Zoller M. CD44: Can a cancer-initiating cell profit from an abundantly expressed molecule? Nature Reviews. 2011 Apr;**11**(4):254-267

[63] Solis MA, Chen YH, Wong TY, Bittencourt VZ, Lin YC, Huang LL. Hyaluronan regulates cell behavior: A potential niche matrix for stem cells. Biochemistry Research International. 2012;**2012**:346972

[64] Prochazka L, Tesarik R, Turanek J. Regulation of alternative splicing of CD44 in cancer. Cellular Signalling. 2014 Oct;**26**(10):2234-2239

[65] Fan X, Long A, Goggins M, Fan X, Keeling PW, Kelleher D. Expression of CD44 and its variants on gastric epithelial cells of patients with *Helicobacter pylori* colonisation. Gut. 1996 Apr;**38**(4):507-512

[66] Okayama H, Kumamoto K, Saitou K, Hayase S, Kofunato Y, Sato Y, et al. CD44v6, MMP-7 and nuclear Cdx2 are significant biomarkers for prediction of lymph node metastasis in primary gastric cancer. Oncology Reports. 2009 Oct;**22**(4):745-755

[67] Mayer B, Jauch KW, Gunthert U, Figdor CG, Schildberg FW, Funke I, et al. De-novo expression of CD44 and survival in gastric cancer. Lancet. 1993 Oct 23;**342**(8878):1019-1022

[68] Wang L, Li HG, Wen JM, Peng TS, Zeng H, Wang LY. Expression of CD44v3, erythropoietin and VEGF-C in gastric adenocarcinomas: correlations with clinicopathological features. Tumori. 2014 May-Jun;**100**(3):321-327

[69] da Cunha CB, Oliveira C, Wen X, Gomes B, Sousa S, Suriano G, et al. De novo expression of CD44 variants in sporadic and hereditary gastric cancer. Laboratory Investigation; A Journal of Technical Methods and Pathology. 2010 Nov;**90**(11):1604-14

[70] Ishimoto T, Oshima H, Oshima M, Kai K, Torii R, Masuko T, et al. CD44+ slow-cycling tumor cell expansion is triggered by cooperative actions of Wnt and prostaglandin E2 in gastric tumorigenesis. Cancer Science. 2011 Mar;**101**(3):673-678

[71] Han ME, Jeon TY, Hwang SH, Lee YS, Kim HJ, Shim HE, et al. Cancer spheres from gastric cancer patients provide an ideal model system for cancer stem cell research. Cellular and Molecular Life Sciences. 2011 Nov;**68**(21):3589-3605

[72] Chen W, Zhang X, Chu C, Cheung WL, Ng L, Lam S, et al. Identification of CD44+ cancer stem cells in human gastric cancer. Hepato-Gastroenterology. 2013 Jun;**60**(124):949-954

[73] Zhang C, Li C, He F, Cai Y, Yang H. Identification of CD44+CD24+ gastric cancer stem cells. Journal of Cancer Research and Clinical Oncology. 2011 Nov;**137**(11):1679-1686

[74] Yoon C, Park DJ, Schmidt B, Thomas NJ, Lee HJ, Kim TS, et al. CD44 expression denotes a subpopulation of gastric cancer cells in which Hedgehog signaling promotes chemotherapy resistance. Clinical Cancer Research. 2014 Aug 01;**20**(15):3974-3988

[75] Nishikawa S, Konno M, Hamabe A, Hasegawa S, Kano Y, Ohta K, et al. Aldehyde dehydrogenase high gastric cancer stem cells are resistant to chemotherapy. International Journal of Oncology. 2013 Apr;**42**(4):1437-1442

[76] Fukuda K, Saikawa Y, Ohashi M, Kumagai K, Kitajima M, Okano H, et al. Tumor initiating potential of side population cells in human gastric cancer. International Journal of Oncology. 2009 May;**34**(5):1201-1207

[77] Ehata S, Johansson E, Katayama R, Koike S, Watanabe A, Hoshino Y, et al. Transforming growth factor-beta decreases the cancer-initiating cell population within diffuse-type gastric carcinoma cells. Oncogene. 2011 Apr 07;**30**(14):1693-1705

[78] She JJ, Zhang PG, Wang X, Che XM, Wang ZM. Side population cells isolated from KATO III human gastric cancer cell line have cancer stem cell-like characteristics. World Journal of Gastroenterology. 2012 Sep 07;**18**(33):4610-4617

[79] Chiang AC, Massague J. Molecular basis of metastasis. The New England Journal of Medicine. 2008 Dec 25;**359**(26):2814-2823

[80] Chaffer CL, Weinberg RA. A perspective on cancer cell metastasis. Science (New York, NY). 2011 Mar 25;**331**(6024):1559-1564

[81] Baud J, Varon C, Chabas S, Chambonnier L, Darfeuille F, Staedel C. *Helicobacter pylori* initiates a mesenchymal transition through ZEB1 in gastric epithelial cells. PLoS One. 2013;**8**(4):e60315

[82] Chen T, Yang K, Yu J, Meng W, Yuan D, Bi F, et al. Identification and expansion of cancer stem cells in tumor tissues and peripheral blood derived from gastric adenocarcinoma patients. Cell Research. 2012 Jan;**22**(1):248-258

[83] Staedel C, Varon C, Nguyen PH, Vialet B, Chambonnier L, Rousseau B, et al. Inhibition of gastric tumor cell growth using seed-targeting LNA as specific, long-lasting microRNA inhibitors. Molecular Therapy. 2015;**4**:e246

Section 3

Molecular Heterogeneity of Gastric Cancer

Chapter 6

Clinical Implications of Molecular Heterogeneity of Gastric Cancer

Petra Hudler and Radovan Komel

Additional information is available at the end of the chapter

http://dx.doi.org/10.5772/intechopen.69775

Abstract

Gastric cancer incidence has been steadily declining in countries with low frequencies of gastric carcinoma since early 1930s. In areas with higher incidences, the decline has been less obvious and slower. Nevertheless, gastric adenocarcinoma remains one of the most common causes of cancer-related death worldwide. The poor outcome has been attributed to late detection of the condition, particularly in Americas and Europe, aggressive pathogenesis and lack of symptoms during early stages of the tumor development. In addition, sporadic stomach cancer mostly affects elderly individuals. In the majority of countries with low incidence, the average age at the disease presentation is above 65. Therefore, gastric adenocarcinoma, among other diseases associated with old age, raises health concerns in countries with changing demographic age profiles that show a trend of an increase in the proportion of the population aged over 60. The low 5-year survival rate of patients underscores the critical need for the development of more accurate diagnostic tools and safe targeted chemotherapeutics. However, the heterogeneity of molecular changes represents one of the most pressing issues in the current research of gastric cancer, impeding the translation of genetic aberrations into novel applications for medical practice.

Keywords: antineoplastic agent, cancer, chemotherapy, clinical trials, gastric adenocarcinoma, gastroesophageal junction adenocarcinoma, molecular heterogeneity, monoclonal antibodies, small-molecule inhibitor, targeted therapy

1. Introduction

The incidence of gastric cancer (GC) has been declining globally in the last decades. This slow, yet steady decrease in incidence and mortality rates has been attributed to improved medical treatment of peptic ulcers and chronic gastritis, development of protocols for *Helicobacter pylori* eradication, lifestyle changes, and introduction of safer food preservation methods [1, 2]. However, it is also important to note that the total incidence of most common gastric malignancy, adenocarcinoma, varies by geographic areas up to 20-fold between the highest and the lowest risk populations. The high risk areas are in certain Asian regions, such as Japan, China and Korea, followed by Eastern Europe and some countries in South America [3]. Low-risk populations are located in North America, India, the Philippines, most countries in Africa, some Western European countries and Australia [4]. Up to 10% of GCs arise as a consequence of inherited cancer predisposition syndromes, such as Li-Fraumeni syndrome, Lynch syndrome, Peutz-Jeghers syndrome, hereditary breast and ovarian cancer, MUTYH-associated adenomatous polyposis (MAP), familial adenomatous polyposis (FAP), juvenile polyposis syndrome and PTEN hamartoma tumor syndrome (Cowden syndrome) [5, 6]. Genetic counselling and mutation analyses, regular endoscopic surveillance and screening of the at-risk family members and risk-reduction surgery of stomach have greatly improved management of patients with hereditary mutations predisposing to the development of hereditary GC [5, 7]. However, approximately 90% of GCs are sporadic and typically occur in elderly population [6, 8]. Despite improvements in the diagnostic procedures, most cases of sporadic GCs are still detected at advanced stages due to the lack of specific symptoms associated with the early phases of tumor development. Consequently, high mortality rates attributable to advanced GC contribute significantly to the public health burden worldwide. The estimated overall 5-year relative survival rates of patients with advanced GC in developed countries are still low, around 30% [9]. An additional reason for concern is the demographic transition to the older population accounting for the significant proportion of population in developed countries [10]. This demographic shift will have an impact on health services, as the number of people over the age of 65, who comprise the highest risk group for the development of sporadic GC, has been steadily increasing in these countries. The challenge most countries are facing at the present time is how to improve the healthy life expectancy with regard to early detection of chronic and degenerative diseases, including cancers.

2. From basic research to clinical needs

Research efforts have identified several risk factors, including environmental factors as well as epigenetic and genetic aberrations, which could be implicated in the initiation and progression of gastric malignancies. Advances in high-throughput technologies and bioinformatic systematic analyses have been complementing our knowledge of an intricate network of genetic and epigenetic changes associated with stomach carcinogenesis. Unfortunately, only a few of common mutations could be associated with the development of sporadic gastric adenocarcinomas, which is the most common type of GC in the non-Asian world regions. In addition, breakthroughs in next-generation sequencing and SNP profiling microarrays have revealed another dimension, contributing to the heterogeneity of cancers. Genetic background, which affects the susceptibility for developing GC, could also be responsible for differences in responses to drugs and outcome measures evaluating survival, efficacy and safety of novel biological therapeutics in distinct populations.

Discovery-oriented research performed in different world populations revealed that molecular aberrations found in sporadic GCs do not correlate well with macroscopic and microscopic classifications that are currently used in clinical practice for diagnosis and for rough assessment of the postoperative therapeutic management protocols [11]. For example, pathohistological Lauren classification, which is the most widely used diagnostic feature in clinical setting in Western countries, recognizes two main subtypes, intestinal and diffuse types of GC. Intestinal type of gastric adenocarcinoma is associated with intestinal metaplasia and tubular structures, whereas diffuse-type carcinomas mostly consist of discohesive cells and/or signet ring cells. Two additional subtypes fall into this classification, if the tumors do not fit into two major subtypes clearly. Approximately 14% of tumors, exhibiting characteristics of intestinal and diffuse morphology, are classified as mixed type, whereas roughly 10% of gastric tumors, which display uncommon features, are allocated into indeterminate category [11–16]. It should also be noted that all adenocarcinomas show heterogeneity at the histological level. For example, even if tumors were histologically classified as intestinal or diffuse type, they are in fact often a mixture of several coexisting tissue types, including more or less well-developed tubular structures, poorly cohesive cells and signet ring cells, though one of these cell types usually predominates [17]. In the past, researchers have been focused on determining distinct gene aberrations that could have been associated with these subtypes in order to constitute reliable biomarker panels, which would correlate with histological subtypes and indicate the likely course of disease progression. However, accumulating molecular data on GC aberrations revealed immense intertumor and intratumor heterogeneity of GCs [9, 18–21].

In recent years, molecular classifications, based on the results from high-throughput technologies, revealed the existence of different molecular subtypes regardless of pathohistological subtypes [17, 22–24]. The advantage of these novel classifications is that distinct aberrant molecular changes that characterize different subtypes could be exploited to develop novel treatment approaches. For example, the EBV subtype, recognized in the TCGA study, is defined by frequent amplification of *JAK2*, *CD274* (*PD-L1*) and *PDCD1LG2* (*PD-L2*) together with DNA hypermethylation and *PIK3CA* mutations [22]. Thus, patients with aberrations in PD-1 signaling pathways could benefit from addition of pembrolizumab or other antibodies targeting PD-1 axis [25]. Frequent occurrence of characteristic CpG island methylator phenotypes (CIMP) in GCs, particularly in association with *H. pylori* or Epstein-Barr virus infection, could lead to introduction of epigenetic modulators into standard treatment regimens used against early and advanced forms of adenocarcinomas [22]. Deciphering molecular heterogeneity of malignant gastric tumors and subsequent translation of this information into precision medicine or eventually into personalized medicine is the subject of several ongoing collaborative projects, such as The Cancer Genome Atlas (TCGA) based at the National Cancer Institute, the Cancer Genome Project at the Wellcome Trust Sanger Institute, and the International Cancer Genome Consortium, based at Ontario Institute for Cancer Research [22, 26–28].

However, the novelties of molecular classifications brought additional obstacles in translational research. It has become evident that there is a gap between real clinical needs and current genetic research. The resources being put into high-throughput identification of genetic and epigenetic changes accelerated the understanding of the molecular mechanisms underlying human diseases; however, the progression of this knowledge to patient benefit is lagging behind. In particular, surgical resection of stomach is still the main curative approach in the treatment of gastric cancer [29]. Although different types of nonsurgical treatment modalities, including chemotherapy, radiation therapy, chemoradiation, as well as targeted therapies, have been evaluated in clinical studies and have been subsequently integrated in clinical setting, these regimens have not been internationally standardized and remain in the form of guidelines and recommendations [30]. In recent years, several roadmaps and initiatives have been established, with the aim to advance the knowledge transfer, promote collaborations between different scientific disciplines and medical environment, and determine the main obstacles, which hinder the progression and implementation of effective health care solutions [31–33]. The main recognized barriers have been associated with (i) the explosion of molecular research conducted by highly specialized scientists, (ii) the fragmented fields of biomedical research, (iii) the dynamics of basic research with regard to promotion, obtaining funding and grants, which resulted in separation of basic and clinically relevant research, (iv) differences in education and training, (v) lack of communication between clinicians and researchers and (vi) the separation of methodologies and infrastructure available in clinical environment and specialized molecular research laboratories [32, 33]. In addition, complex regulatory issues, associated with research ethical procedures and approvals and clearances of innovative biomedical devices or approaches, have been recognized as limiting factors in translational research [34]. One of the most pressing medical research problems in heterogeneous diseases, such as GC, issuing from the accumulating research data, is the biological elucidation of molecular changes and how they affect processes and metabolic pathways in malignant cells. Although several molecular targets have been identified in complex diseases, only a few targeted therapies and other novel treatment approaches have been found to be effective in the management of malignant diseases. Another concern, which also has roots in underlying molecular changes driving the malignant phenotype, is the development of drug resistance, which results in therapeutic failure. Although multidisciplinary research efforts have identified main pathways as well as some specific genetic determinants implicated in this phenomenon, innate or acquired resistance of cancer cells remains a significant challenge of translational medicine [33, 34].

3. Targeted management of gastric cancer

Gastrointestinal malignancies are highly aggressive and currently used standard therapies showed only a modest effect on improving survival and preventing recurrence [35]. Targeted therapies, based on antibodies or small molecule compounds, targeting specific molecular aberrations associated with gastric tumors, could offer improved outcomes and potentially fewer adverse effects. In general, antibody-based therapies are aimed against specific targets on the cell surface, whereas the design of small molecules is focused on their capacity to penetrate the cell membranes and target molecules inside cells.

3.1. Monoclonal antibodies

A number of monoclonal antibodies targeting different proteins, including EGFR, PD-1 (CD279), VEGF growth factor family, MET, and IGF-1R, are currently being tested and evaluated in clinical trials (**Table 1**) [36–39].

Target	Anticancer agent	Approval status in EU or USA
EGFR	Cetuximab	Advanced colorectal cancers with wild-type *KRAS*, EGFR-expressing
		Squamous cell carcinoma of the head and neck
	Matuzumab	Discontinued, no benefits
	Nimotuzumab	High-grade glioma[b] (orphan status withdrawn in 2008)
		Pancreatic cancer[b]
	Panitumumab	Metastatic colorectal cancer with wild-type *KRAS*
CD3, EpCAM	Catumaxomab	Gastric cancer[b]
HER2	Ado-Trastuzumab emtansine (T-DM1)[a]	Advanced or metastatic breast cancer, HER2-positive
	Pertuzumab	Breast cancer, HER2-positive
	Trastuzumab	Breast cancer, HER2-positive
		Gastric cancer, HER2-positive
		Gastroesophageal junction adenocarcinoma, HER2-positive
IGF1R/IGF1/IGF2	Robatumumab	Terminated due to business reasons
HGF/MET	Margetuximab	Clinical trial (NCT02689284), recruiting participants, promising preliminary results
	Onartuzumab	Clinical trial (NCT01662869), MET-positive gastric cancer
	Rilotumumab	Gastric cancer (orphan status)[b], (HGF-positive)
PD-1	Atezolizumab	Locally advanced or metastatic urothelial carcinoma[c]
		Metastatic nonsmall cell lung cancer[c]
	Durvalumab	Bladder cancer (in review for approval)[c]
	Nivolumab	Nonsmall cell lung cancer
		Renal cell carcinoma
		Hodgkin disease
		Melanoma, BRAF V600 wild-type or BRAFV600 mutation-positive
		Recurrent or metastatic squamous cell carcinoma of the head and neck[c]
	Pembrolizumab	Unresectable or metastatic melanoma
		Metastatic squamous cell carcinoma of the head and neck[c]
		Metastatic nonsmall cell lung cancer
VEGFR/VEGF	Bevacizumab	Metastatic colorectal cancer
		Nonsquamous nonsmall cell lung cancer
		Glioblastoma[c]
		Metastatic renal cell carcinoma with interferon alfa[c]
		Cervical cancer
		Platinum-resistant recurrent epithelial ovarian, fallopian tube or primary peritoneal cancer
		Metastatic breast cancer[b]
		Metastatic kidney cancer[b]

Target	Anticancer agent	Approval status in EU or USA
	Ramucirumab	Advanced gastric cancer
		Nonsmall cell lung cancer
		Metastatic colorectal cancer

[a]Antibody-drug conjugate (ADC) of stably linked trastuzumab and potent microtubule inhibitor emtansine.
[b]Only in Europe.
[c]Only in USA.

Table 1. Antineoplastic monoclonal antibodies, currently being evaluated in clinical trials for the treatment of gastric cancer.

The Phase III ToGA study (NCT01041404), which evaluated the addition of trastuzumab to chemotherapy for treatment of advanced gastric cancer and gastroesophageal junction (GEJ) cancer, was one of the first studies that clearly demonstrated the benefits of targeted therapy in a selected group of patients [40, 41]. Trastuzumab is a monoclonal antibody directed against HER2 (ERBB2, HER2/neu). Overexpression of HER2 was observed in approximately 10–20% of gastric and GEJ cancer patients in different populations [42]. In ToGA study, the patients, who were eligible for the treatment, were selected after evaluation of HER2 expression in tumor tissues using immunohistochemistry (IHC) or fluorescence in situ hybridization (FISH). The median overall survival was significantly improved in patients who received trastuzumab and cisplatin-based chemotherapy in comparison with patients, who received only chemotherapy. In addition, further studies showed that the quality of life in HER2-positive patients, receiving trastuzumab in combination with chemotherapy, was improved and the toxicity burden was comparable to chemotherapy-alone arm [43]. It was also observed that the time to deterioration and quality-adjusted time without symptoms of disease or toxicity were prolonged in the trastuzumab-chemotherapy arm. Additional post hoc exploratory analyses investigated the correlations between HER2 overexpression and clinical and epidemiological features of patients [44]. Interestingly, HER2 overexpression levels were similar in patients from Europe and Asia, whereas they were lower in patients from Central/South America. Overexpression or amplification of HER2 was more common in intestinal GCs than diffuse or mixed types of GC, which was in concordance with other studies [45, 46]. In addition, GEJ tumors showed higher rate of HER2 overexpression or amplification than stomach tumors, indicating that GEJ adenocarcinoma differs in etiology and pathogenesis from distal stomach tumors. Evaluation of HER2 staining performance indicated great variability and the researchers concluded that ideally six to eight specimens should be collected in order to obtain accurate estimation of HER2-positivity. HER2 testing and trastuzumab treatment have been integrated in clinical settings in several developed countries.

Ramucirumab is a monoclonal antibody, targeting angiogenesis-related protein VEGFR2. It has been or is being evaluated in more than 20 clinical trials (NCT01246960, NCT01170663, NCT01983878, NCT02661971, NCT02314117, NCT00917384, NCT02934464 and so on) [47]. First published results demonstrated promising results for this biological drug, indicating that combination of ramucirumab with paclitaxel or platinum-containing or fluoropyrimidine-containing chemotherapy increases overall survival, progression-free survival as well as quality of life when compared to chemotherapy-only arm [48–50]. In 2014, FDA approved the addition of ramucirumab to paclitaxel as the treatment for patients with advanced GC or GEJ adenocarcinoma as well as its use as monotherapy for patients who did not respond to the first-line therapy with platinum- or fluoropyrimidine-containing chemotherapy [51]. However, another Phase II study (NCT01246960), evaluating addition of ramucirumab to combined leucovorin, 5-fluorouracil and oxaliplatin chemotherapy (FOLFOX), did not show an improvement of outcome measures, progression-free survival and overall survival, in participants with gastric, esophageal and GEJ cancers [52].

Based on previous more or less promising results in the treatment of glioblastoma, colon, breast and lung cancers targeting angiogenesis with monoclonal antibody bevacizumab directed against VEGFA, Avagast clinical study was launched with the aim to evaluate the benefit of bevacizumab for GC patients [53–61]. Bevacizumab was added to the first-line chemotherapy, consisting of cisplatin and capecitabine or fluorouracil (FU) [54]. The subsequent unadjusted analyses demonstrated improved overall response rate and progression-free survival in the bevacizumab-cisplatin-FU arm. Unadjusted overall survival rate did not reach statistical significance. The toxicity of the tested treatment was comparable with the placebo-cisplatin-FU chemotherapy as well as with previous findings in patients with colon cancer receiving similar treatment. Subgroup analyses demonstrated differences in the efficacy of bevacizumab addition to chemotherapy between examined populations. Efficacy was increased in Pan-American and possibly European populations (the results were not clear), whereas Asian patients appeared to have no benefit from treatment with bevacizumab. The research group also observed regional differences in median overall survival and progression-free survival, which could be attributed to different factors, such as different distributions of tumor histological types in the examined populations, differences in administering subsequent therapies and so on [54]. In a similar study, Avatar, which included patients from the China, the researchers also confirmed that patients receiving bevacizumab plus capecitabine-cisplatin did not show an improvement in overall survival and progression-free survival, when compared to placebo arm [62]. Although the response rate was higher in bevacizumab arm, the difference was not significant. Inconsistencies in overall survival of patients receiving bevacizumab in addition to chemotherapy, prompted further research, focused on evaluating plasma and tumor biomarkers and clinical outcomes [63]. High plasma VEGFA levels were associated with better overall survival, progression-free survival and overall response rate in the group of patients with high plasma VEGFA levels, receiving bevacizumab-cisplatin-FU therapy, in comparison with patients with low plasma VEGFA levels. Interestingly, the beneficial effect of bevacizumab in these patients with regard to two measured indicators, overall survival and progression-free response, was more prominent in non-Asian patients, whereas in Asian patients, the effect was not significant. In addition, a weak association between low levels of tumor neuropilin-1 expression and better overall survival, progression-free survival and overall response rate was observed in a group of patients, receiving bevacizumab, compared to patients who had high expression of neuropilin-1. In conclusion, both VEGFA and neuropilin-1 are promising predictive biomarkers for selection of patients who would benefit from addition of bevacizumab to standard chemotherapy, although, as researchers noted, more thorough investigations to further characterize these markers are needed [63].

A preliminary investigation Phase 1b KEYNOTE-012 (NCT01848834) of selected patients with GC or esophageal cancer who were PD-1L positive showed that this population of patients could benefit from treatment with pembrolizumab, a monoclonal IgG4 antibody designed to block the interaction between PD-1 (CD279) and its ligands PD-L1 (CD274) and PD-L2 [64]. PD-1L is one of two known ligands for PD-1 receptor that is implicated in downregulation of the immune system by terminating T cell activation [65]. PD-1L has been relatively frequently (from 25 to 65%) found overexpressed in gastric epithelial cells as well as in tumor infiltrating cells [66–69]. Activation of PD-1 axis is associated with tumor-induced immune suppression [70]. PD-1 overexpression has been less well characterized. Investigation of the expression of several immune checkpoint molecules, including PD-1 in peripheral blood mononuclear cells of patients with gastric adenocarcinoma prior to and after the surgery, showed that expression of PD-1 was upregulated on $CD4^+$ and $CD8^+$ T cells after surgery, reaching peaks on the days 1 and 7 after surgery, respectively [71]. The frequencies of $PD\text{-}1^+CD4^+$ and $PD\text{-}1^+CD8^+$ cells reached preoperative levels after approximately 30 days after the surgery, indicating that surgery stress suppresses immune activity and could promote immune evasion of tumor and metastatic cells [71]. In particular, this mechanism could affect the ability of circulating tumor cells, which are shed from primary tumor mass, to evade immune system and establish secondary tumor niches. Another study also confirmed significantly higher expression of PD-1 on T cells obtained from blood and tumor tissues in patients with GC, when compared to normal gastric tissues from controls [72]. In KEYNOTE-012 study, the overall response rate to treatment with pembrolizumab was 32% in Asian patients and 30% in non-Asian patients. The researchers also observed that significant associations existed between progression-free survival, overall response rate and PD-1L expression. Further analyses showed that overall response was 22% for all enrolled patients, although all responses were partial responses. It should be noted that this study was preliminary, the number of tested patients was small and the majority of patients had prior to enrolment in this study received two or more systemic or adjuvant therapies. The researchers also observed that although no treatment-related deaths occurred, four patients had to terminate the treatment due to immune-mediated toxic effects [25]. Further studies are currently being carried out in order to assess the safety, tolerability and antitumor activity of pembrolizumab in patients with GC (NCT02335411, NCT02370498, NCT02494583, and NCT02443324). In addition, the downregulation of activated T cells immediately after surgery through PD-1 signaling pathway, as demonstrated in one study [71], could be further explored to assess the benefit of administering PD-1 blocking antibodies prior to or immediately after surgery.

Rilomet-1 (NCT01697072) study attempted to evaluate the addition of rilotumumab to standard cisplatin and capecitabine chemotherapy as a first-line therapy for patients with advanced MET-positive GC or GEJ adenocarcinoma [73, 74]. Rilotumumab is a human monoclonal antibody against c-MET (HGFR) factor. HGF is the only known ligand for HGFR or c-MET, a tyrosine kinase receptor, which has been found to be frequently overexpressed in tumor gastric tissues [75–80]. Although the first results were promising, showing trends toward improved survival of patients, all trials with this compound were later terminated, due to unexpected deaths of patients in the rilotumumab-chemotherapy arm compared with the chemotherapy-alone arm in one of the trials [81].

3.2. Small-molecule compounds

In 2010, FDA approved lapatinib, a small-molecule tyrosine kinase inhibitor of EGFR and HER2, for the treatment of HER2-positive breast cancer. Studies on gastric cell lines confirmed its antiproliferative activity [82]. Several clinical trials attempted to evaluate its effectivity and toxicity in patients with HER2-positive GC (NCT02015169, NCT00313599, NCT00447226, NCT00103324, NCT00680901, NCT00486954, NCT01123473 and so on). Currently, the results are still inconclusive, due to termination of some of these studies or negative results regarding the lapatinib efficacy. For example, in Phase II study (NCT01145404), which recruited HER2-positive patients with advanced GC, who have previously failed first-line platinum-based therapy, lapatinib addition to capecitabine or lapatinib monotherapy did not show improvements in overall survival and response rates and the study was prematurely terminated [83]. Nevertheless, interesting conclusions could be drawn from the observations from two larger studies involving lapatinib testing. A multinational randomized clinical trial, TRIAL-013/LOGiC (NCT00680901), investigated the benefit of the lapatinib addition to capecitabine-oxaliplatin (CapeOx) chemotherapy, administered to HER2-positive patients with locally advanced, unresectable, or metastatic gastric, esophageal, or GEJ cancer [45]. A total of 545 eligible patients were evaluated, and lapatinib efficacy analyses were performed in a group consisting of 454 patients with FISH confirmed amplification of HER2 (primary efficacy population, PEP). The underlying reason for this stratification was based on the results of previous studies performed on breast cancer patients, which showed that lapatinib administration benefits only a selected population of patients with HER2 amplification, regardless of the status of HER2 expression, determined with IHC [84]. Although the lapatinib addition to CapeOX did not improve overall survival in PEP and neither in the group of total eligible patients, there was significant improvement of progression-free survival in PEP. Additional analyses revealed that lapatinib was more effective in Asian patients and younger patients. In addition, lapatinib was less effective in patients, who had undergone gastrectomy with pylorus removed, than in patients with intact pylorus [45]. Based on these results, the authors did not recommend the use of lapatinib in combination with CapeOx in patients with HER2-positive GC [45]. In a TyTAN Phase III (NCT00486954) clinical trial, which included Asian patients, lapatinib addition to paclitaxel chemotherapy also did not significantly improve median overall survival and progression-free survival [85]. Lapatinib benefit was observed a small group of patients, whose gastric tumors were both FISH positive and had a score of 3+ in IHC evaluation. In addition, population stratification analyses showed that Chinese patients in the lapatinib arm had significantly improved overall survival and progression-free survival. Preliminary pharmacokinetic analyses performed as a part of trial revealed that lapatinib or lapatinib-paclitaxel administration could result in different plasma concentrations of the drugs. Furthermore, both AUC_{0-24} (area under the concentration-time curve from time 0 to 24 h) and maximum plasma concentration of lapatinib were lower in patients with pylorus removed than in patients with intact pylorus [85].

The underlying causes of clinical outcomes associated with lapatinib administration and HER2 gene amplification levels were further thoroughly investigated in TRIAL-013/LOGiC cohort of patients [86]. Another group of upper gastrointestinal cancers, consisting of 419

(86%) gastric, 43 (8.8%) GEJ, and 26 (5.3%) esophageal cancers, obtained from commercial providers, was subsequently included for HER2 testing and analyses. This group was used to evaluate the concordance between different HER2 assay methods, which were performed in two central laboratories and local laboratory. The researchers observed high agreement rates between two different FISH methods, FDA-approved Dako HER2 IQFISH pharmDx FISH assay and PathVysion HER2 FISH assay (Abbott Molecular, Inc.), for detecting HER2 amplification. The concordance rate was also high (95%) between two central laboratories when evaluating results of FISH assays, whereas the concordance between local and central laboratories was 87%. Expression of HER2 was tested using the FDA-approved IHC test HercepTest (Dako Biotechnology). Comparison of local laboratory and central laboratory HER2 testing using IHC assay for the assessment of HER2 status in patients assigned to TRIO-013/LOGiC trial showed that the concordance rate was less than 50%. Comparison of agreement between IHC and FISH assays in central laboratories showed 88% overall agreement for cases from the commercially obtained upper gastrointestinal carcinomas and 91% for the TRIO-013/LOGiC cohort. Additional analyses confirmed the findings of Hecht and colleagues [45] that progression-free survival as well as overall survival was significantly higher in selected groups of patients, such as Asian patients and younger patients [45, 86]. These findings correlated well with the fact that these patients had higher levels of HER2 gene amplification. Interestingly, other studies also reported similar outcomes in GC patients with high HER2 amplification status when treated with monoclonal antibody trastuzumab [87, 88]. These findings pointed out clinically important aspect, which could underlie the discrepancy between studies and clinical trials, evaluating the benefit of anti-HER2 targeted chemotherapies. First, HER2 expression patterns differ between GC and breast cancer and furthermore, in GC the expression patterns are frequently heterogeneous [44, 46, 86, 88]. The optimal cutoff for selecting patients with GC who would benefit from addition of lapatinib to chemotherapy should be evaluated in further studies; however, at present, the results indicated that the cutoff value, based on FISH assays, could be the ratios 5.01–10.0 and >10.0 [86]. Second, it was also recognized that other alterations could affect the treatment with lapatinib. For example, it was established that in trastuzumab-resistant breast and esophagogastric cancers, MET amplification could contribute to intrinsic or treatment-acquired resistance to trastuzumab [89, 90]. Studies of breast and lung cancers have indicated that overexpression of other tyrosine kinases, including IGF-1R, other members of HER family, and EphA2, could lead to development of resistance mechanisms against anti-HER2 drugs, by bypassing anti-HER2 inhibition of MAPK and PI3K/Akt signaling pathways [91, 92]. Therefore, additional studies, focusing on molecular biomarkers for selection of eligible patients for anti-HER2 therapy, could improve the efficacy and safety of small molecular HER2 inhibitors as well as the safety of anti-HER2 antibodies.

Several other small molecule inhibitors, which have been approved for use in treatment of other cancers, are being tested in clinical studies. For example, sunitinib, which inhibits cellular signaling by targeting PDGFRs and VEGFRs, has been evaluated as safe for treatment of GC patients in a few Phase I studies; however, Phase II studies have not confirmed its efficacy and benefit [93–96]. The safety and benefit of apatinib, which selectively inhibits VEGFR2, have been shown in Phase II and Phase III clinical trials [97, 98]. However, recent reports from other studies have raised concerns regarding the toxicity of apatinib, since it has shown toxicity in previous studies on patients with metastatic triple-negative breast cancer [99].

4. Conclusion

In recent years, only two targeted therapeutics, trastuzumab and ramucirumab, have been approved in Western countries for treatment of advanced GC, which is less than the number of approved biological drugs for use in other common cancers. Several reasons could be responsible for that. First, although the explosion of knowledge on molecular mechanisms involved in human diseases has led to novel perspectives in medical treatment and diagnostic procedures, it appears that the enormous amount of molecular and biological information and the complexity of bioinformatic approaches, used to decipher the experimental data, in reality impede the transition from basic research to clinical applications. Second, clinical trials as well as basic research, utilizing novel high-throughput techniques, revealed great heterogeneity among populations. The consequences of interracial differences are particularly evident in the field of developing novel small-molecule drugs and antibodies. Genetic background in populations appears to account for unequal effectiveness and different safety profiles of targeted therapies in different population [100]. In addition, intratumor heterogeneity found within individuals further complicates the development of effective drugs. There is common consensus that novel molecular determinants should be investigated in order to establish genetic profiles, which would enable the identification of the patient subpopulations, in which the treatment with targeted anti-cancer agents would be most effective and beneficial. The first milestone in this process involves determination of different genetic landscapes of GCs across the world, followed by tight collaborations between researchers, healthcare practitioners and pharmaceutical companies. In addition, bioinformatic exploitation of biomedical data collected in databases and utilization and aggregation of already available research data from clinical studies and basic research could provide additional opportunities to identify disease-specific genetic profiles and establish suitable prognosis prediction models, which could guide personalized treatment management.

Author details

Petra Hudler* and Radovan Komel

*Address all correspondence to: petra.hudler@mf.uni-lj.si

Faculty of Medicine, Medical Centre for Molecular Biology, Institute of Biochemistry, University of Ljubljana, Slovenia

References

[1] Jin Z, Jiang W, Wang L. Biomarkers for gastric cancer: Progression in early diagnosis and prognosis (Review). Oncology Letters. 2015;**9**(4):1502-1508. DOI: 10.3892/ol.2015.2959

[2] Ang TL, Fock KM. Clinical epidemiology of gastric cancer. Singapore Medical Journal. 2014;**55**(12):621-628. DOI: 10.11622/smedj.2014174

[3] Dikshit RP, Mathur G, Mhatre S, Yeole BB. Epidemiological review of gastric cancer in India. Indian Journal of Medical and Paediatric Oncology. 2011;**32**(1):3-11. DOI: 10.4103/0971-5851.81883

[4] Ma J, Shen H, Kapesa L, Zeng S. Lauren classification and individualized chemotherapy in gastric cancer. Oncology Letters. 2016;**11**(5):2959-2964. DOI: 10.3892/ol.2016.4337

[5] van der Post RS, Vogelaar IP, Carneiro F, Guilford P, Huntsman D, Hoogerbrugge N, Caldas C, Schreiber KE, Hardwick RH, Ausems MG, Bardram L, Benusiglio PR, Bisseling TM, Blair V, Bleiker E, Boussioutas A, Cats A, Coit D, DeGregorio L, Figueiredo J, Ford JM, Heijkoop E, Hermens R, Humar B, Kaurah P, Keller G, Lai J, Ligtenberg MJ, O'Donovan M, Oliveira C, Pinheiro H, Ragunath K, Rasenberg E, Richardson S, Roviello F, Schackert H, Seruca R, Taylor A, Ter Huurne A, Tischkowitz M, Joe ST, van Dijck B, van Grieken NC, van Hillegersberg R, van Sandick JW, Vehof R, van Krieken JH, Fitzgerald RC. Hereditary diffuse gastric cancer: Updated clinical guidelines with an emphasis on germline CDH1 mutation carriers. Journal of Medical Genetics. 2015;**52**(6):361-374. DOI: 10.1136/jmedgenet-2015-103094

[6] Pinheiro H, Oliveira C, Seruca R, Carneiro F. Hereditary diffuse gastric cancer—Pathophysiology and clinical management. Best Practice and Research Clinical Gastroenterology. 2014;**28**(6):1055-1068. DOI: 10.1016/j.bpg.2014.09.007

[7] Hansford S, Kaurah P, Li-Chang H, Woo M, Senz J, Pinheiro H, Schrader KA, Schaeffer DF, Shumansky K, Zogopoulos G, Santos TA, Claro I, Carvalho J, Nielsen C, Padilla S, Lum A, Talhouk A, Baker-Lange K, Richardson S, Lewis I, Lindor NM, Pennell E, MacMillan A, Fernandez B, Keller G, Lynch H, Shah SP, Guilford P, Gallinger S, Corso G, Roviello F, Caldas C, Oliveira C, Pharoah PD, Huntsman DG. Hereditary diffuse gastric cancer syndrome: CDH1 mutations and beyond. JAMA Oncology. 2015;**1**(1):23-32. DOI: 10.1001/jamaoncol.2014.168

[8] Balducci L. Systemic treatment of gastric and esophageal adenocarcinoma in elderly patients. The Journal of Gastrointestinal Oncology. 2015;**6**(1):75-78. DOI: 10.3978/j.issn.2078-6891.2014.093

[9] Hudler P. Challenges of deciphering gastric cancer heterogeneity. World Journal of Gastroenterology. 2015;**21**(37):10510-10527. DOI: 10.3748/wjg.v21.i37.10510

[10] Izekenova AK, Kumar AB, Abikulova AK. Trends in ageing of the population and the life expectancy after retirement: A comparative country-based analysis. Journal of Research in Medical Sciences. 2015;**20**(3):250-252

[11] Berlth F, Bollschweiler E, Drebber U, Hoelscher AH, Moenig S. Pathohistological classification systems in gastric cancer: Diagnostic relevance and prognostic value. World Journal of Gastroenterology. 2014;**20**(19):5679-5684. DOI: 10.3748/wjg.v20.i19.5679

[12] Stelzner S,Emmrich P. The mixed type in Lauren's classification of gastric carcinoma. Histologic description and biologic behavior. General and Diagnostic Pathology. 1997;**143**(1):39-48

[13] Sun-Mi L, Kyoung-Mee K, Jae YR. Gastric carcinoma: Morphologic classifications and-molecular changes. In Lazar D, editor. Gastric Carcinoma – New Insights into Current Management. Rijeka: InTech; 2013. DOI: 10.5772/54617

[14] Lauren P. The two histological main types of gastric carcinoma: Diffuse and so-called intestinal-type carcinoma. An attempt at a histo-clinical classification. Acta Pathologica Et Microbiologica Scandinavica. 1965;**64**:31-49

[15] Dominguez RL, Crockett SD, Lund JL, Suazo LP, Heidt P, Martin C, Morgan DR. Gastric cancer incidence estimation in a resource-limited nation: Use of endoscopy registry methodology. Cancer Causes and Control. 2013;**24**(2):233-239. DOI: 10.1007/s10552-012-0109-5

[16] Lopez-Carrillo L, Vega-Ramos B, Costa-Dias R, Rascon-Pacheco RA. Histological types of gastric cancer in Mexico. The International Journal of Epidemiology. 1997;**26**(6):1166-1171

[17] Lin X, Zhao Y, Song WM, Zhang B. Molecular classification and prediction in gastric cancer. Computational and Structural Biotechnology Journal. 2015;**13**:448-458. DOI: 10.1016/j.csbj.2015.08.001

[18] Burrell RA, McGranahan N, Bartek J, Swanton C. The causes and consequences of genetic heterogeneity in cancer evolution. Nature. 2013;**501**(7467):338-345. DOI: 10.1038/nature12625

[19] Hudler P, Repse S, Juvan R, Komel R. A genomic approach to investigate expression profiles in Slovenian patients with gastric cancer. Oncology Letters. 2011;**2**:1003-1014. DOI: 10.3892/ol.2011.362

[20] Gerashchenko TS, Denisov EV, Litviakov NV, Zavyalova MV, Vtorushin SV, Tsyganov MM, Perelmuter VM, Cherdyntseva NV. Intratumor heterogeneity: Nature and biological significance. Biochemistry (Moscow). 2013;**78**(11):1201-1215. DOI: 10.1134/S0006297913110011

[21] Greaves M, Maley CC. Clonal evolution in cancer. Nature. 2012;**481**(7381):306-313. DOI: 10.1038/nature10762

[22] The Cancer Genome Atlas Research Network. Comprehensive molecular characterization of gastric adenocarcinoma. Nature. 2014;**513**(7517):202-209. DOI: 10.1038/nature13480

[23] Cristescu R, Lee J, Nebozhyn M, Kim KM, Ting JC, Wong SS, Liu J, Yue YG, Wang J, Yu K, Ye XS, Do IG, Liu S, Gong L, Fu J, Jin JG, Choi MG, Sohn TS, Lee JH, Bae JM, Kim ST, Park SH, Sohn I, Jung SH, Tan P, Chen R, Hardwick J, Kang WK, Ayers M, Hongyue D, Reinhard C, Loboda A, Kim S, Aggarwal A. Molecular analysis of gastric cancer identifies subtypes associated with distinct clinical outcomes. Nature Medicine. 2015;**21**(5):449-456. DOI: 10.1038/nm.3850

[24] Lei Z, Tan IB, Das K, Deng N, Zouridis H, Pattison S, Chua C, Feng Z, Guan YK, Ooi CH, Ivanova T, Zhang S, Lee M, Wu J, Ngo A, Manesh S, Tan E, Teh BT, So JB, Goh LK,

Boussioutas A, Lim TK, Flotow H, Tan P, Rozen SG. Identification of molecular subtypes of gastric cancer with different responses to PI3-kinase inhibitors and 5-fluorouracil. Gastroenterology. 2013;**145**(3):554-565. DOI: 10.1053/j.gastro.2013.05.010

[25] Muro K, Chung HC, Shankaran V, Geva R, Catenacci D, Gupta S, Eder JP, Golan T, Le DT, Burtness B, McRee AJ, Lin C-C, Pathiraja K, Lunceford J, Emancipator K, Juco J, Koshiji M, Bang Y-J. Pembrolizumab for patients with PD-L1-positive advanced gastric cancer (KEYNOTE-012): A multicentre, open-label, phase 1b trial. The Lancet Oncology. 2016;**17**(6):717-726. DOI: 10.1016/s1470-2045(16)00175-3

[26] Zhang J, Baran J, Cros A, Guberman JM, Haider S, Hsu J, Liang Y, Rivkin E, Wang J, Whitty B, Wong-Erasmus M, Yao L, Kasprzyk A. International Cancer Genome Consortium Data Portal—A one-stop shop for cancer genomics data. Database (Oxford). 2011;**2011**:bar026. DOI: 10.1093/database/bar026

[27] Tomczak K, Czerwinska P, Wiznerowicz M. The Cancer Genome Atlas (TCGA): An immeasurable source of knowledge. Contemporary oncology (Poznań). 2015;**19**(1A):A68–A77. DOI: 10.5114/wo.2014.47136

[28] Forbes SA, Beare D, Boutselakis H, Bamford S, Bindal N, Tate J, Cole CG, Ward S, Dawson E, Ponting L, Stefancsik R, Harsha B, Kok CY, Jia M, Jubb H, Sondka Z, Thompson S, De T, Campbell PJ. COSMIC: Somatic cancer genetics at high-resolution. Nucleic Acids Research. 2017;**45**(D1):D777–D783. DOI: 10.1093/nar/gkw1121

[29] Marano L, Polom K, Patriti A, Roviello G, Falco G, Stracqualursi A, De Luca R, Petrioli R, Martinotti M, Generali D, Marrelli D, Di Martino N, Roviello F. Surgical management of advanced gastric cancer: An evolving issue. European Journal of Surgical Oncology. 2016;**42**(1):18-27. DOI: 10.1016/j.ejso.2015.10.016

[30] Park SC, Chun HJ. Chemotherapy for advanced gastric cancer: Review and update of current practices. Gut and Liver. 2013;**7**(4):385-393. DOI: 10.5009/gnl.2013.7.4.385

[31] Cohrs RJ, Martin T, Ghahramani P, Bidaut L, Higgins PJ, Shahzad A. Translational medicine definition by the European Society for Translational Medicine. New Horizons in Translational Medicine. 2015;**2**(3):86-88. DOI: 10.1016/j.nhtm.2014.12.002

[32] Emmert-Buck MR. Translational research: From biological discovery to public benefit (or not). Advances in Biology. 2014;**2014**:20. DOI: 10.1155/2014/278789

[33] Homer-Vanniasinkam S,Tsui J. The continuing challenges of translational research: Clinician-scientists' perspective. Cardiology Research and Practice. 2012;**2012**:246710. DOI: 10.1155/2012/246710

[34] Fudge N, Sadler E, Fisher HR, Maher J, Wolfe CD, McKevitt C. Optimising translational research opportunities: A systematic review and narrative synthesis of basic and clinician scientists' perspectives of factors which enable or hinder translational research. PLoS One. 2016;**11**(8):e0160475. DOI: 10.1371/journal.pone.0160475

[35] Goel G, Sun W. Advances in the management of gastrointestinal cancers—An upcoming role of immune checkpoint blockade. Journal of Hematology and Oncology. 2015;**8**:86. DOI: 10.1186/s13045-015-0185-6

[36] Lazar DC, Taban S, Cornianu M, Faur A, Goldis A. New advances in targeted gastric cancer treatment. World Journal of Gastroenterology. 2016;**22**(30):6776-6799. DOI: 10.3748/wjg.v22.i30.6776

[37] Molife LR, Fong PC, Paccagnella L, Reid AH, Shaw HM, Vidal L, Arkenau HT, Karavasilis V, Yap TA, Olmos D, Spicer J, Postel-Vinay S, Yin D, Lipton A, Demers L, Leitzel K, Gualberto A, de Bono JS. The insulin-like growth factor-I receptor inhibitor figitumumab (CP-751,871) in combination with docetaxel in patients with advanced solid tumours: Results of a phase Ib dose-escalation, open-label study. The British Journal of Cancer. 2010;**103**(3):332-339. DOI: 10.1038/sj.bjc.6605767

[38] Schulte N, Ebert MP, Hartel N. Gastric cancer: New drugs—New strategies. Gastrointestinal Tumors. 2014;**1**(4):180-194. DOI: 10.1159/000380786

[39] Xu W, Yang Z, Lu N. Molecular targeted therapy for the treatment of gastric cancer. Journal of Experimental and Clinical Cancer Research. 2016;**35**:1. DOI: 10.1186/s13046-015-0276-9

[40] Bang YJ, Van Cutsem E, Feyereislova A, Chung HC, Shen L, Sawaki A, Lordick F, Ohtsu A, Omuro Y, Satoh T, Aprile G, Kulikov E, Hill J, Lehle M, Ruschoff J, Kang YK. Trastuzumab in combination with chemotherapy versus chemotherapy alone for treatment of HER2-positive advanced gastric or gastro-oesophageal junction cancer (ToGA): A phase 3, open-label, randomised controlled trial. Lancet. 2010;**376**(9742):687-697. DOI: 10.1016/S0140-6736(10)61121-X

[41] Boku N. HER2-positive gastric cancer. Gastric Cancer. 2014;**17**(1):1-12. DOI: 10.1007/s10120-013-0252-z

[42] Grillo F, Fassan M, Sarocchi F, Fiocca R, Mastracci L. HER2 heterogeneity in gastric/gastroesophageal cancers: From benchside to practice. World Journal of Gastroenterology. 2016;**22**(26):5879-5887. DOI: 10.3748/wjg.v22.i26.5879

[43] Satoh T, Bang YJ, Gotovkin EA, Hamamoto Y, Kang YK, Moiseyenko VM, Ohtsu A, Van Cutsem E, Al-Sakaff N, Urspruch A, Hill J, Weber HA, Chung HC. Quality of life in the trastuzumab for gastric cancer trial. Oncologist. 2014;**19**(7):712-719. DOI: 10.1634/theoncologist.2014-0058

[44] Van Cutsem E, Bang YJ, Feng-Yi F, Xu JM, Lee KW, Jiao SC, Chong JL, Lopez-Sanchez RI, Price T, Gladkov O, Stoss O, Hill J, Ng V, Lehle M, Thomas M, Kiermaier A, Ruschoff J. HER2 screening data from ToGA: Targeting HER2 in gastric and gastroesophageal junction cancer. Gastric Cancer. 2015;**18**(3):476-484. DOI: 10.1007/s10120-014-0402-y

[45] Hecht JR, Bang YJ, Qin SK, Chung HC, Xu JM, Park JO, Jeziorski K, Shparyk Y, Hoff PM, Sobrero A, Salman P, Li J, Protsenko SA, Wainberg ZA, Buyse M, Afenjar K, Houe V, Garcia A, Kaneko T, Huang Y, Khan-Wasti S, Santillana S, Press MF, Slamon D. Lapatinib in combination with capecitabine plus oxaliplatin in human epidermal growth factor receptor 2-positive advanced or metastatic gastric, esophageal, or gastroesophageal adenocarcinoma: TRIO-013/LOGiC—A randomized phase III trial. Journal of Clinical Oncology. 2016;**34**(5):443-451. DOI: 10.1200/JCO.2015.62.6598

[46] Namikawa T, Munekage E, Munekage M, Maeda H, Yatabe T, Kitagawa H, Sakamoto K, Obatake M, Kobayashi M, Hanazaki K. Evaluation of a trastuzumab-containing treatment regimen for patients with unresectable advanced or recurrent gastric cancer. Molecular *and* Clinical Oncology. 2016;**5**(1):74-78. DOI: 10.3892/mco.2016.892

[47] ClinicalTrials.gov. [Internet] 2017. Available from: https://clinicaltrials.gov/ [Accessed: January 19, 2017]

[48] Al-Batran SE, Van Cutsem E, Oh SC, Bodoky G, Shimada Y, Hironaka S, Sugimoto N, Lipatov ON, Kim TY, Cunningham D, Rougier P, Muro K, Liepa AM, Chandrawansa K, Emig M, Ohtsu A, Wilke H. Quality-of-life and performance status results from the phase III RAINBOW study of ramucirumab plus paclitaxel versus placebo plus paclitaxel in patients with previously treated gastric or gastroesophageal junction adenocarcinoma. Annals of Oncology. 2016;**27**(4):673-679. DOI: 10.1093/annonc/mdv625

[49] Fuchs CS, Tomasek J, Yong CJ, Dumitru F, Passalacqua R, Goswami C, Safran H, dos Santos LV, Aprile G, Ferry DR, Melichar B, Tehfe M, Topuzov E, Zalcberg JR, Chau I, Campbell W, Sivanandan C, Pikiel J, Koshiji M, Hsu Y, Liepa AM, Gao L, Schwartz JD, Tabernero J. Ramucirumab monotherapy for previously treated advanced gastric or gastro-oesophageal junction adenocarcinoma (REGARD): An international, randomised, multicentre, placebo-controlled, phase 3 trial. Lancet. 2014;**383**(9911):31-39. DOI: 10.1016/S0140-6736(13)61719-5

[50] Wilke H, Muro K, Van Cutsem E, Oh SC, Bodoky G, Shimada Y, Hironaka S, Sugimoto N, Lipatov O, Kim TY, Cunningham D, Rougier P, Komatsu Y, Ajani J, Emig M, Carlesi R, Ferry D, Chandrawansa K, Schwartz JD, Ohtsu A. Ramucirumab plus paclitaxel versus placebo plus paclitaxel in patients with previously treated advanced gastric or gastro-oesophageal junction adenocarcinoma (RAINBOW): A double-blind, randomised phase 3 trial. The Lancet Oncology. 2014;**15**(11):1224-1235. DOI: 10.1016/S1470-2045(14)70420-6

[51] Young K, Smyth E, Chau I. Ramucirumab for advanced gastric cancer or gastro-oesophageal junction adenocarcinoma. Therapeutic advances in gastroenterology. 2015;**8**(6):373-383. DOI: 10.1177/1756283X15592586

[52] Yoon HH, Bendell JC, Braiteh FS. Ramucirumab (RAM) plus FOLFOX as front-line therapy (Rx) for advanced gastric or esophageal adenocarcinoma (GE-AC): Randomized, double-blind, multicenter phase 2 trial. Journal of Clinical Oncology. 2014;**32**(5 Suppl). abstr 4004

[53] Ducreux M, Adenis A, Pignon JP, Francois E, Chauffert B, Ichante JL, Boucher E, Ychou M, Pierga JY, Montoto-Grillot C, Conroy T. Efficacy and safety of bevacizumab-based combination regimens in patients with previously untreated metastatic colorectal cancer: Final results from a randomised phase II study of bevacizumab plus 5-fluorouracil, leucovorin plus irinotecan versus bevacizumab plus capecitabine plus irinotecan (FNCLCC ACCORD 13/0503 study). European Journal of Cancer. 2013;**49**(6):1236-1245. DOI: 10.1016/j.ejca.2012.12.011

[54] Ohtsu A, Shah MA, Van Cutsem E, Rha SY, Sawaki A, Park SR, Lim HY, Yamada Y, Wu J, Langer B, Starnawski M, Kang YK. Bevacizumab in combination with chemotherapy

as first-line therapy in advanced gastric cancer: A randomized, double-blind, placebo-controlled phase III study. Journal of Clinical Oncology. 2011;**29**(30):3968-3976. DOI: 10.1200/JCO.2011.36.2236

[55] Zhang G, Huang S, Wang Z. A meta-analysis of bevacizumab alone and in combination with irinotecan in the treatment of patients with recurrent glioblastoma multiforme. Journal of Clinical Neuroscience. 2012;**19**(12):1636-1640. DOI: 10.1016/j.jocn.2011.12.028

[56] Friedman HS, Prados MD, Wen PY, Mikkelsen T, Schiff D, Abrey LE, Yung WK, Paleologos N, Nicholas MK, Jensen R, Vredenburgh J, Huang J, Zheng M, Cloughesy T. Bevacizumab alone and in combination with irinotecan in recurrent glioblastoma. Journal of Clinical Oncology. 2009;**27**(28):4733-4740. DOI: 10.1200/JCO.2008.19.8721

[57] Reck M, von Pawel J, Zatloukal P, Ramlau R, Gorbounova V, Hirsh V, Leighl N, Mezger J, Archer V, Moore N, Manegold C. Phase III trial of cisplatin plus gemcitabine with either placebo or bevacizumab as first-line therapy for nonsquamous non-small-cell lung cancer: AVAil. Journal of Clinical Oncology. 2009;**27**(8):1227-1234. DOI: 10.1200/JCO.2007.14.5466

[58] Reck M, von Pawel J, Zatloukal P, Ramlau R, Gorbounova V, Hirsh V, Leighl N, Mezger J, Archer V, Moore N, Manegold C. Overall survival with cisplatin-gemcitabine and bevacizumab or placebo as first-line therapy for nonsquamous non-small-cell lung cancer: Results from a randomised phase III trial (AVAiL). Annals of Oncology. 2010;**21**(9):1804-1809. DOI: 10.1093/annonc/mdq020

[59] Miller K, Wang M, Gralow J, Dickler M, Cobleigh M, Perez EA, Shenkier T, Cella D, Davidson NE. Paclitaxel plus bevacizumab versus paclitaxel alone for metastatic breast cancer. The New England Journal of Medicine. 2007;**357**(26):2666-2676. DOI: 10.1056/NEJMoa072113

[60] Cella D, Wang M, Wagner L, Miller K. Survival-adjusted health-related quality of life (HRQL) among patients with metastatic breast cancer receiving paclitaxel plus bevacizumab versus paclitaxel alone: Results from Eastern Cooperative Oncology Group Study 2100 (E2100). Breast Cancer Research and Treatment. 2011;**130**(3):855-861. DOI: 10.1007/s10549-011-1725-6

[61] Hurwitz H, Fehrenbacher L, Novotny W, Cartwright T, Hainsworth J, Heim W, Berlin J, Baron A, Griffing S, Holmgren E, Ferrara N, Fyfe G, Rogers B, Ross R, Kabbinavar F. Bevacizumab plus irinotecan, fluorouracil, and leucovorin for metastatic colorectal cancer. The New England Journal of Medicine. 2004;**350**(23):2335-2342. DOI: 10.1056/NEJMoa032691

[62] Shen L, Li J, Xu J, Pan H, Dai G, Qin S, Wang L, Wang J, Yang Z, Shu Y, Xu R, Chen L, Liu Y, Yu S, Bu L, Piao Y. Bevacizumab plus capecitabine and cisplatin in Chinese patients with inoperable locally advanced or metastatic gastric or gastroesophageal junction cancer: Randomized, double-blind, phase III study (AVATAR study). Gastric Cancer. 2015;**18**(1):168-176. DOI: 10.1007/s10120-014-0351-5

[63] Van Cutsem E, de Haas S, Kang Y-K, Ohtsu A, Tebbutt NC, Ming Xu J, Peng Yong W, Langer B, Delmar P, Scherer SJ, Shah MA. Bevacizumab in combination with chemotherapy as first-line therapy in advanced gastric cancer: A biomarker evaluation from the AVAGAST randomized phase III trial. Journal of Clinical Oncology. 2012;**30**(17):2119-2127. DOI: 10.1200/jco.2011.39.9824

[64] Muro K, Bang Y, Shankaran V, Geva R, Catenacci DVT, Gupta S, Eder JP, Berger R, Gonzalez EJ, Pulini J, Ray AB, Dolled-Filhart M, Emancipator K, Pathiraja K, Shu X, Koshiji MR, Cheng J, Chung HC. LBA15A phase 1b study of pembrolizumab (PEMBRO; MK-3475) in patients (pts) with advanced gastric cancer. Annals of Oncology. 2014;**25**(Suppl 4):mdu438.15-mdu438.15. DOI: 10.1093/annonc/mdu438.15

[65] de Guillebon E, Roussille P, Frouin E, Tougeron D. Anti program death-1/anti program death-ligand 1 in digestive cancers. The World Journal of Gastrointestinal Oncology. 2015;**7**(8):95-101. DOI: 10.4251/wjgo.v7.i8.95

[66] Eto S, Yoshikawa K, Nishi M, Higashijima J, Tokunaga T, Nakao T, Kashihara H, Takasu C, Iwata T, Shimada M. Programmed cell death protein 1 expression is an independent prognostic factor in gastric cancer after curative resection. Gastric Cancer. 2016;**19**(2):466-471. DOI: 10.1007/s10120-015-0519-7

[67] Geng Y, Wang H, Lu C, Li Q, Xu B, Jiang J, Wu C. Expression of costimulatory molecules B7-H1, B7-H4 and Foxp3+ tregs in gastric cancer and its clinical significance. The International Journal of Clinical Oncology. 2015;**20**(2):273-281. DOI: 10.1007/s10147-014-0701-7

[68] Wu C, Zhu Y, Jiang J, Zhao J, Zhang XG, Xu N. Immunohistochemical localization of programmed death-1 ligand-1 (PD-L1) in gastric carcinoma and its clinical significance. Acta Histochemica. 2006;**108**(1):19-24. DOI: 10.1016/j.acthis.2006.01.003

[69] Zhang M, Dong Y, Liu H, Wang Y, Zhao S, Xuan Q, Zhang Q. The clinicopathological and prognostic significance of PD-L1 expression in gastric cancer: A meta-analysis of 10 studies with 1,901 patients. Scientific Reports. 2016;**6**:37933. DOI: 10.1038/srep37933

[70] Dolan DE,Gupta S. PD-1 pathway inhibitors: Changing the landscape of cancer immunotherapy. Cancer Control. 2014;**21**(3):231-237

[71] Takaya S, Saito H, Ikeguchi M. Upregulation of immune checkpoint molecules, PD-1 and LAG-3, on $CD4^+$ and $CD8^+$ T cells after gastric cancer surgery. Yonago Acta Medica. 2015;**58**(1):39-44

[72] Saito H, Kuroda H, Matsunaga T, Osaki T, Ikeguchi M. Increased PD-1 expression on $CD4^+$ and $CD8^+$ T cells is involved in immune evasion in gastric cancer. Journal of Surgical Oncology. 2013;**107**(5):517-522. DOI: 10.1002/jso.23281

[73] Doshi S, Gisleskog PO, Zhang Y, Zhu M, Oliner KS, Loh E, Perez Ruixo JJ. Rilotumumab exposure-response relationship in patients with advanced or metastatic gastric cancer. Clinical Cancer Research. 2015;**21**(11):2453-2461. DOI: 10.1158/1078-0432.CCR-14-1661

[74] Iveson T, Donehower RC, Davidenko I, Tjulandin S, Deptala A, Harrison M, Nirni S, Lakshmaiah K, Thomas A, Jiang Y, Zhu M, Tang R, Anderson A, Dubey S, Oliner KS, Loh E. Rilotumumab in combination with epirubicin, cisplatin, and capecitabine as first-line treatment for gastric or oesophagogastric junction adenocarcinoma: An open-label, dose de-escalation phase 1b study and a double-blind, randomised phase 2 study. The Lancet Oncology. 2014;**15**(9):1007-1018. DOI: 10.1016/S1470-2045(14)70023-3

[75] Gherardi E, Birchmeier W, Birchmeier C, Vande Woude G. Targeting MET in cancer: Rationale and progress. Nature Reviews Cancer. 2012;**12**(2):89-103. DOI: 10.1038/nrc3205

[76] Pyo JS, Kang G, Cho H. Clinicopathological significance and diagnostic accuracy of c-met expression by immunohistochemistry in gastric cancer: A meta-analysis. Journal of Gastric Cancer. 2016;**16**(3):141-151. DOI: 10.5230/jgc.2016.16.3.141

[77] Nakajima M, Sawada H, Yamada Y, Watanabe A, Tatsumi M, Yamashita J, Matsuda M, Sakaguchi T, Hirao T, Nakano H. The prognostic significance of amplification and overexpression of c-met and c-erb B-2 in human gastric carcinomas. Cancer. 1999;**85**(9):1894-1902

[78] Huang TJ, Wang JY, Lin SR, Lian ST, Hsieh JS. Overexpression of the c-met protooncogene in human gastric carcinoma—Correlation to clinical features. Acta Oncologica. 2001;**40**(5):638-643

[79] Rajcevic U, Hudler P, Mijovski G, Gorjanc G, Hoelzl G, Repse S, Juvan R, Kovac M, Huber CG, Komel R. Assessment of differential expression of oncogenes in adenocarcinoma of stomach with fluorescent labeling and simultaneous amplification of gene transcripts. Radiology and Oncology. 2007;**41**(4):174-182

[80] Wu CW, Li AF, Chi CW, Chung WW, Liu TY, Lui WY, P'Eng F K. Hepatocyte growth factor and Met/HGF receptors in patients with gastric adenocarcinoma. Oncology Reports. 1998;**5**(4):817-822

[81] Amgen Announces Termination Of All Amgen-Sponsored Clinical Studies of Rilotumumab In Advanced Gastric Cancer. [Internet] 2014. Available from: http://investors.amgen.com/phoenix.zhtml?c=61656&p=irol-newsArticle&ID=1992492 [Accessed: January 21, 2017]

[82] Wainberg ZA, Anghel A, Desai AJ, Ayala R, Luo T, Safran B, Fejzo MS, Hecht JR, Slamon DJ, Finn RS. Lapatinib, a dual EGFR and HER2 kinase inhibitor, selectively inhibits HER2-amplified human gastric cancer cells and is synergistic with trastuzumab in vitro and in vivo. Clinical Cancer Research. 2010;**16**(5):1509-1519. DOI: 10.1158/1078-0432.CCR-09-1112

[83] Lorenzen S, Riera Knorrenschild J, Haag GM, Pohl M, Thuss-Patience P, Bassermann F, Helbig U, Weissinger F, Schnoy E, Becker K, Stocker G, Ruschoff J, Eisenmenger A, Karapanagiotou-Schenkel I, Lordick F. Lapatinib versus lapatinib plus capecitabine as second-line treatment in human epidermal growth factor receptor 2-amplified metastatic gastro-oesophageal cancer: A randomised phase II trial of the Arbeitsgemeinschaft Internistische Onkologie. European Journal of Cancer. 2015;**51**(5):569-576. DOI: 10.1016/j.ejca.2015.01.059

[84] Press MF, Finn RS, Cameron D, Di Leo A, Geyer CE, Villalobos IE, Santiago A, Guzman R, Gasparyan A, Ma Y, Danenberg K, Martin AM, Williams L, Oliva C, Stein S, Gagnon R, Arbushites M, Koehler MT. HER-2 gene amplification, HER-2 and epidermal growth factor receptor mRNA and protein expression, and lapatinib efficacy in women with metastatic breast cancer. Clinical Cancer Research. 2008;**14**(23):7861-7870. DOI: 10.1158/1078-0432.CCR-08-1056

[85] Satoh T, Xu RH, Chung HC, Sun GP, Doi T, Xu JM, Tsuji A, Omuro Y, Li J, Wang JW, Miwa H, Qin SK, Chung IJ, Yeh KH, Feng JF, Mukaiyama A, Kobayashi M, Ohtsu A, Bang YJ. Lapatinib plus paclitaxel versus paclitaxel alone in the second-line treatment of HER2-amplified advanced gastric cancer in Asian populations: TyTAN--a randomized, phase III study. Journal of Clinical Oncology. 2014;**32**(19):2039-2049. DOI: 10.1200/JCO.2013.53.6136

[86] Press MF, Ellis CE, Gagnon RC, Grob TJ, Buyse M, Villalobos I, Liang Z, Wu S, Bang YJ, Qin SK, Chung HC, Xu J, Park JO, Jeziorski K, Afenjar K, Ma Y, Estrada MC, Robinson DM, Scherer SJ, Sauter G, Hecht JR, Slamon DJ. HER2 status in advanced or metastatic gastric, esophageal, or gastroesophageal adenocarcinoma for entry to the TRIO-013/LOGiC trial of lapatinib. Molecular Cancer Therapeutics. 2017;**16**(1):228-238. DOI: 10.1158/1535-7163.MCT-15-0887

[87] Gomez-Martin C, Plaza JC, Pazo-Cid R, Salud A, Pons F, Fonseca P, Leon A, Alsina M, Visa L, Rivera F, Galan MC, Del Valle E, Vilardell F, Iglesias M, Fernandez S, Landolfi S, Cuatrecasas M, Mayorga M, Jose Paules M, Sanz-Moncasi P, Montagut C, Garralda E, Rojo F, Hidalgo M, Lopez-Rios F. Level of HER2 gene amplification predicts response and overall survival in HER2-positive advanced gastric cancer treated with trastuzumab. Journal of Clinical Oncology. 2013;**31**(35):4445-4452. DOI: 10.1200/JCO.2013.48.9070

[88] Ock CY, Lee KW, Kim JW, Kim JS, Kim TY, Lee KH, Han SW, Im SA, Kim WH, Bang YJ, Oh DY. Optimal patient selection for trastuzumab treatment in HER2-positive advanced gastric cancer. Clinical Cancer Research. 2015;**21**(11):2520-2529. DOI: 10.1158/1078-0432.CCR-14-2659

[89] Kwak EL, Ahronian LG, Siravegna G, Mussolin B, Godfrey JT, Clark JW, Blaszkowsky LS, Ryan DP, Lennerz JK, Iafrate AJ, Bardelli A, Hong TS, Corcoran RB:. Molecular heterogeneity and receptor coamplification drive resistance to targeted therapy in MET-amplified esophagogastric cancer. Cancer Discovery. 2015;**5**(12):1271-1281. DOI: 10.1158/2159-8290.CD-15-0748

[90] Shattuck DL, Miller JK, Carraway KL, Sweeney C. Met receptor contributes to trastuzumab resistance of Her2-overexpressing breast cancer cells. Cancer Research. 2008;**68**(5):1471-1477. DOI: 10.1158/0008-5472.CAN-07-5962

[91] Luque-Cabal M, Garcia-Teijido P, Fernandez-Perez Y, Sanchez-Lorenzo L, Palacio-Vazquez I. Mechanisms behind the resistance to trastuzumab in HER2-amplified breast cancer and strategies to overcome it. Clinical Medicine Insights: Oncology. 2016;**10**(Suppl 1):21-30. DOI: 10.4137/CMO.S34537

[92] Finocchiaro G, Toschi L, Gianoncelli L, Baretti M, Santoro A. Prognostic and predictive value of MET deregulation in non-small cell lung cancer. The Annals of Translational Medicine. 2015;**3**(6):83. DOI: 10.3978/j.issn.2305-5839.2015.03.43

[93] Bang YJ, Kang YK, Kang WK, Boku N, Chung HC, Chen JS, Doi T, Sun Y, Shen L, Qin S, Ng WT, Tursi JM, Lechuga MJ, Lu DR, Ruiz-Garcia A, Sobrero A. Phase II study of sunitinib as second-line treatment for advanced gastric cancer. Investigational New Drugs. 2011;**29**(6):1449-1458. DOI: 10.1007/s10637-010-9438-y

[94] Boku N, Muro K, Machida N, Hashigaki S, Kimura N, Suzuki M, Lechuga M, Miyata Y. Phase I study of sunitinib plus S-1 and cisplatin in Japanese patients with advanced or metastatic gastric cancer. Investigational New Drugs. 2014;**32**(2):261-270. DOI: 10.1007/s10637-013-9948-5

[95] Lee KW, Park SR, Oh DY, Park YI, Khosravan R, Lin X, Lee SY, Roh EJ, Valota O, Lechuga MJ, Bang YJ. Phase I study of sunitinib plus capecitabine/cisplatin or capecitabine/oxaliplatin in advanced gastric cancer. Investigational New Drugs. 2013;**31**(6):1547-1558. DOI: 10.1007/s10637-013-0032-y

[96] Yi JH, Lee J, Park SH, Park JO, Yim DS, Park YS, Lim HY, Kang WK. Randomised phase II trial of docetaxel and sunitinib in patients with metastatic gastric cancer who were previously treated with fluoropyrimidine and platinum. The British Journal of Cancer. 2012;**106**(9):1469-1474. DOI: 10.1038/bjc.2012.100

[97] Li J, Qin S, Xu J, Guo W, Xiong J, Bai Y, Sun G, Yang Y, Wang L, Xu N, Cheng Y, Wang Z, Zheng L, Tao M, Zhu X, Ji D, Liu X, Yu H. Apatinib for chemotherapy-refractory advanced metastatic gastric cancer: Results from a randomized, placebo-controlled, parallel-arm, phase II trial. Journal of Clinical Oncology. 2013;**31**(26):3219-3225. DOI: 10.1200/JCO.2013.48.8585

[98] Li J, Qin S, Xu J, Xiong J, Wu C, Bai Y, Liu W, Tong J, Liu Y, Xu R, Wang Z, Wang Q, Ouyang X, Yang Y, Ba Y, Liang J, Lin X, Luo D, Zheng R, Wang X, Sun G, Wang L, Zheng L, Guo H, Wu J, Xu N, Yang J, Zhang H, Cheng Y, Wang N, Chen L, Fan Z, Sun P, Yu H. Randomized, double-blind, placebo-controlled phase III trial of apatinib in patients with chemotherapy-refractory advanced or metastatic adenocarcinoma of the stomach or gastroesophageal junction. Journal of Clinical Oncology Journal. 2016;**34**(13):1448-1454. DOI: 10.1200/JCO.2015.63.5995

[99] Hu X, Zhang J, Xu B, Jiang Z, Ragaz J, Tong Z, Zhang Q, Wang X, Feng J, Pang D, Fan M, Li J, Wang B, Wang Z, Sun S, Liao C. Multicenter phase II study of apatinib, a novel VEGFR inhibitor in heavily pretreated patients with metastatic triple-negative breast cancer. The International Journal of Cancer. 2014;**135**(8):1961-1969. DOI: 10.1002/ijc.28829

[100] Stepanov VA. Genomes, populations and diseases: Ethnic genomics and personalized medicine. Acta Naturae. 2010;**2**(4):15-30

Section 4

Molecular Biological Mechanism Involved in Patients with Gatric Cancer

Chapter 7

Molecular Prognostic Factors in Gastric Cancer

Daniela Lazar, Sorina Taban, Marioara Cornianu,
Alexandra Faur, Ioan Romosan and Adrian Goldis

Additional information is available at the end of the chapter

http://dx.doi.org/10.5772/intechopen.69737

Abstract

Gastric cancer represents a major health problem worldwide. Literature data have demonstrated that gastric tumors present a high molecular heterogeneity, responsible for the process of carcinogenesis and dissemination. By revealing the molecular subtype of the tumor, it is possible to assess its behavior, the outcome of the patient, and the treatment approach, according to its genetic and epigenetic profile. This chapter aims to highlight some of the many different genetic mutations, epigenetic alterations, as well as aberrant signaling pathways involved in the pathogenesis of stomach cancers, each of these molecular abnormalities acting in a specific stage of the disease. Moreover, the manuscript describes the novel therapeutic agents that target some of these aberrant molecular signaling pathways. Unfortunately, only a few agents are currently part of the standard treatment of gastric cancer, while most of the others remain to prove their therapeutic efficacy in the setting of clinical trials. By discovering the different molecular subtypes of gastric cancer, as well as numerous classes of targeted molecular agents, in the future, we would be able to perform an individualized treatment, associated with maximum efficiency and less costs.

Keywords: gastric cancer, molecular classification, gene expressions-based prognostic scoring system, molecular biomarkers, molecular targeted treatment

1. Introduction

Despite a decline in the incidence in past decades, gastric cancer remains a major health problem globally [1, 2], being the fifth most common type of cancer worldwide, with almost one million new cases estimated to have occurred in 2012, according to Globocan [3]. Furthermore, stomach cancer represents the third leading cause of cancer death in both sexes worldwide (723,000 deaths) [3].

According to the World Health Organization classification, the vast majority of gastric cancers are adenocarcinomas, divided into papillary, tubular, mucinous (colloid), and poorly cohesive carcinomas (including signet-ring cell carcinoma and other variants) [4]. Although it was proposed a long time ago (1965), the Lauren classification is still widely used in clinical practice and subdivides gastric carcinomas into intestinal and diffuse types, associated with different pathogenesis, ways of spreading, and outcome [5]. Unfortunately, these two classification systems have little clinical impact, making the development of classifiers that can define prognosis and guide patient's treatment as an urgent need.

Literature data have demonstrated that the development of gastric cancer is associated in the majority of cases with infectious agents such as the Gram-negative spiral bacterium *Helicobacter pylori* (most often) [6] and Epstein-Barr virus (EBV) (about 9% of all cases of gastric cancer) [7]. Only a small percentage of gastric cancer patients (hereditary cases) are associated with germline mutation in E-cadherin (CDH1) [8] or mismatch repair genes (Lynch syndrome) [9]. In contrast to the familial clustering of gastric cancer, sporadic mismatch repair-deficient gastric tumors present epigenetic silencing of hMLH1 and p16 in the context of a CpG island methylator phenotype (CIMP) [10].

Due to a lack of early specific clinical features, most patients with gastric cancer are diagnosed in advanced stages, resulting in poor 5-year survival rates [11], with a median survival of less than 1 year in case of metastatic stage IV patients [12–14]. Nowadays, survival has gained only minor improvement despite the advances in diagnostic techniques, the multidisciplinary therapeutic management, and the development of novel molecular targeted treatment agents.

Unfortunately, despite modern treatments, less than a quarter of gastric cancer patients survive longer than 5 years after surgery. Gastric cancer represents a complex disease, showing major differences in their tumor cell behavior and responses to chemotherapy.

Recent data have demonstrated that gastric tumors present a high molecular heterogeneity involved both in the process of carcinogenesis and cancer spread. By identifying the specific molecular patterns of the tumor, it is possible to assess its behavior, the prognosis of the patient, and also to decide the most appropriate treatment, a much more personalized one. It is well known that in the pathogenesis of stomach cancers many different genetic mutations, epigenetic alterations, as well as dysregulated signaling pathways are involved, each of these molecular abnormalities acting in a different stage of the disease.

Currently, novel therapeutic agents that target some of these aberrant molecular signaling pathways are already part of the standard treatment of gastric cancer, while others remain to prove their therapeutic efficacy in the setting of clinical trials [15].

2. Oncogenic pathway combinations predict outcome of gastric cancer patients

Gastric cancers are molecularly heterogeneous tumors, showing different dysregulated oncogenic pathways such as E2F, K-RAS, p53, and Wnt/β-catenin signaling that occur with varying frequencies in these types of tumors [16, 17]. In contrast to the previous studies that have focused on single pathways [18–20], experimental evidence indicates that, in most cases, carcinogenesis is dictated by complex interactions between multiple pro- and anti-oncogenic signaling pathways [21].

Unlike previous gastric tumor microarray researches relating different gene expression patterns to specific histological features or anatomical location [22], Ooi et al. [23] have succeeded in subdividing gastric cancers into molecularly homogenous subgroups that enable personalizing patient treatments and improving prognosis. It was for the first time when, by using multiple patterns of oncogenic pathway activation, a novel cancer classification approach has been developed, namely a genomic taxonomy of gastric cancer. They developed an in silico technique to define activation levels of different oncogenic pathways implemented in context of complex tumor profiles and validated this classification approach using proof-of-concept examples from breast cancer. Afterward, they have applied this method to gastric tumors and evaluated 11 oncogenic pathways previously known to be involved in gastric tumorigenesis [16–20, 24–27]. They have assessed over 300 primary stomach cancers coming from three independent patient cohorts. The researchers have discovered three oncogenic pathways, nuclear factor-kB (NF-κB), Wnt/β-catenin, and proliferation/stem cell, which were dysregulated in over 70% of gastric cancers and validated the patient stratification in vitro using gastric cancer cell lines. Patient classification by oncogenic pathway combinations revealed significant survival differences, suggesting a major role for pathway combinations in determining gastric cancer behavior. Therefore, gastric cancer can be taxonomized into biologically, molecularly, and clinically significant subtypes.

The authors defined concomitant activation of different oncogenic pathways, such as of E2F, MYC, p21 (repression), and the "proliferation/stem cell" pathway, most likely due to increased cellular proliferation in tumor cells [28], and in stem cells (embryonic stem cells (ESCs)) [29]. Co-activation of different pathways demonstrates the ability of the cancer cell to dictate the activity of multiple pathways.

The study showed that NF-κB signaling may be elevated in a significant proportion of gastric cancers probably due to *H. pylori* infection [30]; therefore, targeted NF-κB inhibitors may represent an appropriate treatment for gastric tumors. Pathway-based taxonomies may be useful in developing potential pathway inhibitors and novel targeted therapies that would be studied on prestratifying patients using molecular or pathologic criteria.

3. Molecular classification of gastric cancers by "The Cancer Genome Atlas (TCGA)" project

The goals of "The Cancer Genome Atlas (TCGA)" project were to develop a molecular classification of gastric cancer with clinical impact and to detect the major dysregulated pathways of distinct subtypes of gastric cancer [31].

The researchers have analyzed fresh frozen gastric adenocarcinoma primary tumor tissue from 295 patients with no prior chemo- or radiotherapy, using six genomic and molecular platforms including genome/exome/methylome DNA sequencing, RNA sequencing, and protein arrays. Germline DNA from blood/nonmalignant gastric mucosa was used as a control for detecting somatic alterations. Nonmalignant gastric samples were also collected for DNA methylation ($n = 527$) and expression ($n = 529$) assessment.

Tumors were first subgrouped by EBV-positivity (9%), then by MSI-high status (named MSI; 22%), and the remaining tumors were classified by degree of aneuploidy into genomically stable cancers (20%) or those exhibiting chromosomal instability (CIN; 50%).

This project revealed that the vast majority of the diffuse histological subtype belongs to the genomically stable group. CIN tumors were mostly located in the gastroesophageal junction/cardia, whereas most of the EBV-positive tumors were located in the gastric fundus or body. Genomically, stable tumors were diagnosed at an earlier age compared to MSI tumors; most EBV-positive cases were male (81%), in concordance with previous results [32].

As previously reported [33], all EBV-positive tumors exhibited extreme CIMP, distinct from that in the MSI subtype [10] (CDKN2A promoter hypermethylation versus MLH1 hypermethylation) [34]. Furthermore, in concordance with prior data [35, 36], the study revealed a strong predilection for PIK3CA mutation in EBV positive tumors, with nonsilent PIK3CA mutations found in 80% of this subgroup ($P < 0.001$), that could be targeted using PI(3)-kinase inhibition.

By assessing 63 hypermutated tumors, there were identified 37 significantly mutated genes including TP53, KRAS, ARID1A, PIK3CA, ERBB3, PTEN, and HLA-B. The analysis of genes mutated within MSI subgroup of gastric cancers revealed alterations in major histocompatibility complex class I genes, a beneficial event for hypermutated tumors by dysregulating antigen presentation to the immune system.

Through the analysis of the 215 nonhypermutated cancers, there were identified 25 significantly mutated genes, including TP53, ARID1A, KRAS, PIK3CA, and RNF43, genes involved in the β-catenin pathway, the TGF-b pathway, RASA1, and ERBB2 (therapeutic target).

In addition to PIK3CA mutations, EBV-positive tumors had frequent ARID1A and BCOR (encoding an anti-apoptotic protein) gene mutations. TP53 mutations were detected in 71% of CIN tumors. The genomically stable subtype presented a high frequency of CDH1somatic mutations and inactivating ARID1A mutations. RHOA mutations were detected almost exclusively in genomically stable tumors. In its activated form, RHOA controls cellular motility [37, 38] and activates STAT3 to initiate tumorigenesis [39, 40]. It seems that the activation of RHOA-driven pathways contribute to the invasive phenotype of diffuse gastric cancer.

Oncogenic signaling pathways, including candidate therapeutic targets such as receptor tyrosine kinases (RTKs), RAS, and PI(3)-kinase signaling were characterized. EBV-positive tumors contained PIK3CA mutations and recurrent JAK2 and ERBB2 amplifications. MSI cases presented some mutations in PIK3CA, ERBB3, ERBB2, and EGFR [41]. The genomically stable subtype expressed recurrent RHOA and CLDN 18 events. CIN tumors showed genomic amplifications of RTKs that may be therapeutically blocked. Recurrent amplification of the gene encoding ligand VEGFA and frequent amplifications of cell cycle mediators highlight the role of the VEGFR2 targeting antibody (the already approved agent ramucirumab) [42] and suggest the possible efficacy of cyclin-dependent kinases.

All the subtypes (to a lesser degree the genomically stable tumors) showed increased expression of components involved in the mitotic process, such as AURKA/B and E2F, DNA damage response pathways, targets of MYC activation, and FOXM1 and PLK1 signaling pathways. In addition, the genomically stable subtype exhibited elevated expression of cell adhesion pathways, the B1/B3 integrins, syndecan-1 mediated signaling, and angiogenesis-related pathways, suggesting more potential therapeutic targets, including the aurora kinases (AURKA/B) and polo-like (PLK) family members. The elevated IL-12-mediated signaling expression, along with evidence of PD-L1/2 overexpression in EBV-positive tumors, suggests the importance of immune checkpoint inhibitors evaluation in this subtype of gastric cancer [31].

Therefore, the four major genomic subtypes defined by "The Cancer Genome Atlas (TCGA)" may provide a guide to molecular targeted agents that should be assessed in clinical trials for distinct populations of gastric cancer patients.

4. Gene-expression signatures as markers for cancer grades and stages

Cui et al. [43] developed for the first time a computational study aimed to identify a set of genes whose expression patterns can distinguish among gastric cancers of different grades, with the aim of developing a gene expression-based grading system for gastric cancer.

A total of 452 genes were found to be differentially expressed in the 54 gastric cancer specimens studied. It was revealed that genes whose expression changes correlated with the degree of differentiation are highly enriched among secreted/membrane proteins, involved in signaling pathways (ErbB, FAS, NOD-like receptor, PPAR and Wnt signaling), as well as cell adhesion molecules (CAMs) and tight junctions.

The researchers identified a 19-gene group that can distinguish between well versus poorly differentiated tumors (overall agreement at 79.2%), based on the expression fold change in cancer versus control tissues. The protein products of these 19 genes mentioned above are involved in cell growth, differentiation (IL17RB, SMYD1, SHCBP1), and motility (ACTG2), angiogenesis (ADIPOQ), tumorigenesis (ECRG4), matrix protein synthesis (COL3A1, COL6A3), and extracellular communication.

Moreover, there is a 198-gene group which can distinguish among the four different cancer grades (well-, moderate-, poorly-, and un-differentiated) and the control group according to their gene expression (74.2% accuracy). In addition, the functions of the 198-gene group involve cell division, immune response control, signal transduction, and transcription.

There were also analyzed grade-specific gene signatures. LAPTM4B gene has demonstrated a high classification accuracy for tumor and control samples in the well-differentiated group (AUC = 0.97), a gene known to be essential for cell growth and survival; its up-regulation has been previously found to be correlated with the degree of differentiation of hepatocellular carcinoma [15]. Similarly, they have also identified single gene discriminators for each grade group.

Cui et al. have identified two multigene signatures that can distinguish early stage (stages I and II) and advanced stage gastric cancer (stages III and IV), namely a 10-gene group (CPS

1+DEFA5+DES+DMN+GFRA3+MUC17+OR9G1+REEP3+TMED6+TTN) and a 9-gene group (DPT+EIF1AX+FAM26D+IFITM2+ LOC401498+OR2AE1+PRRG1+REEP3+RTKN2). The overall classification accuracy obtained on the three groups, early, advanced stomach cancer, and control, was 71.4%. Among the early-stage signature genes, there are signaling and immune-related genes that may represent the early changes of tissue cells during carcinogenesis. A few genes were found to be in both the cancer grading and staging signatures (e.g., CPS1, DES, GFRA3, TMED6, and DPT), indicating some functional connection between cancer differentiation and progression. LANCL3, MFAP2, and PPA1 were genes highly correlated with different pathological stages, showing consistent upregulation or downregulation along with tumor progression.

There were found 62 genes with consistent differential expression in gastric cancer versus control tissues, related to extracellular processes such as CAMs, tight junction, cytokine-cytokine receptor interaction, and ECM receptor interaction, the plasminogen activation cascade, as well as signaling pathways (Wnt and Integrin signaling) related to the control of cell growth and proliferation.

The study revealed that the differential expression patterns of 15 genes are highly specific to gastric cancer (e.g., GKN2, CLDN7, THY1, GIF, and PGA4), while most others are general to numerous cancer types, including a few members of the collagen gene family, the carcinoembryonic antigen-related cell adhesion molecule, matrix metalloproteinases, topoisomerase, and secreted phosphoprotein. Only three genes, CLDN7, CLDN1, and DPT, were significantly differentiated in all grades and stages of gastric neoplasia; the consistent expression of dysregulation across all the cancer subgroups may indicate their involvement in major biological pathways leading to cancer development and progression. Dermatopontin (DPT) represents an extracellular matrix protein that creates a link between the dermal fibroblast cell surface and its extracellular matrix, previously found to be downregulated in both uterine leiomyomas and keloids [44].

5. Gene expression-based prognostic scoring systems

Data from literature revealed the important role of the molecular biological characteristics of gastric cancer in the prognosis of the patients and determination of a most suitable clinical therapy for these patients. There are some dysregulated gene expressions found to be associated with the prognosis, such as the overexpressions of HER2 [45] and p53 genes [46]. Also, the hypoxia inducible factor-1 alpha (HIF-1α) seems to be related to the early development of gastric tumor [47].

Takeno et al. [48] elaborated a gastric cancer regulatory network with CDKNIA as the node and examined the expression levels of seven genes in different stages of gastric cancer (iMMP7, SPARC, SOD2, INHBA, IGFBP7, NEK6, and LUM). Their results showed that these seven genes were activated as the disease progressed, suggesting the association of these genes with cancer development.

Wang et al. [49] proposed the hypothesis that molecular features are determining the tumor behavior and can be used to establish prognostic scoring system. Based on the Cancer Genome Atlas (TCGA) data and using different multivariate clustering techniques to identify the key genes for prognostic classification of these analyses, they created a 53-gene expression prognostic scoring system and successfully implemented it to predict overall survival (OS) in the TCGA and the GSE15459 data (Gastric Cancer Project 2008).

These prognostic scores are able to distinguish between patients with good prognosis and bad prognosis, respectively. These genes include TNFAIP2 [50], FGFR4 [51, 52], CXCL10 [53], CEP55 [54], CXCL1 [55], LIMK1 [56], LAMC2 [57], APOE [58], INHBA [59], OSMR [60], APOC1 [61], KLF4 [62], MMP14 [63], ADH1C [64], COL6A3 [65], CCT2 [66], NOL8 [67], EPHB4 [68], and MCM2 [69]. The high expression of FGFR4 protein was previously reported to be associated with a poor prognosis in patients with advanced gastric tumors [51], while the FGFR4 Gly388Arg polymorphism proved to be a useful prognostic marker for early gastric cancer patients [52]. CEP55 functions in cell cycle regulation; knockdown of CEP55 led to diminished proliferation in gastric cancer cell lines acting on the PI3K/AKT signaling pathway and the expression of cyclin-related proteins, suggesting a potential role of CEP55 as a target used in gastric cancer treatment [54]. Some studies show that MCM2 expression levels are a useful tool for the diagnosis and prognosis of gastric tumors [69] and that SNPs in miRNA-binding sites may represent susceptibility markers for gastric cancer [50]. Chemokine (C-X-C motif) ligand (CXCL1) seems to play a major role in tumor metastasis; it has been previously reported that its expression is associated with hepatocellular carcinoma survival [55]. The study of Wang showed that CXCL1 is also involved in gastric cancer overall survival. ATP-binding cassette E1 (ABCE1) known to play a crucial role in the metastasis of lung cancers, and therefore, a potential therapeutic target in this setting [70], was also elevated in gastric tumors and predicted the prognosis of patients.

6. The role of molecular biomarkers in the treatment of gastric cancer

Besides the few standard chemotherapeutic agents having efficiency in the treatment of gastric cancer, molecular targeted therapy for gastric cancer is limited, including mainly agents acting on the HER2 and vascular endothelial growth factor (VEGF) pathways [71].

On the other hand, until present, the only used markers for gastric cancer in clinical practice are carcinoembryonic antigens, CA 19-9 [72] and CA-72 [73], with questionable efficacy. Nowadays, there are multiple molecular biomarkers that had shown their accuracy as diagnostic or prognostic tools but still need further validation for implementing in the routine clinical practice, predicting the response to chemotherapy, posttreatment survival, or disease recurrence.

6.1. Molecular biomarkers predicting the treatment response

The future of cancer treatment aims for a personalized medicine, treating the patient according to his genetic and epigenetic profile, and identifying the occurrence of chemoresistance using specific markers in order to obtain maximum treatment efficiency with lower costs [74]. Heretofore, the vast majority of data regarding predictive biomarkers derive from small retrospective studies; therefore, these biomarkers cannot be used for the moment in clinical practice, outside the setting of clinical trials.

6.1.1. Genetic markers

Lin et al. [75] described the link between integrated genomic signatures, the biological functions, and the background molecular pathways [76]. There were developed prediction models of activity for eight anticancer drugs [76], along with clinical responses to 5-FU (cDNA microarray analysis) [77] and resistance-related genes such as dihydropyrimidine dehydrogenase (DPD) and HB-EGF-like growth factor genes [78]. Also, it was reported that metallothionein-IG and heparin-binding epidermal growth factor-like growth factor (HB-EGF), glutathione-S-transferase, and cyclooxygenase-2 genes were cisplatin-resistance-related and genes such as ADAM22, CYR61, FN1, SPHK1, and GNAI1 were linked to doxorubicin response [79]. Furthermore, in some studies, the genetic polymorphism was linked to the response of 5-FU, cisplatin [80], and paclitaxel [81].

Cristescu et al. described four molecular subtypes of gastric tumors related to disease progression and prognosis: the mesenchymal-like type with highest recurrence frequency, microsatellite-unstable tumors that are hyper-mutated and are associated with the best overall prognosis, tumor protein 53 (TP53)-active and TP53-inactive types that have intermediate prognosis and recurrence [82].

As already mentioned, researchers from "The Cancer Genome Atlas (TCGA)" project proposed a molecular classification dividing gastric tumors into four subtypes, useful for stratifying patients and choosing the appropriate targeted treatment: (1) Epstein-Barr virus positive tumors: PIK3CA mutations, DNA hypermethylation, and amplification of JAK2, CD274, and PDCD1LG2; (2) microsatellite unstable tumors: increased mutation rates, including genes encoding targetable proteins involved in oncogenic signaling pathways; (3) genomically stable tumors: mutations of RHO-family GTPase-activating proteins; (4) tumors with chromosomal instability: marked aneuploidy and amplification of receptor tyrosine kinases [41].

6.1.2. Epigenetic markers

MicroRNA was linked by some studies to the resistance to trastuzumab [83], the pathologic response to neoadjuvant chemotherapy [81], and the chemotherapeutic response of cisplatin/fluorouracil [84].

Long noncoding RNAs (lncRNAs) are potential biomarkers for gastric cancer especially using minimally invasive routes (blood, gastric secretions) [85]. The lncRNA MRUL (Multidrug resistence (MDR)-related and upregulated lncRNA) originated from tissue samples was associated with multidrug chemotherapeutic resistance [86].

Methylation-related biomarkers: methylation of Bcl-2/adenovirus E1B 19 kDa-interacting protein 3 and death-associated protein kinase (DAPK) correlate with poor response to fluoropyrimidine-based chemotherapy [87]; decreased methylation of the bone morphogenetic protein 4 (BMP4) correlates with cisplatin resistance, and the regain of treatment response may be achieved using targeted inhibition of BMP4 [88]. Also, the increased expression of Reprimo (a highly glycosylated cellular protein) due to methylation was associated with a lower response to cisplatin/5-FU chemotherapy [89].

6.1.3. Protein markers

Cellular enzymatic activity: Cellular enzymatic activity was correlated with the chemotherapeutic resistance, thymidylate synthetase (TS) and DPD being associated with tumor sensitivity to 5-FU-based regimens [90].

Cellular proteins: Serum level of alpha-1-microglobulin/bikunin precursor (AMBP) protein, as well as increased expression of β-tubulin III protein, was demonstrated to predict lower chemotherapeutic response to paclitaxel-capecitabine schemes [91, 92]; regenerating gene family member 4 (Reg IV or REG4) predicted resistance to 5-FU-based regimens [93]; forkhead box M1 (FOXM1) transcription factor seems to predict resistance to docetaxel [94]; and dysregulated ribosomal proteins were found to enhance vincristine, adriamycin, and 5-FU resistance [95].

6.2. Molecular aberrations as potential therapeutic targets

Although a great number of targeted therapies belonging to different classes of drugs have been investigated in both preclinical and clinical trials for the treatment of gastric cancer, their use in clinical practice is still limited for the moment.

6.2.1. Anti-HER2 therapies

The HER2 receptor belongs to the EGFR/HER family, having an important role in signal transduction, cell growth, and differentiation [96]. Recent data have revealed HER2 overexpression in 7-34% of patients with gastroesophageal adenocarcinomas and an efficiency of anti-HER2 therapies for both in vitro and in vivo gastric cancer models [97].

6.2.1.1. Monoclonal antibodies targeting HER-2

Trastuzumab (Herceptin) is a humanized anti-HER2 monoclonal antibody; its efficacy for gastric cancer being demonstrated in a phase III trial (ToGA) that randomized naive patients with metastatic or locally advanced unresectable gastric adenocarcinoma with overexpressed HER2 to chemotherapy associated with trastuzumab versus classic chemotherapy [98]. The results of this study demonstrated that adding trastuzumab to standard chemotherapy could increase the OS of these patients to more than 1 year. Currently, the combination of trastuzumab with capecitabine/5-fluorouracil and cisplatin is recommended for the treatment of patients with HER2-positive metastatic adenocarcinoma of the stomach, defined as an immunohistochemical (IHC) 3 positive result or an IHC 2 and fluorescence in situ hybridization (FISH) double positive result.

There are several other ongoing studies of trastuzumab treatment in advanced gastric cancer, such as the HELOISE trial, the phase II study NCT01130337, the TOXAG study, the HERFLOT study, and the phase III trial RTOG 1010. Two phase II clinical trials confirmed the efficacy of trastuzumab combined with XELOX (capecitabine/oxaliplatin) or SP (S-1/cisplatin), respectively, for advanced gastric cancer treatment [99, 100].

The second generation of anti-HER2 agents includes Pertuzumab, which binds to a distinct site on the HER2 receptor. This drug is currently being investigated in the phase III JACOB study in patients with HER2-positive metastatic or locally advanced gastric cancer. [101]. Trastuzumab emtansine (TDM-1) is another second-generation agent currently assessed in a second-line phase II/III trial in advanced gastric cancer [102].

6.2.1.2. Tyrosine kinase inhibitors (TKIs) of HER2

Lapatinib is an oral TKI of EGFR and HER2, which was studied in combination with standard chemotherapy in patients with HER2-positive advanced gastric adenocarcinomas in the phase III LOGIC study [45] and in the phase III Asian TyTAN trial without demonstrating an improvement in OS. Currently, the MAGIC-B study is evaluating the addition of lapatinib to perioperative epirubicin, cisplatin, and capecitabine (ECX) chemotherapy in patients with HER2 (+) gastric cancers [103].

6.2.2. EGFR inhibition

EGFR overexpression is found in 30-50% of gastroesophageal tumors, associated with a more aggressive behavior [104].

6.2.2.1. Anti-EGFR monoclonal antibodies

Cetuximab (Erbitux) is a chimeric monoclonal anti-EGFR antibody. Unfortunately, clinical trials, including the phase III EXPAND trial did not demonstrate a PFS or OS benefit for cetuximab as first-line chemotherapy in the treatment of gastric cancer [105, 106].

Panitumumab is a fully human monoclonal anti-EGFR antibody without a demonstrated efficacy in naive patients with advanced esophagogastric cancer according to the results of clinical trials including the REAL-3 study [107, 108].

Nimotuzumab is a recombinant humanized monoclonal antibody that was evaluated in a double-blind phase II trial [109] including patients with advanced gastric cancer who received nimotuzumab plus irinotecan versus irinotecan alone, showing no difference in PFS or OS between these two groups. Nevertheless, the EGFR2+/3+ subgroups presented a significant benefit when treated with nimotuzumab.

6.2.2.2. TKIs of EGFR

Gefitinib is an oral EGFR TKI currently assessed in a phase I/II study, in combination with chemoradiation, in subjects with resectable gastric cancer [110], in a phase II study in patients with unresectable and/or metastatic gastric carcinomas, and also in a phase III trial in patients with advanced gastro-esophageal junction cancers after progression on chemotherapy [111]. The results of these studies could define the role of this agent in gastric cancer treatment.

Erlotinib (Tarceva) is an oral EGFR TKI, shown to be active in a phase II trial only in patients with gastro-esophageal cancer, but not in those with gastric cancer [112].

6.2.3. VEGF/VEGF receptor inhibition

Angiogenesis is an essential event in tumor growth and spread. VEGF has demonstrated a major role in tumor angiogenesis, growth, and metastasis in numerous tumors, including gastric cancer [113], therefore, being considered an essential therapeutic target. Data revealed that VEGF expression correlates with the clinical stage and prognosis of gastric cancer [114].

6.2.3.1. Anti-VEGF monoclonal antibodies

Bevacizumab (Avastin) efficacy as a first-line treatment in combination with cisplatin-based chemotherapy for advanced gastric cancer was evaluated in the phase III AVAGAST trial (Avastin in gastric cancer) [115], which demonstrated a median PFS and overall response rate significantly improved in the bevacizumab group, but without a significant benefit in OS. Another phase III study, AVATAR, also found that bevacizumab combined with capecitabine/cisplatin chemotherapy did not significantly improve OS in patients with advanced gastric cancer [116]. Possibly, the negative results of these studies might have resulted from not having selected the most molecularly suitable gastric cancer patients.

The MAGIC-B study is currently assessing the role of bevacizumab for perioperative chemotherapy in resectable adenocarcinoma of the stomach, [117]. Hopefully, this trial will allow for the detection of predictive biomarkers that could identify the subset of patients with the greatest potential benefit from the use of perioperative VEGF-A inhibitory monoclonal antibody [118].

Currently, the safety and efficacy of adding bevacizumab to taxane-based chemotherapeutic regimens irinotecan [119] or anti-Her2-targeted treatment in advanced/metastatic gastric cancer is being evaluated in several clinical trials with pending results [120].

6.2.3.2. Anti-VEGF receptor monoclonal antibodies

Ramucirumab is a human monoclonal antibody that inhibits VEGFR-2. It was approved by the FDA as a single agent in gastric cancer after progression on a platinum- or fluoropyrimidine-containing regimen, based on the phase III REGARD study (second-line ramucirumab monotherapy for advanced gastric adenocarcinoma), which found significantly longer OS for ramucirumab versus best supportive care (BSC) [42]. Furthermore, the results of a phase III clinical trial of ramucirumab plus paclitaxel versus placebo plus paclitaxel in the second-line treatment of metastatic gastric adenocarcinoma (RAINBOW trial) revealed significantly longer PFS and OS for the ramucirumab group [121], also leading to approval by the FDA of ramucirumab in combination with paclitaxel as a second-line therapy. Therefore, ramucirumab is for the moment, the only antiangiogenic agent that has been approved for the treatment of gastric carcinoma [122].

Endostar is a novel recombinant human endostatin, which was investigated [123] combined with SOX (S-1/oxaliplatin) for the first-line treatment of patients with advanced gastric cancer; the results showed significantly better PFS for the group including Endostar. More studies for the efficacy of Endostatin in stomach cancer settings are needed.

6.2.3.3. TKIs of VEGF

Apatinib is an anti-VEGF-2 small molecule TKI evaluated in China [124]. Phase II and III studies have shown that apatinib was the first discovered anti-VEGF-2 molecule TKI with benefits for Asian patients with advanced gastric cancer [125], representing a significant progress for third-line treatment, although it prolonged OS by less than 2 months. Further studies are needed to assess the efficacy and safety of this agent in Caucasians. Based on these positive results, apatinib was approved by the Chinese Food and Drug Administration (CFDA) for metastatic adenocarcinoma of the stomach after second-line chemotherapy progression [126].

Sunitinib represents an oral multitargeted TKI of VEGFR, PDGFR, c-KIT (stem cell factor receptor), rearranged during transfection, and FMS-like tyrosine kinase-3 receptor; when administrated in a phase III trial as second-line monotherapy in patients with advanced gastric cancer, it showed a median OS of 6.8 months [127]. The efficacy of sunitinib in advanced gastric cancer was also confirmed by other studies [128].

Sorafenib (Nexavar) is a multitargeted TKI. A phase II study using sorafenib combined with docetaxel and cisplatin as a second-line treatment for gastric cancer patients obtained very long median PFS and median OS [129], although other clinical trials have been terminated early because of low response rates [130].

Pazopanib is an oral agent that inhibits angiogenesis through multiple pathways (VEGFR, PDGFR, and c-KIT), which is currently under investigation in two phase II trials in patients with advanced gastric tumors: the PaFLO trial (FLO ± pazopanib as first-line treatment) [131] and another trial associating pazopanib with capecitabine and oxaliplatin [132].

Regorafenib is an oral multikinase; a phase II trial investigating the efficacy of regorafenib in the treatment of refractory advanced esophagogastric cancer demonstrated a significantly longer median PFS (11 wk versus 3.9 wk) and OS (25 wk versus 19.4 wk) for the regorafenib group versus the placebo group [133] but with serious drug-related toxicity. The role of regorafenib in advanced gastric cancer will be better assessed by the ongoing phase I and II trials.

6.2.4. IGF-1 inhibition

IGF-1 receptor (IGF-1R) is a transmembrane tyrosine kinase receptor promoting tumor angiogenesis, growth, and metastasis in several cancers, including gastroesophageal tumors [134].

Figitumumab is a humanized IgG2 monoclonal antibody against IGF-1R. Some phase I clinical trials have assessed the overall safety and pharmacokinetic profile of figitumumab administrated in patients with advanced solid tumors [135]. Its role in gastric cancer treatment requires further studies.

6.2.5. Fibroblast growth factor TKIs

Fibroblast growth factor (FGF) and its signaling receptors have a major role in cell proliferation, differentiation, and transformation [136].

Although AZD2171 (AZD), a potent oral FGF TKIs, led to tumor inhibition in animal models of gastric cancer, unfortunately, the results of a phase II study [137] showed no statistically significant difference in PFS for FGFR2 amplified gastric cancer patients treated with AZD.

A phase I, first in-human study of JNJ-42756493 (a pan-FGFR TKI) was initiated in advanced solid tumor patients, including gastric cancer, showing that this agent had excellent pharmaceutical properties and safety profile [138].

Ki23057 is an oral TKI broad-range FGF TKI that inhibits the proliferation of gastric scirrhous cancer cells presenting FGFR2 gene amplification. The study of Qiu et al. found that the FGFR2 inhibitor Ki23057 might be therapeutically promising for treating drug-resistant gastric cancer cells, especially when used in combination with other chemotherapeutic drugs. [139].

We expect the results of the ongoing phase I and II clinical trials using TKI such as dovitinib, brivanib, and INCB054828 (FGF inhibitors) in patients with advanced gastric cancer to add new informations regarding the role of FGF inhibitors in this type of tumor [140].

6.2.6. *Hepatocyte growth factor/c-MET (mesenchymal-epithelial transition factor receptor) inhibitors*

C-MET and its signal pathway activation determine gastric cancer cell proliferation, survival, and migration [141].

6.2.6.1. *Anti-HGF/c-MET monoclonal antibodies*

Rilotumumab is a human monoclonal antibody directed against HGF, demonstrated to show efficacy in locally advanced/metastatic gastric cancer patients with MET overexpression by immunohistochemistry (phase II study). Unfortunately, due to the increased toxicity of the agent and treatment-related deaths in the RILOMET-1 trial, all of the clinical trials investigating the role of rilotumumab in gastric tumors, including the phase III RILOMET-1 (with ECX) and RILOMET-2 (with cisplatin and capecitabine) studies, were interrupted.

Onartuzumab is a humanized antibody directed against MET that is also being investigated in a first-line, phase III trial in MET-positive, HER2-negative gastroesophageal patients in combination with mFOLFOX6. The results of this study revealed unfortunately that this treatment could not prolong OS [142].

6.2.6.2. *Anti-HGF/c-MET tyrosine kinase*

Foretonib is an oral molecule inhibitor of c-MET and VEGFR-2A, which was investigated in a phase II study as a single agent in patients with metastatic gastric cancer, demonstrating good tolerability but only minimal antitumor efficacy [143].

6.2.7. *PI3 kinase/mammalian target of the rapamycin pathway inhibition*

Upregulation of the PI3k/Akt/mTOR pathway was associated with poor prognosis and could be implicated in the chemoresistance of gastric cancer [144].

Everolimus is an oral mTOR inhibitor demonstrated to have efficiency in both phase I and phase II studies, which have shown that everolimus monotherapy had a good response rate for advanced gastric cancer patients in the second-line setting [145, 146]. Unfortunately, the phase III GRANITE-1 trial investigating the everolimus monotherapy as a second-/third-line in patients with advanced gastric cancer did not show OS benefit, only the association of severe adverse reactions [147]. Therefore, the use of this agent in the treatment of gastric cancer needs further investigations.

Rapamycin has shown efficiency in preclinical studies and animal models against gastric cancer, increasing also the effectiveness of chemotherapeutic drugs [148]; nevertheless, its use in gastric cancer does not have enough support yet.

6.2.8. PARP inhibitors

These agents were demonstrated to prevent the cancer cell's single stranded break repair mechanism, leading to tumor cell death [149].

A phase II trial in metastatic/recurrent gastroesophageal cancer studied the effectiveness of administrating the PARP inhibitor olaparib as a second-line treatment [150], demonstrating improved OS. There is also an ongoing phase III study of second-line treatment using paclitaxel with or without olaparib in advanced gastric cancer patients [151].

Veliparib was developed to increase the effectiveness of DNA-damaging therapies, such as chemo- or radiotherapy. A study of the efficacy of veliparib associated with the FOLFIRI regimen in gastric cancer is pending results [152].

6.2.9. Immunotherapy/immuno-checkpoint blockade

Because it was revealed that tumors evade host immune recognition [153], immunotherapy has emerged as a novel field of antitumor treatment, which acts by using the blockage mechanism of the inhibitory immune regulatory pathways. New agents targeting immune checkpoints, programmed cell death-1 (PD-1) and programmed cell death-ligand 1 (PD-L1), have been recently investigated.

Ipilimumab blocks the inhibitory receptor called cytotoxic T-lymphocyte-associated antigen 4 (CTLA-4). Unfortunately, a phase II trial assessing the efficacy of ipilimumab after first-line chemotherapy in unresectable locally advanced or metastatic gastric cancer patients revealed no statistically significant improvement in OS [154].

Nivolumab blocks the interactions between PD-1 and PD-L1 stimulated immune function in vitro, showing antitumor activity in preclinical models. A phase I/II study of nivolumab monotherapy versus nivolumab combined with ipilimumab in patients with advanced or metastatic solid tumors, including gastric cancer, is still ongoing [155]. Interim results revealed that nivolumab monotherapy demonstrated encouraging antitumor activity in heavily pretreated gastric cancer patients [156]. Furthermore, a phase III trial is currently assessing the tolerability and efficacy of nivolumab in patients with unresectable advanced or recurrent gastric cancer refractory to standard chemotherapy [157].

Pembrolizumab is an agent that blocks the binding of PD-1 to PDL-1, demonstrated to have good tolerability, as well as anti-tumor activity in a phase 1 study including recurrent and metastatic gastric adenocarcinoma patients with PD-L1 (+) tumors [158]. Other phase I-III trials are investigating this agent in advanced gastric cancer [159, 160], with the aim of investigating the molecular subtypes of gastric tumors through integrative genomic analysis [161]. Some phase I/II studies are assessing its efficacy in combination with other classes of agents (anti-HER2 or anti-VEGFR monoclonal antibodies, multitargeted TKIs) [162–165].

Durvalumab, an anti-PDL-1 drug, has shown some activity in gastric cancer treatment [166]. The combination of durvalumab and tremelimumab (anti-CTLA-4) plus first-line chemotherapy is currently being investigated in advanced solid tumors (including gastric cancers) [167, 168].

6.2.10. Guanylyl cyclase C inhibitors

Guanylyl cyclase C (GCC) is a transmembrane cell surface receptor, expressed both on normal intestinal tissue and on the tumor cells of gastrointestinal neoplasias. MLN0264 consists of a human monoclonal antibody targeting GCC, demonstrating good tolerability of the drug and promising results in a phase I trial in patients with gastrointestinal malignancies expressing GCC [169, 170]. Phase I-II studies of MLN 0264 in previously treated patients with metastatic/recurrent gastric GCC (+) cancers are currently recruiting patients [171, 172].

6.2.11. Inhibitors of the tumor cell cycle

In gastric tumors, there is an alteration of cell cycle regulatory mechanisms [173]. Flavopiridol is a cyclin-dependent kinase inhibitor, unfortunately demonstrated to have low efficacy and serious adverse effects in gastric cancer [174]. Because of its low activity as a single agent, it must be investigated in combination with other chemotherapeutics.

6.2.12. Agents inducing tumor cell apoptosis

The induction of tumor cell apoptosis seems to be a promising target in cancer treatment. NF-κB expression showed to be positively correlated with the degree of the tumor and is negatively correlated with cancer prognosis.

Bortezomib is a highly potent proteasome inhibitor that acts by inhibiting activation of the NF-κB signaling pathway. Preclinical studies have demonstrated an effect of growth inhibition of this agent in combination with standard chemotherapy for gastric cancer [175, 176]. However, phase II studies assessing the efficacy of bortezomib either alone or in combination with irinotecan or paclitaxel plus carboplatin showed no positive results [177–179].

6.2.13. Matrix metalloproteinase inhibitors

The aberrant synthesis of matrix metalloproteinase (MMPs) leads to local tumor invasion by destroying the extracellular matrix and the basement membrane. Literature data have previously associated the high expression of some MMPs with a poor prognosis of gastric cancer [180, 181].

Marimastat is a broad-spectrum MMP. There was a study in patients with nonresectable gastric adenocarcinoma that revealed the first indication of a survival benefit for an MMP inhibitor, supporting a possible role for this agent as a maintenance treatment following chemotherapy [182].

7. Conclusion

Gastric cancer represents a major health problem worldwide, with most of the patients being diagnosed in advanced stages of the disease, associated with poor prognosis. Gastric tumors are molecularly heterogeneous; therefore, it is of major importance to identify the molecular subtype of the tumor and specific molecular biomarkers in order to assess the prognosis of the patient.

Furthermore, it is essential to identify molecular biomarkers that could predict treatment response according to the genetic and epigenetic profile of the patients and also to identify the occurrence of chemoresistance using specific markers, in order to obtain maximum response. The discovery of the molecular background of gastric cancer leads to the development of novel molecular targeted treatments. Heretofore, among the multitude of classes of agents targeting different signaling pathways, such as VEGF, EGFR, HER-2, IGF, immunotherapy, and mTOR pathways, only anti-HER2 monoclonal antibody trastuzumab and anti-VEGFR antibody ramucirumab have been approved for the treatment of advanced gastric cancer. Also, Apatinib, an anti-VEGFR2 TKI demonstrated efficiency in Chinese gastric cancer patients, receiving approval for treatment in this setting. Moreover, there are other classes of agents such as immunotherapy drugs (e.g., Pembrolizumab) that showed encouraging results in clinical trials, but we have still to wait for the final results until implementing them in clinical practice.

Therefore, further clinical studies are needed to demonstrate the effectiveness of molecular targeted treatments in order to have a personalized treatment approach and to improve the outcome of gastric cancer patients.

Author details

Daniela Lazar[1*], Sorina Taban[2], Marioara Cornianu[2], Alexandra Faur[3], Ioan Romosan[4] and Adrian Goldis[1]

*Address all correspondence to: lazar_daniela@yahoo.com

1 Department of Gastroenterology, University of Medicine and Pharmacy "Victor Babeş" Timisoara, Romania

2 Department of Pathology, University of Medicine and Pharmacy "Victor Babeş" Timisoara, Romania

3 Department of Anatomy and Embryology, University of Medicine and Pharmacy "Victor Babeş" Timisoara, Romania

4 Department of Internal Medicine, University of Medicine and Pharmacy "Victor Babeş" Timişoara, Romania

References

[1] Ferro A, Peleteiro B, Malvezzi M, Bosetti C, Bertuccio P, Levi F, Negri E, La Vecchia C, Lunet N. Worldwide trends in gastric cancer mortality (1980-2011), with predictions to 2015, and incidence by subtype. European Journal of Cancer 2014;**50**:1330-1344. PMID: 24650579 DOI: 10.1016/j.ejca.2014.01.029

[2] Jemal A, Bray F, Center MM, Ferlay J, Ward E, Forman D. Global cancer statistics. CA: A Cancer Journal for Clinicians 2011;**61**:69-90. PMID: 21296855 DOI: 10.3322/caac.20107

[3] Globocan 2012. Estimated cancer incidence, mortality and prevalence worldwide in 2012. Available from: http://globocan.iarc.fr./Pages/fact sheets cancer.aspx

[4] WHO Classification of Tumours of the Digestive System. 4th ed. International Agency for Research on Cancer; 2010

[5] Lauren, P. The two histological main types of gastric carcinoma: Diffuse and so-called intestinal-type carcinoma.Acta Pathologica et Microbiologica Scandinavica 1965;**64**:31-49. PMID:14320675

[6] Uemura N, Okamoto S, Yamamoto S, Matsumura N, Yamaguchi S, Yamakido M, Taniyama K, Sasaki N, Schlemper RJ. Helicobacter pyloriinfection and the development of gastric cancer. New England Journal of Medicine. 2001;**345**:784-789. DOI: 10.1056/NEJMoa001999

[7] Fuentes-Pananá EM, Morales-Sánchez A. Epstein-Barr Virus-associated Gastric Cancer and Potential Mechanisms of Oncogenesis. Current Cancer Drug Targets. 2016 Sep 26. [Epub ahead of print] PMID: 27677953

[8] Richards FM, McKee SA, Rajpar MH, Cole TR, Evans DG, Jankowski JA, McKeown C, Sanders DS, Maher ER. Germline E-cadherin gene (CDH1) mutations predispose to familial gastric cancer and colorectal cancer. Human Molecular Genetics. 1999;**8**:607-610. PMID:10072428

[9] Keller G, Grimm V, Vogelsang H, Bischoff P, Mueller J, Siewert JR, Hofler H. Analysis for microsatellite instability and mutations of the DNA mismatch repair genehMLH1in familial gastric cancer. International Journal of Cancer. 1996;**68**:571-576. DOI: 10.1002/(SICI)1097-0215(19961127)68:5<571::AID-IJC3>3.0.CO;2-W

[10] Toyota M, Ahuja N, Suzuki H, Itoh F, Ohe-Toyota M, Imai K, Baylin SB, Issa J-PJ. Aberrant methylation in gastric cancer associated with the CpG island methylator phenotype. Cancer Research. 1999;**59**:5438-5442. PMID: 10554013

[11] Correa P. Is gastric cancer preventable? Gut. 2004;**53**:1217-1219. PMID: 15306570 DOI: 10.1136/gut.2004.039834

[12] Cervantes A, Roda D, Tarazona N, Roselló S, Pérez-Fidalgo JA. Current questions for the treatment of advanced gastric cancer. Cancer Treatment Reviews. 2013;39:60-67. PMID: 23102520 DOI: 10.1016/j.ctrv.2012.09.007

[13] Siegel R, Ma J, Zou Z, Jemal A. Cancer statistics, 2014. CA: A Cancer Journal for Clinicians. 2014;**64**:9-29. PMID: 24399786 DOI: 10.3322/caac.21208

[14] Jemal A, Siegel R, Ward E, Hao Y, Xu J, Thun MJ. Cancer statistics, 2009. CA: A Cancer Journal for Clinicians. 2009;**59**:225-249. PMID: 19474385

[15] Kothari N, Almhanna K. Current status of novel agents in advanced gastroesophageal adenocarcinoma. Journal of Gastrointestinal Oncology. 2015;**6**:60-74. PMID: 25642339 DOI: 10.3978/j.issn.2078-6891.2014.098

[16] Suzuki T, Yasui W, Yokozaki H, Naka K, Ishikawa T, Tahara E. Expression of the E2F family in human gastrointestinal carcinomas. International Journal of Cancer. 1999;**81**:535-538. DOI: 10.1002/(SICI)1097-0215(19990517)81:4<535::AID-IJC5>3.0.CO;2-4

[17] Zheng H, Takahashi H, Murai Y, Cui Z, Nomoto K, Miwa S, Tsuneyama K, Takano Y. Pathobiological characteristics of intestinal and diffuse-type gastric carcinoma in Japan: An immunostaining study on the tissue microarray. Journal of Clinical Pathology. 2007;**60**:273-277. PMCID: PMC1860577 DOI: 10.1136/jcp.2006.038778

[18] Hiyama T, Haruma K, Kitadai Y, Masuda H, Miyamoto M, Tanaka S, Yoshihara M, Shimamoto F, Chayama K. K-ras mutation in helicobacter pylori-associated chronic gastritis in patients with and without gastric cancer. International Journal of Cancer. 2002;**97**:562-566. PMID: 11807778

[19] Cheng X, Wang Z, Chen X, Sun Y, Kong Q, Liu J, Li H. Correlation of Wnt-2 expression andb-catenin intracellular accumulation in Chinese gastric cancers: Relevance with tumour dissemination. Cancer Letters. 2005;**223**:339-347. PMID:15896469 DOI:10.1016/j.canlet.2004.11.013

[20] Sasaki N, Morisaki T, Hashizume K, Yao T, Tsuneyoshi M, Noshiro H, Nakamura K, Yamanaka T, Uchiyama A, Tanaka M, Katano M. Nuclear factor-kappaB p65 (RelA) transcription factor is constitutively activated in human gastric carcinoma tissue. Clinical Cancer Research. 2001;**7**:4136-4142. PMID:11751513

[21] Hanahan D, Weinberg RA. The hallmarks of cancer. Cell. 2000;**100**:57-70. PMID: 10647931 DOI: 10.1016/S0092-8674(00)81683-9

[22] Tay ST, Leong SH, Yu K, Aggarwal A, Tan SY, Lee CH, Wong K, Visvanathan J, Lim D, Wong WK, Soo KC, Kon OL, Tan P. A combined comparative genomic hybridization and expression microarray analysis of gastric cancer reveals novel molecular subtypes. Cancer Research. 2003;**63**: 3309-3316. PMID:12810664

[23] Ooi CH, Ivanova T, Wu J, Lee M, Tan IB, Tao J, Ward L, Koo JH, Gopalakrishnan V, Zhu Y, Cheng LL, Lee J, Rha SY, Chung HC, Ganesan K, So J, Soo KC, Lim D, Chan WH, Wong WK, Bowtell D, Yeoh KG, Grabsch H, Boussioutas A, Tan P. Oncogenic pathway combinations predict clinical prognosis in gastric cancer. PLoS Genetics. 2009;**5**(10):e1000676. PMID:19798449 PMCID: PMC2748685 DOI:10.1371/journal.pgen.1000676

[24] Xie HL, Su Q, He XS, Liang XQ, Zhou JG, Yin Song Y, Li YQ. Expression of p21(WAF1) and p53 and polymorphism of p21(WAF1) gene in gastric carcinoma. World Journal of Gastroenterology. 2004;**10**:1125-1131. PMCID: PMC4656346 DOI: 10.3748/wjg.v10.i8.1125

[25] Humar B, Fukuzawa R, Blair V, Dunbier A, More H, Charlton A, Yang HK, Kim WH, Reeve AE, Martin I, Guilford P. Destabilized adhesion in the gastric proliferative zone and c-SRC kinase activation mark the development of early diffuse gastric cancer. Cancer Research. 2007;**67**:2480-2489. DOI: 10.1158/0008-5472.CAN-06-3021

[26] Choi JH, Kwon HJ, Yoon BI, Kim JH, Han SU, Joo HJ, Kim DY. Expression profile of histone deacetylase 1 in gastric cancer tissues. Japanese Journal of Cancer Research. 2001;**92**:1300-1304. PMID:11749695

[27] Katoh M. Dysregulation of stem cell signaling network due to germline mutation, SNP, Helicobacter pylori infection, epigenetic change and genetic alteration in gastric cancer. Cancer Biology & Therapy. 2007;**6**:832-839. DOI:10.4161/cbt.6.6.4196

[28] Coller HA, Grandori C, Tamayo P, Colbert T, Lander ES, Eisenman RN, Golub TR. Expression analysis with oligonucleotide microarrays reveals that MYC regulates genes involved in growth, cell cycle, signaling, and adhesion. Proceedings of the National Academy of Sciences of the United States of America. 2000;**97**:3260-3265. PMID:10737792 PMCID: PMC16226

[29] Orford KW, Scadden DT. Deconstructing stem cell self-renewal: Genetic insights into cell-cycle regulation. Nature Reviews. Genetics. 2008;**9**:115-128. PMID:18202695 DOI:10.1038/nrg2269

[30] Hirata Y, Maeda S, Ohmae T, Shibata W, Yanai A, Ogura K, Yoshida H, Kawabe T, Omata M. Helicobacter pylori induces IkB kinase α nuclear translocation and chemokine production ingastric epithelial cells. Infection and Immunity. 2006;**74**(3):1452-1461. DOI: 10.1128/IAI.74.3.1452-1461.2006

[31] Bass AJ, Thorsson V, Shmulevich I, Reynolds SM, Miller M, Bernard B, Hinoue T, from The Cancer Genome Atlas Research Network. Comprehensive molecular characterization of gastric adenocarcinoma. Nature. 2014 Sep 11;**513**(7517):202-209. PMID:25079317 PMCID: PMC4170219 DOI: 10.1038/nature13480

[32] Murphy G, Pfeiffer R, Camargo MC, Rabkin CS. Meta-analysis shows that prevalence of Epstein-Barr virus-positive gastric cancer differs based on sex and anatomic location.Gastroenterology. 2009;**137**:824-833. PMID: 19445939 PMCID: PMC3513767 DOI:10.1053/j.gastro.2009.05.001

[33] Matsusaka K, Kaneda A, Nagae G, Ushiku T, Kikuchi Y, Hino R, Uozaki H, Seto Y, Takada K, Aburatani H, Fukayama M. Classification of Epstein-Barr virus-positive gastric cancers by definition of DNA methylation epigenotypes. Cancer Research. 2011;**71**:7187-7197. PMID:21990320 DOI:10.1158/0008-5472.CAN-11-1349

[34] Geddert H, Zur Hausen A, Gabbert HE, Sarbia M. EBV-infection in cardiac and non-cardiac gastric adenocarcinomas is associated with promoter methylation of p16, p14 and APC, but not hMLH1. Analytical Cellular Pathology. 2010;**33**:143-149. PMCID: PMC4605817 DOI: 10.3233/ACP-CLO-2010-0540

[35] Lee J, van Hummelen P, Go C, Palescandolo E, Jang J, Park HY, Kang SY, Park JO, Kang WK, MacConaill L, Kim KM. High-throughput mutation profiling identifies frequent somatic mutations in advanced gastric adenocarcinoma. PLoS One. 2012;**7**:e38892. DOI: http://dx.doi.org/10.1371/journal.pone.0038892

[36] Sukawa Y, Yamamoto H, Nosho K, Kunimoto H, Suzuki H, Yasushi A, Nakazawa M, Nobuoka T, Kawayama M, Mikami M, Matsuno T, Sasegawa T, Hirata K, Imai K, Shinomura Y. Alterations in the human epidermal growth factor receptor 2-phosphatidylinositol 3-kinase-v-Akt pathway in gastric cancer. World Journal of Gastroenterology. 2012;**18**:6577-6586. PMCID: PMC3516204 DOI: 10.3748/wjg.v18.i45.6577

[37] Ridley AJ, Schwartz MA, Burridge K, Firtel RA, Ginsberg MH, Borisy G, Parsons JT, Horwitz AR. Cell migration: Integrating signals from front to back. Science. 2003;**302**:1704-1709. PMID:14657486 DOI: 10.1126/science.1092053

[38] Thumkeo D, Watanabe S, Narumiya S. Physiological roles of Rho and Rho effectors in mammals. European Journal of Cell Biology. 2013;**92**:303-315. DOI: http://dx.doi.org/10.1016/j.ejcb.2013.09.002

[39] Aznar S. et al. Simultaneous tyrosine and serine phosphorylation of STAT3 transcription factor is involved in Rho A GTPase oncogenic transformation. Molecular Biology of Cell. 2001;**12**:3282-3294. PMCID: PMC60173

[40] Yu H, Jove R. The STATs of cancer—New molecular targets come of age. Nature Reviews Cancer. 2004;**4**:97-105. PMID:14964307 DOI:10.1038/nrc1275

[41] The Cancer Genome Atlas Network. Comprehensive molecular characterization of human colon and rectal cancer. Nature. 2012;**487**:330-337. http://www.impactjournals.com/oncotarget/index.php?journal=oncotarget&page=article&op=view&path%5B%5D=1781&path%5B%5D=2086

[42] Fuchs CS, Tomasek J, Yong CJ, Dumitru F, Passalacqua R, Goswami C, Safran H, dos Santos LV, Aprile G, Ferry DR, Melichar B, Tehfe M, Topuzov E, Zalcberg JR, Chau I, Campbell W, Sivanandan C, Pikiel J, Koshiji M, Hsu Y, Liepa AM, Gao L, Schwartz JD, Tabernero J.. Ramucirumab monotherapy for previously treated advanced gastric or gastro-oesophageal junction adenocarcinoma (REGARD): An international, randomised, multicentre, placebo-controlled, phase 3 trial. Lancet. 2014;**383**:31-39. PMID: 24094768 DOI: 10.1016/S0140-6736(13)61719-5

[43] Cui J, Li F, Wang G, Fang X, Puett JD, Xu Y. Gene-expression signatures can distinguish gastric cancer grades and stages. PLoS One. 2011;**6**(3):e17819. PMID: 21445269 PMCID: PMC3060867 DOI:10.1371/journal.pone.0017819

[44] Catherino WH, Leppert PC, Stenmark MH, Payson M, Potlog-Nahari C, Nieman LK, Segars JH. Reduced dermatopontin expression is a molecular link between uterine leiomyomas and keloids. Genes Chromosomes Cancer. 2004;**40**:204-217. PMID: 15139000 PMCID: PMC4152899 DOI: 10.1002/gcc.20035

[45] Hecht JR, Bang YJ, Qin SK, Chung HC, Xu JM, Park JO, Jeziorski K, Shparyk Y, Hoff PM, Sobrero A, Salman P, Li J, Protsenko SA, Wainberg ZA, Buyse M, Afenjar K, Houé V, Garcia A, Kaneko T, Huang Y, Khan-Wasti S, Santillana S, Press MF, Slamon D. Lapatinib in combination with capecitabine plus oxaliplatin in human epidermal growth factor receptor 2-positive advanced or metastatic gastric, esophageal, or gastroesophageal adenocarcinoma: TRIO-013/LOGiC-a randomized Phase III trial. Journal of Clinical Oncology. 2016;**34**:443-451. PMID:26628478 DOI: 10.1200/JCO.2015.62.6598

[46] Mattioni M, Soddu S, Porrello A, D'Alessandro R, Spila A, Guadagni F. Serum anti-p53 antibodies as a useful marker for prognosis of gastric carcinoma. The International Journal of Biological Markers. 2006;**22**:302-306. PMID:18161662

[47] Cabuk D, Basaran G, Celikel C, Dane F, Yumuk PF, Iyikesici MS, Ekenel M, Turhal NS. Vascular endothelial growth factor, hypoxia-inducible factor 1 alpha and CD34 expressions in early-stage gastric tumors: Relationship with pathological factors and prognostic impact on survival. Oncology. 2007;**72**:111-117. PMID:18025805 DOI: 10.1159/111118

[48] Takeno A, Takemasa I, Doki Y, Yamasaki M, Miyata H, Takiguchi S, Fujiwara Y, Matsubara K, Monden M. Integrative approach for differentially overexpressed genes in gastric cancer by combining large-scale gene expression profiling and network analysis. British Journal of Cancer. 2008;**99**:1307-1315. DOI:10.1038/sj.bjc.6604682

[49] Wang P, Wang Y, Hang B, Zou X, Mao JH. A novel gene expression-based prognostic scoring system to predict survival in gastric cancer. Oncotarget. 2016;**7**(34):55343-55351. DOI: 10.18632/oncotarget.10533

[50] Xu Y, Ma H, Yu H, Liu Z, Wang L-E, Tan D, Muddasani R, Lu V, Ajani JA, Wang Y, Wei Q. The miR-184 bindingsite rs8126 T> C polymorphism in TNFAIP2 is associated with risk of gastric cancer. PLoS One. 2013;**8**:e64973. PMID: 23724109 PMCID: PMC3665554 DOI: 10.1371/journal.pone.0064973

[51] Ye YW, Zhang X, Zhou Y, Wu J, Zhao C, Yuan L, Wang G, Du C, Wang C, Shi Y. The correlations between the expression of FGFR4 protein and clinicopathological parameters as well as prognosis of gastric cancer patients. Journal of Surgical Oncology. 2012;**106**:872-879. PMID: 22585711 DOI:10.1002/jso.23153

[52] Shen YY, Lu YC, Shen DP, Liu YJ, Su XY, Zhu GS, Yin XL, Ni XZ. Fibroblast growth factor receptor 4 Gly388Arg polymorphism in Chinese gastric cancer patients. World Journal of Gastroenterology. 2013;**19**:4568-4575. PMCID: PMC3725383 DOI: 10.3748/wjg.v19.i28.4568

[53] Rajkumar T, Vijayalakshmi N, Gopal G, Sabitha K, Shirley S, Raja UM, Ramakrishnan SA. Identification and validation of genes involved in gastric tumorigenesis. Cancer Cell International.2010;**10**:45.PMID:21092330PMCID:PMC3004887DOI:10.1186/1475-2867-10-45

[54] Tao J, Zhi X, Tian Y, Li Z, Zhu Y, Wang W, et al. CEP55 contributes to human gastric carcinoma by regulating cell proliferation. Tumor Biology. 2014;**35**:4389-4399. PMID:24390615 DOI:10.1007/s13277-013-1578-1

[55] Xiang Z, Jiang DP, Xia GG, Wei ZW, Chen W, He Y, Zhang CH. CXCL1 expression is correlated with Snail expression and affects the prognosis of patients with gastric cancer. Oncology Letters. 2015;**10**:2458-2464. DOI: 10.3892/ol.2015.3614

[56] You T, Gao W, Wei J, Jin X, Zhao Z, Wang C, Li Y. Overexpression of LIMK1 promotes tumor growth and metastasis in gastric cancer. Biomedicine & Pharmacotherapy. 2015;**69**:96-101. PMID: 25661344 DOI: 10.1016/j.biopha.2014.11.011

[57] Yamamoto H, Kitadai Y, Yamamoto H, Oue N, Ohdan H, Yasui W, Kikuchi A. Laminin gamma2 mediates Wnt5a induced invasion of gastric cancer cells. Gastroenterology. 2009;**137**:242. PMID:19582886

[58] Sakashita K, Tanaka F, Zhang X, Mimori K, Kamohara Y, Inoue H, Sawada T, Hirakawa K, Mori M. Clinical significance of ApoE expression in human gastric cancer. Oncology Reports. 2008;**20**:1313-1319. DOI: 10.3892/or_00000146

[59] Oshima T, Yoshihara K, Aoyama T, Hasegawa S, Sato T, Yamamoto N, Akito N, Shiozawa M, Yoshikawa T, Numata K, Rino Y, Kunisaki C, Tanaka K, Akaike M, Imada T, Masuda M. Relation of INHBA gene expression to outcomes in gastric cancer after curative surgery. Anticancer Research. 2014;**34**:2303-2309

[60] Junnila S, Kokkola A, Karjalainen-Lindsberg ML, Puolakkainen P, Monni O. Genome-wide gene copy number and expression analysis of primary gastric tumors and gastric cancer cell lines. BMC Cancer. 2010;**10**:73. PMID:20187983 PMCID:PMC2837868 DOI:10.1186/1471-2407-10-73

[61] Oue N, Hamai Y, Mitani Y, Matsumura S, Oshimo Y, Aung PP, Kuraoka K, Nakayama H, Yasui W. Gene expression profile of gastric carcinoma identification of genes and tags potentially involved in invasion, metastasis, and carcinogenesis by serial analysis of gene expression. Cancer Research. 2004;**64**:2397-2405. PMID:15059891

[62] Zhang L, Kim S, Ding W, Tong Y, Zhang X, Pan M, Chen S. Arsenic sulfide inhibits cell migration and invasion of gastric cancer in vitro and in vivo. Drug Design, Development and Therapy. 2015;**9**:5579-5590. PMID:26487802 PMCID:PMC4607060 DOI:10.2147/DDDT.S89805

[63] Dong Y, Chen G, Gao M, Tian X. Increased expression of MMP14 correlates with the poor prognosis of Chinese patients with gastric cancer. Gene. 2015;**563**:29-34. PMID:25748728 DOI: 10.1016/j.gene.2015.03.003

[64] Duell EJ, Sala N, Travier N, Muñoz X, Boutron-Ruault MC, Clavel-Chapelon F, Barricarte A, Arriola L, Navarro C, Sánchez-Cantalejo E, Quirós JR, Krogh V, Vineis P, et al. Genetic variation in alcohol dehydrogenase (ADH1A, ADH1B, ADH1C, ADH7) and aldehyde dehydrogenase (ALDH2), alcohol consumption and gastric cancer risk in the European Prospective Investigation into Cancer and Nutrition (EPIC) cohort. Carcinogenesis. 2012;**33**:361-367. PMID:22144473 DOI: 10.1093/carcin/bgr285

[65] Xie X, Liu X, Zhang Q, Yu J. Overexpression of collagen VI $\alpha3$ in gastric cancer. Oncology Letters 2014;**7**:1537-1543. DOI: 10.3892/ol.2014.1910

[66] Malta-Vacas J, Nolasco S, Monteiro C, Soares H, Brito M. Translation termination and protein folding pathway genes are not correlated in gastric cancer. Clinical Chemistry and Laboratory Medicine. 2009;**47**:427-431. DOI:10.1515/CCLM.2009.091

[67] Jinawath N, Furukawa Y, Nakamura Y. Identification of NOL8, a nucleolar protein containing an RNA recognition motif (RRM), which was overexpressed in diffuse-type gastric cancer. Cancer Science. 2004;**95**:430-435. PMID:15132771

[68] Liersch-Löhn B, Slavova N, Buhr HJ, Bennani-Baiti IM. Differential protein expression and oncogenic gene network link tyrosine kinase ephrin B4 receptor to aggressive gastric and gastroesophageal junction cancers. International Journal of Cancer. 2016;**138**:1220-31. DOI: 10.1002/ijc.29865

[69] Yang C, Wen Y, Li H, Zhang D, Zhang N, Shi X, Jiang B, Ma X, Yang P, Tang H, Peng Z, Yang Y. Overexpression of minichromosome maintenance 2 predicts poor prognosis in patients with gastric cancer. Oncology Reports. 2012;**27**:135-142. PMID:21947329 DOI: 10.3892/or.2011.1473

[70] Tian Y, Tian X, Han X, Chen Y, Song CY, Jiang WJ, Tian DL. ABCE1 plays an essential role in lung cancer progression and metastasis. Tumor Biology. 2016;**37**(6):8375-82. [Epub ahead of print].

[71] Matboli M, El-Nakeep S, Hossam N, Habieb A, Azazy AEM, Ebrahim AE, Nagy Z, Abdel-Rahman O. Exploring the role of molecular biomarkers as a potential weapon against gastric cancer: A review of the literature. World Journal of Gastroenterology. 2016;**22**(26):5896-5908. DOI: 10.3748/wjg.v22.i26.5896

[72] Pectasides D, Mylonakis A, Kostopoulou M, Papadopoulou M, Triantafillis D, Varthalitis J, Dimitriades M, Athanassiou A. CEA, CA 19-9, and CA-50 in monitoring gastric carcinoma. American Journal of Clinical Oncology. 1997;**20**:348-353. PMID: 9256887

[73] Aloe S, D'Alessandro R, Spila A, Ferroni P, Basili S, Palmirotta R, Carlini M, Graziano F, Mancini R, Mariotti S, Cosimelli M, Roselli M, Guadagni F. Prognostic value of serum and tumor tissue CA 72-4 content in gastric cancer. International Journal of Biological Markers. 2003;**18**:21-27. PMID: 12699059

[74] Cho JY. Molecular diagnosis for personalized target therapy in gastric cancer. Journal of Gastric Cancer. 2013;**13**:129-135. PMID: 24156032 DOI: 10.5230/jgc.2013.13.3.129

[75] Lin X, Zhao Y, Song WM, Zhang B. Molecular classification and prediction in gastric cancer. Computational and Structural Biotechnology Journal. 2015;**13**:448-458. PMID: 26380657 DOI: 10.1016/j.csbj.2015.08.001

[76] Tanaka T, Tanimoto K, Otani K, Satoh K, Ohtaki M, Yoshida K, Toge T, Yahata H, Tanaka S, Chayama K, Okazaki Y, Hayashizaki Y, Hiyama K, Nishiyama M. Concise prediction models of anticancer efficacy of 8 drugs using expression data from 12 selected genes. International Journal of Cancer. 2004;**111**:617-626. PMID: 15239142 DOI: 10.1002/ijc.20289

[77] Sève P, Mackey J, Isaac S, Trédan O, Souquet PJ, Pérol M, Lai R, Voloch A, Dumontet C. Class III beta-tubulin expression in tumor cells predicts response and outcome in patients with nonsmall cell lung cancer receiving paclitaxel. Molecular Cancer Therapeutics. 2005;**4**:2001-2007. PMID: 16373715 DOI: 10.1158/1535-7163.MCT-05-0244

[78] Suganuma K, Kubota T, Saikawa Y, Abe S, Otani Y, Furukawa T, Kumai K, Hasegawa H, Watanabe M, Kitajima M, Nakayama H, Okabe H. Possible chemoresistance-related genes for gastric cancer detected by cDNA microarray. Cancer Science. 2003;**94**:355-359. PMID: 12824904

[79] Liu H, Li N, Yao L, Jiang L, Bao G, Li J, Ma Q, Liu Z. Prediction of doxorubicin sensitivity in gastric cancers based on a set of novel markers. Oncology Reports. 2008;**20**:963-969. PMID: 18813841

[80] Bashash M, Shah A, Hislop G, Treml M, Bretherick K, JanooGilani R, Leach S, Le N, Bajdik C, Brooks-Wilson A. Genetic polymorphisms at TIMP3 are associated with survival of adenocarcinoma of the gastroesophageal junction. PLoS One. 2013;**8**:e59157. PMID: 23527119 DOI: 10.1371/journal.pone.0059157

[81] Liu K, Qian T, Tang L, Wang J, Yang H, Ren J. Decreased expression of microRNA let-7i and its association with chemotherapeutic response in human gastric cancer. World Journal of Surgical Oncology. 2012;**10**:225. PMID: 23107361 DOI: 10.1186/1477-7819-10-225

[82] Cristescu R, Lee J, Nebozhyn M, Kim KM, Ting JC, Wong SS, Liu J, Yue YG, Wang J, Yu K, Ye XS, Do IG, Liu S, Gong L, Fu J, Jin JG, Choi MG, Sohn TS, Lee JH, Bae JM, Kim ST, Park SH, Sohn I, Jung SH, Tan P, Chen R, Hardwick J, Kang WK, Ayers M, Hongyue D, Reinhard C, Loboda A, Kim S, Aggarwal A. Molecular analysis of gastric cancer identifies subtypes associated with distinct clinical outcomes. Nature Medicine. 2015;**21**:449-456. PMID: 25894828 DOI: 10.1038/nm.3850

[83] Eto K, Iwatsuki M, Watanabe M, Ida S, Ishimoto T, Iwagami S, Baba Y, Sakamoto Y, Miyamoto Y, Yoshida N, Baba H. The microRNA-21/PTEN pathway regulates the sensitivity of HER2-positive gastric cancer cells to trastuzumab. Annals of Surgical Oncology. 2014;**21**:343-350. PMID: 24154840 DOI: 10.1245/s10434-013-3325-7

[84] Huang D, Wang H, Liu R, Li H, Ge S, Bai M, Deng T, Yao G, Ba Y. miRNA27a is a biomarker for predicting chemosensitivity and prognosis in metastatic or recurrent gastric cancer. Journal of Cellular Biochemistry. 2014;**115**:549-556. PMID: 24122958 DOI: 10.1002/jcb.24689

[85] Yang Z, Guo X, Li G, Shi Y, Li L. Long noncoding RNAs as potential biomarkers in gastric cancer: Opportunities and challenges. Cancer Letters. 2016;**371**:62-70. PMID: 26577810 DOI: 10.1016/j.canlet.2015.11.011

[86] Wang Y, Zhang D, Wu K, Zhao Q, Nie Y, Fan D. Long noncoding RNA MRUL promotes ABCB1 expression in multidrug-resistant gastric cancer cell sublines. Molecular and Cellular Biology. 2014;**34**:3182-3193. PMID: 24958102 DOI: 10.1128/MCB.01580-13

[87] Sugita H, Iida S, Inokuchi M, Kato K, Ishiguro M, Ishikawa T, Takagi Y, Enjoji M, Yamada H, Uetake H, Kojima K, Sugihara K. Methylation of BNIP3 and DAPK indicates lower response to chemotherapy and poor prognosis in gastric cancer. Oncology Reports. 2011;**25**:513-518. PMID: 21152877 DOI: 10.3892/or.2010.1085

[88] Ivanova T, Zouridis H, Wu Y, Cheng LL, Tan IB, Gopalakrishnan V, Ooi CH, Lee J, Qin L, Wu J, Lee M, Rha SY, Huang D, Liem N, Yeoh KG, Yong WP, Teh BT, Tan P. Integrated epigenomics identifies BMP4 as a modulator of cisplatin sensitivity in gastric cancer. Gut. 2013;**62**:22-33. PMID: 22535375 DOI: 10.1136/gutjnl-2011-301113

[89] Ooki A, Yamashita K, Yamaguchi K, Mondal A, Nishimiya H, Watanabe M. DNA damage-inducible gene, reprimo functions as a tumor suppressor and is suppressed by promoter methylation in gastric cancer. Molecular Cancer Research. 2013;**11**:1362-1374. PMID: 23982217 DOI: 10.1158/1541-7786.MCR-13-0091

[90] Ishikawa Y, Kubota T, Otani Y, Watanabe M, Teramoto T, Kumai K, Takechi T, Okabe H, Fukushima M, Kitajima M. Dihydropyrimidine dehydrogenase and messenger RNA levels in gastric cancer: Possible predictor for sensitivity to 5-fluorouracil. Japanese Journal of Cancer Research. 2000;**91**:105-112. PMID: 10744051

[91] Huang H, Han Y, Gao J, Feng J, Zhu L, Qu L, Shen L, Shou C. High level of serum AMBP is associated with poor response to paclitaxel-capecitabine chemotherapy in advanced gastric cancer patients. Medical Oncology. 2013;**30**:748. PMID: 24135868 DOI: 10.1007/s12032-013-0748-8

[92] Yu J, Gao J, Lu Z, Li Y, Shen L. Serum levels of TUBB3 correlate with clinical outcome in Chinese patients with advanced gastric cancer receiving first-line paclitaxel plus capecitabine. Medical Oncology. 2012;**29**:3029-3034. PMID: 22766748 DOI: 10.1007/s12032-012-0292-y

[93] Mitani Y, Oue N, Matsumura S, Yoshida K, Noguchi T, Ito M, Tanaka S, Kuniyasu H, Kamata N, Yasui W. Reg IV is a serum biomarker for gastric cancer patients and predicts response to 5-fluorouracil-based chemotherapy. Oncogene 2007;**26**:4383-4393. PMID: 17237819 DOI: 10.1038/sj.onc.1210215

[94] Okada K, Fujiwara Y, Takahashi T, Nakamura Y, Takiguchi S, Nakajima K, Miyata H, Yamasaki M, Kurokawa Y, Mori M, Doki Y. Overexpression of forkhead box M1 transcription factor (FOXM1) is a potential prognostic marker and enhances chemoresistance for docetaxel in gastric cancer. Annals of Surgical Oncology. 2013;**20**:1035-1043. PMID: 23054116 DOI: 10.1245/s10434-012-2680-0

[95] Shi Y, Zhai H, Wang X, Han Z, Liu C, Lan M, Du J, Guo C, Zhang Y, Wu K, Fan D. Ribosomal proteins S13 and L23 promote multidrug resistance in gastric cancer cells by suppressing drug-induced apoptosis. Experimental Cell Research. 2004;**296**:337-346. PMID: 15149863 DOI: 10.1016/j.yexcr.2004.02.009

[96] Coussens L, Yang-Feng TL, Liao YC, Chen E, Gray A, McGrath J, Seeburg PH, Libermann TA, Schlessinger J, Francke U. Tyrosine kinase receptor with extensive homology to EGF receptor shares chromosomal location with neu oncogene. Science. 1985;**230**:1132-1139. PMID: 2999974 DOI: 10.1126/science.2999974

[97] Stintzing S, Jung A, Rossius L, Modest DP, von Weikersthal LF, Decker T, Kiani A, Al-Batran SE, Vehling-Kaiser U, Heintges T, Moehler M, Scheithauer W, Kirchner T, Heinemann V. Mutations within the EGFR signaling pathway: Influence on efficacy in FIRE-3-A randomized phase III study of FOLFIRI plus cetuximab or bevacizumab as first-line treatment for wild-type (WT) KRAS (exon 2) metastatic colorectal cancer (mCRC) patients. Journal of Clinical Oncology. 2014;**32**(Suppl 3):abstr 445

[98] Bang YJ, Van Cutsem E, Feyereislova A, Chung HC, Shen L, Sawaki A, Lordick F, Ohtsu A, Omuro Y, Satoh T, Aprile G, Kulikov E, Hill J, Lehle M, Rüschoff J, Kang YK. Trastuzumab in combination with chemotherapy versus chemotherapy alone for treatment of HER2-positive advanced gastric or gastro-oesophageal junction cancer (ToGA): A phase 3, open-label, randomised controlled trial. Lancet. 2010;**376**:687-697. PMID: 20728210 DOI: 10.1016/S0140-6736(10)61121-X

[99] Clinical trials.gov. A Study of the Combination of Oxaliplatin, Capecitabine and Herceptin (Trastuzumab) and Chemoradiotherapy in the Adjuvant Setting in Operated Patients with HER2 Gastric or Gastro-esophageal Junction Cancer (TOXAG Study). Available from: http://www.clinicaltrials.gov/show/NCT01748773

[100] Ryu MH, Yoo C, Kim JG, Ryoo BY, Park YS, Park SR, Han HS, Chung IJ, Song EK, Lee KH, Kang SY, Kang YK. Multicenter phase II study of trastuzumab in combination with capecitabine and oxaliplatin for advanced gastric cancer. European Journal of Cancer. 2015;**51**:482-488. PMID: 25661103 DOI: 10.1016/j.ejca.2014.12.015

[101] Hoff P, Tabernero J, Shen L. P-0111 pertuzumab, trastuzumab and chemotherapy in HER2-positive metastatic gastric or gastrooesophageal junction cancer: An international phase III study (JACOB). Annals of Oncology. 2013;**24**:iv67. DOI: 10.1093/annonc/mdt203.109

[102] Clinical trials.gov. A Study of Trastuzumab Emtansine versus Taxane in Patients with Advanced Gastric Cancer. Available from: http://clinicaltrials.gov/show/NCT01641939

[103] Satoh T, Xu RH, Chung HC, Sun GP, Doi T, Xu JM, Tsuji A, Omuro Y, Li J, Wang JW, Miwa H, Qin SK, Chung IJ, Yeh KH, Feng JF, Mukaiyama A, Kobayashi M, Ohtsu A, Bang YJ. Lapatinib plus paclitaxel versus paclitaxel alone in the secondline treatment of HER2-amplified advanced gastric cancer in Asian populations: TyTAN—A randomized, phase III study. Journal of Clinical Oncology. 2014;**32**:2039-2049. PMID: 24868024 DOI: 10.1200/JCO.2013.53.6136

[104] Lieto E, Ferraraccio F, Orditura M, Castellano P, Mura AL, Pinto M, Zamboli A, De Vita F, Galizia G. Expression of vascular endothelial growth factor (VEGF) and epidermal growth factor receptor (EGFR) is an independent prognostic indicator of worse outcome in gastric cancer patients. Annals of Surgical Oncology. 2008;**15**:69-79. PMID: 17896140

[105] Lordick F, Kang YK, Chung HC, Salman P, Oh SC, Bodoky G, Kurteva G, Volovat C, Moiseyenko VM, Gorbunova V, Park JO, Sawaki A, Celik I, Götte H, Melezínková H, Moehler M. Capecitabine and cisplatin with or without cetuximab for patients with previously untreated advanced gastric cancer (EXPAND): A randomised, open-label phase 3 trial. The Lancet Oncology. 2013;**14**:490-499. PMID: 23594786 DOI: 10.1016/S1470-2045(13)70102-5

[106] Clinical trials.gov. Cetuximab, Cisplatin, and Irinotecan in Treating Patients With Metastatic Esophageal Cancer, Gastroesophageal Junction Cancer, or Gastric Cancer That Did Not Respond to Previous Irinotecan and Cisplatin. Available from: https://www.clinicaltrials.gov/ct2/show/NCT00397904

[107] Waddell T, Chau I, Cunningham D, Gonzalez D, Okines AF, Okines C, Wotherspoon A, Saffery C, Middleton G, Wadsley J, Ferry D, Mansoor W, Crosby T, Coxon F, Smith D, Waters J, Iveson T, Falk S, Slater S, Peckitt C, Barbachano Y. Epirubicin, oxaliplatin, and capecitabine with or without panitumumab for patients with previously untreated advanced oesophagogastric cancer (REAL3): A randomised, open-label phase 3 trial. The Lancet Oncology. 2013;**14**:481-489. PMID: 23594787 DOI: 10.1016/S1470-2045(13)70096-2

[108] Clinical trials.gov. Panitumumab, Paclitaxel, Carboplatin and 5FU in the Treatment of Potentially Resectable Gastroesophageal Adenocarcinoma. Available from: https://www.clinicaltrials.gov/ct2/show/NCT01182610

[109] Satoh T, Lee KH, Rha SY, Sasaki Y, Park SH, Komatsu Y, Yasui H, Kim TY, Yamaguchi K, Fuse N, Yamada Y, Ura T, Kim SY, Munakata M, Saitoh S, Nishio K, Morita S, Yamamoto E, Zhang Q, Kim JM, Kim YH, Sakata Y. Randomized phase II trial of nimotuzumab plus irinotecan versus irinotecan alone as second-line therapy for patients with advanced gastric cancer. Gastric Cancer. 2015;**18**:824-832. PMID: 25185971 DOI: 10.1007/s10120-014-0420-9

[110] Clinical trials.gov. Gefitinib in Combination with Chemoradiation in Resectable Gastric Cancer. Available from: https://www.clinicaltrials.gov/ct2/show?term=gefitinib, gastric cancer&rank=2

[111] Clinical trials.gov. Cisplatin and Irinotecan Chemotherapy, Followed by ZD 1839 (Iressa) in Patients With Esophageal or Gastric Carcinomas. Available from: https://www.clinicaltrials.gov/ct2/show/NCT00215995

[112] Dragovich T, McCoy S, Fenoglio-Preiser CM, Wang J, Benedetti JK, Baker AF, Hackett CB, Urba SG, Zaner KS, Blanke CD, Abbruzzese JL. Phase II trial of erlotinib in gastroesophageal junction and gastric adenocarcinomas: SWOG 0127. Journal of Clinical Oncology. 2006;**24**:4922-4927. PMID: 17050876 DOI: 10.1200/JCO.2006.07.1316

[113] Carmeliet P. Angiogenesis in health and disease. Nature Medicine. 2003;**9**:653-660. PMID: 12778163

[114] Grigore D, Simionescu CE, Stepan A, Mărgăritescu C, Bălăşoiu M, Georgescu CC, Cernea D, Dumitrescu D. Assessment of CD105, α-SMA and VEGF expression in gastric carcinomas. Romanian Journal of Morphology and Embryology. 2013;**54**:701-707. PMID: 24322015

[115] Ohtsu A, Shah MA, Van Cutsem E, Rha SY, Sawaki A, Park SR, Lim HY, Yamada Y, Wu J, Langer B, Starnawski M, Kang YK. Bevacizumab in combination with chemotherapy as firstline therapy in advanced gastric cancer: A randomized, doubleblind, placebo-controlled phase III study. Journal of Clinical Oncology. 2011;**29**:3968-3976. PMID: 21844504 DOI: 10.1200/JCO.2011.36.2236

[116] Shen L, Li J, Xu J, Pan H, Dai G, Qin S, Wang L, Wang J, Yang Z, Shu Y, Xu R, Chen L, Liu Y, Yu S, Bu L, Piao Y. Bevacizumab plus capecitabine and cisplatin in Chinese patients with inoperable locally advanced or metastatic gastric or gastroesophageal junction cancer: Randomized, double-blind, phase III study (AVATAR study). Gastric Cancer. 2015;**18**:168-176. PMID: 24557418 DOI: 10.1007/s10120-014-0351-5

[117] Clinical trials.gov, Cunningham D. Chemotherapy With or Without Bevacizumab or Lapatinib to Treat Operable Oesophagogastric Cancer (ST03). Available from: https://clinicaltrials.gov/ct2/show/NCT00450203

[118] Choi AH, Kim J, Chao J. Perioperative chemotherapy for resectable gastric cancer: MAGIC and beyond. World Journal of Gastroenterology. 2015;**21**:7343-7348. PMID: 26139980 DOI: 10.3748/wjg.v21.i24.7343

[119] Clinical trials.gov. Docetaxel, Cisplatin, Irinotecan and Bevacizumab (TPCA) in Metastatic Esophageal and Gastric Cancer. Available from: https://clinicaltrials.gov/ct2/show/NCT00394433

[120] Clinical trials.gov. Docetaxel, Oxaliplatin, Capecitabine, Bevacizumab and Trastuzumab in Patients with Locally Advanced or Metastatic Gastric Cancer (B-DOCT). Available from: https://clinicaltrials.gov/ct2/show/NCT01359397

[121] Wilke H, Van Cutsem E, Oh SC. RAINBOW: A global, phase 3, randomized, double-blind study of ramucirumab plus paclitaxel versus placebo plus paclitaxel in the treatment of metastatic gastric adenocarcinoma following disease progression on first-line platinum- and fluoropyrimidine containing combination therapy: Results of a multiple Cox regression analysis adjusting for prognostic factors. Journal of Clinical Oncology. 2014;**32**:abstr 4076

[122] Casak SJ, Fashoyin-Aje I, Lemery SJ, Zhang L, Jin R, Li H, Zhao L, Zhao H, Zhang H, Chen H, He K, Dougherty M, Novak R, Kennett S, Khasar S, Helms W, Keegan P, Pazdur R. FDA approval summary: Ramucirumab for gastric cancer. Clinical Cancer Research. 2015;**21**:3372-3376. PMID: 26048277 DOI: 10.1158/1078-0432

[123] Xu R, Ma N, Wang F, Ma L, Chen R, Chen R, Kebinu M, Ma L, Han Z, Ayixiamu M, Su P, Naman Y, Jieensi H, Yang H, Adili A, Aili S, Liu J. Results of a randomized and controlled clinical trial evaluating the efficacy and safety of combination therapy with Endostar and S-1 combined with oxaliplatin in advanced gastric cancer. OncoTargets and Therapy. 2013;**6**:925-929. PMID: 23926435 DOI: 10.2147/OTT.S46487

[124] Geng R, Li J. Apatinib for the treatment of gastric cancer. Expert Opinion on Pharmacotherapy. 2015;**16**:117-122. PMID: 25420417 DOI: 10.1517/14656566.2015.981526

[125] Li J, Qin S, Xu J, Guo W, Xiong J, Bai Y, Sun G, Yang Y, Wang L, Xu N, Cheng Y, Wang Z, Zheng L, Tao M, Zhu X, Ji D, Liu X, Yu H. Apatinib for chemotherapy-refractory advanced metastatic gastric cancer: Results from a randomized, placebo-controlled, parallelarm, phase II trial. Journal of Clinical Oncology. 2013;**31**:3219-3225. PMID:23918952 DOI: 10.1200/JCO.2013.48.8585

[126] Apatinib got CFDA approval. Available from: http://www.inyaohui.com/news/201502/05/5059.html

[127] Bang YJ, Kang YK, Kang WK, Boku N, Chung HC, Chen JS, Doi T, Sun Y, Shen L, Qin S, Ng WT, Tursi JM, Lechuga MJ, Lu DR, Ruiz-Garcia A, Sobrero A. Phase II study of sunitinib as second-line treatment for advanced gastric cancer. Investigational New Drugs. 2011;**29**:1449-1458. PMID: 20461441 DOI: 10.1007/s10637-010-9438-y

[128] Lee KW, Park SR, Oh DY, Park YI, Khosravan R, Lin X, Lee SY, Roh EJ, Valota O, Lechuga MJ, Bang YJ. Phase I study of sunitinib plus capecitabine/cisplatin or capecitabine/oxaliplatin in advanced gastric cancer. Investigational New Drugs. 2013;**31**:1547-1558. PMID: 24091982 DOI: 10.1007/s10637-013-0032-y

[129] Clinical trials.gov. Sorafenib. ICORG 06-41, V4. Available from: https://clinicaltrials.gov/ct2/show/NCT01158287

[130] Clinical trials.gov. Sorafenib as a second line treatment in patients with advanced or metastatic gastric cancer. Available from: http://www.clinicaltrials.gov/ct2/show/NCT00595985

[131] Clinical trials.gov. FLO/- pazopanib as first-line treatment in advanced gastric cancer (PaFLO). Available from: http://clinicaltrials.gov/ct2/show/NCT01503372

[132] Clinical trials.gov. A Study of Pazopanib with CAPEOX in AGC Patients. Available from: http://clinicaltrials.gov/ct2/show/NCT01130805

[133] Pavlakis N, Sjoquist KM, Tsobanis E. INTEGRATE: A randomized phase II double-blind placebo-controlled study of regorafenib (REG) in refractory advanced esophagogastric cancer (AOGC)—A study by the Australasian Gastrointestinal Trials Group (AGITG): Final overall and subgroup results. Annals of Oncology. 2015;**26**(Suppl t4):119

[134] Foulstone E, Prince S, Zaccheo O, Burns JL, Harper J, Jacobs C, Church D, Hassan AB. Insulin-like growth factor ligands, receptors, and binding proteins in cancer. Journal of Pathology 2005;**205**:145-153. PMID: 15641016 DOI: 10.1002/path.1712

[135] Clinical trials.gov. Study of CP-751,871 in Combination with Sunitinib in Patients with Advanced Solid Tumors. Available from: https://www.clinicaltrials.gov/ct2/show/study/NCT00729833

[136] Grose R, Dickson C. Fibroblast growth factor signaling in tumorigenesis. Cytokine and Growth Factor Reviews. 2005;**16**:179-186. PMID: 15863033 DOI: 10.1016/j.cytogfr.2005.01.003

[137] Bang YJ, Van Cutsem E, Mansoor W. A randomized, open label phase II study of AZD4547 (AZD) versus Paclitaxel (P) in previously treated patients with advanced gastric cancer (AGC) with Fibroblast Growth Factor Receptor 2 (FGFR2) polysomy or gene amplification (amp): SHINE study. Journal of Clinical Oncology. 2015;**33**(Suppl):abstr 4014

[138] Dienstmann R, Bahleda R, Adamo B, Rodon J, Varga A, Gazzah A, Platero S, Smit H, Perera T, Zhong B, Stuyckens K, Elsayed Y, Takimoto C, Peddareddigari V, Tabernero J, Luo FR, Soria JR. Abstract CT325: First in human study of JNJ-42756493, a potent pan fibroblast growth factor receptor (FGFR) inhibitor in patients with advanced solid tumors. Proceedings: AACR Annual Meeting. 2014; April 5-9, San Diego, CA. Cancer Research. 2014;**74**:CT325. DOI: 10.1158/1538-7445.AM2014-CT325

[139] Qiu H, Yashiro M, Zhang X, Miwa A, Hirakawa K. A FGFR2 inhibitor, Ki23057, enhances the chemosensitivity of drug resistant gastric cancer cells. Cancer Letters 2011;**307**:47-52. PMID: 21482024 DOI: 10.1016/j.canlet.2011.03.015

[140] Clinical trials.gov. Combination of Brivanib With 5-Fluorouracil/Leucovorin (5 FU/LV) and 5-Fluorouracil/Leucovorin/Irinotecan(FOLFIRI). Available from: https://www.clinicaltrials.gov/ct2/show/NCT01046864

[141] Lordick F. Targeting the HGF/MET pathway in gastric cancer. The Lancet Oncology. 2014;**15**:914-916. PMID: 24965570

[142] Shah MA, Bang YJ, Lordicketal F. MET Gastric: A phase III study of onartuzumab plus mFOLFOX6 in patients with metastatic HER2-negative (HER2-) and MET-positive (MET) adenocarcinoma of the stomach or gastroesophageal junction (GEC). Journal of Clinical Oncology. 2015;**33**(Suppl):abstr 4012

[143] Jhawer M, Kindler HL, Wainberg Z, Ford J, Kunz P, Tang L, McCallum S, Kallender H, Shah MA. Assessment of two dosing schedules of GSK1363089 (GSK089), a dual MET/VEGFR2 inhibitor, in metastatic gastric cancer (GC): Interim results of a multicenter phase II study. Journal of Clinical Oncology. 2009;**27**:abstr 4502

[144] Yu HG, Ai YW, Yu LL, Zhou XD, Liu J, Li JH, Xu XM, Liu S, Chen J, Liu F, Qi YL, Deng Q, Cao J, Liu SQ, Luo HS, Yu JP. Phosphoinositide 3-kinase/Akt pathway plays an important role in chemoresistance of gastric cancer cells against etoposide and doxorubicin induced cell death. International Journal of Cancer. 2008;**122**:433-443. PMID: 17935137 DOI: 10.1002/ijc.23049

[145] Okamoto I, Doi T, Ohtsu A, Miyazaki M, Tsuya A, Kurei K, Kobayashi K, Nakagawa K. Phase I clinical and pharmacokinetic study of RAD001 (everolimus) administered

daily to Japanese patients with advanced solid tumors. Japanese Journal of Clinical Oncology. 2010;**40**:17-23. PMID: 19783551 DOI: 10.1093/jjco/hyp120

[146] Doi T, Muro K, Boku N, Yamada Y, Nishina T, Takiuchi H, Komatsu Y, Hamamoto Y, Ohno N, Fujita Y, Robson M, Ohtsu A. Multicenter phase II study of everolimus in patients with previously treated metastatic gastric cancer. Journal of Clinical Oncology. 2010;**28**:1904-1910. PMID: 20231677 DOI: 10.1200/JCO.2009.26.2923

[147] Ohtsu A, Ajani JA, Bai YX, Bang YJ, Chung HC, Pan HM, Sahmoud T, Shen L, Yeh KH, Chin K, Muro K, Kim YH, Ferry D, Tebbutt NC, Al-Batran SE, Smith H, Costantini C, Rizvi S, Lebwohl D, Van Cutsem E. Everolimus for previously treated advanced gastric cancer: Results of the randomized, double-blind, phase III GRANITE-1 study. Journal of Clinical Oncology. 2013;**31**:3935-3943. PMID: 24043745 DOI: 10.1200/JCO.2012.48.3552

[148] Ha SY, Lee J, Kang SY, Do IG, Ahn S, Park JO, Kang WK, Choi MG, Sohn TS, Bae JM, Kim S, Kim M, Kim S, Park CK, Ignatius Ou SH, Kim KM. MET overexpression assessed by new interpretation method predicts gene amplification and poor survival in advanced gastric carcinomas. Modern Pathology. 2013;**26**:1632-1641. PMID: 23807774 DOI: 10.1038/modpathol.2013.108

[149] Underhill C, Toulmonde M, Bonnefoi H. A review of PARP inhibitors: From bench to bedside. Annals of Oncology. 2011;**22**:268-279. PMID: 20643861 DOI: 10.1093/annonc/mdq322

[150] Bang YJ, Im SA, Lee KW, Cho JY, Song EK, Lee KH, Kim YH, Park JO, Chun HG, Zhang DY, Fielding A, Rowbottom J, Hodgson D, OConnor MJ, Yin X, Kim WH. Olaparib plus paclitaxel in patients with recurrent or metastatic gastric cancer: A randomized, double-blind phase II study. Journal of Clinical Oncology. 2013;**31**:abstr 4013

[151] Clinical trials.gov. Efficacy and Safety Study of Olaparib in Combination With Paclitaxel to Treat Advanced Gastric Cancer. Available from: https://www.clinicaltrials.gov/ct2/show/NCT01924533

[152] Clinical trials.gov. Evaluating the Safety and Tolerability of the Poly-ADP Ribose (PARP) Inhibitor with FOLFIRI in subjects with solid tumor. Available from: https://www.clinicaltrials.gov/ct2/show/NCT01123876

[153] Hamid O, Robert C, Daud A, Hodi FS, Hwu WJ, Kefford R, Wolchok JD, Hersey P, Joseph RW, Weber JS, Dronca R, Gangadhar TC, Patnaik A, Zarour H, Joshua AM, Gergich K, Elassaiss-Schaap J, Algazi A, Mateus C, Boasberg P, Tumeh PC, Chmielowski B, Ebbinghaus SW, Li XN, Kang SP, Ribas A. Safety and tumor responses with lambrolizumab (anti-PD-1) in melanoma. New England Journal of Medicine. 2013;**369**:134-144. PMID: 23724846 DOI: 10.1056/NEJMoa1305133

[154] Clinical trials.gov. An Efficacy Study in Gastric and Gastroesophageal Junction Cancer Comparing Ipilimumab Versus Standard of Care immediately Following First Line Chemotherapy. Available from: https://www.clinicaltrials.gov/ct2/show/NCT01585987

[155] Clinical trials.gov. A Phase 1/2, Open-label Study of Nivolumab Monotherapy or Nivolumab Combined with Ipilimumab in Subjects with Advanced or Metastatic Solid Tumors. Available from: https://www.clinicaltrials.gov/ct2/show/NCT01928394

[156] Le DT, Bendell JC, Calvo E, Kim JW, Ascierto PA, Sharma P, Ott PA, Bono P, Jaeger D, Evans TRJ, De Braud FG, Chau I, Christensen O, Harbison C, Lin CS, Janjigian YY. Safety and activity of nivolumab monotherapy in advanced and metastatic (A/M) gastric or gastroesophageal junction cancer (GC/GEC): Results from the CheckMate-032 study. 2016 Gastrointestinal Cancers Symposium. Journal of Clinical Oncology. 2016;**34**(Suppl4S):abstr 6

[157] Clinical trials.gov. Study of ONO-4538 in Unresectable Advanced or Recurrent Gastric Cancer. Available from: https://www.clinicaltrials.gov/ct2/show/NCT02267343

[158] Muro K, Bang Y, Shankaran V. LBA15 A phase 1b study of pembrolizumab (PEMBRO; MK-3475) in patients (PTS) with advanced gastric cancer. Annals of Oncology. 2014;**25**:1-41. DOI: 10.1093/annonc/mdu438.15

[159] Clinical trials.gov. Study of Pembrolizumab (MK-3475) as FirstLine Monotherapy and Combination Therapy for Treatment of Advanced Gastric or Gastroesophageal Junction Adenocarcinoma (MK-3475-062/KEYNOTE-062). Available from: https://clinicaltrials.gov/ct2/show/NCT02494583

[160] Clinical trials.gov. A Study of Pembrolizumab (MK-3475) in Participants with Recurrent or Metastatic Gastric or Gastroesophageal Junction Adenocarcinoma (MK-3475-059/KEYNOTE-059). Available from: https://clinicaltrials.gov/ct2/show/NCT02335411

[161] Clinical trials.gov. Study of Pembrolizumab in Subjects with Advanced Gastric or Gastroesophageal Junction Adenocarcinoma Who Progressed after First-Line Therapy with Platinum and Fluoropyrimidine: Integration of Molecular Subtypes through Integrative Genomic Analysis. Available from: https://clinicaltrials.gov/ct2/show/NCT02589496

[162] Clinical trials.gov. Combination Margetuximab and Pembrolizumab for Advanced, Metastatic HER2(+) Gastric or Gastroesophageal Junction Cancer. Available from: https://clinicaltrials.gov/ct2/show/NCT02689284

[163] Clinical trials.gov. Pembrolizumab and Monoclonal Antibody Therapy in Advanced Cancer (PembroMab). Available from: https://clinicaltrials.gov/ct2/show/NCT02318901

[164] Clinical trials.gov. A Study of Ramucirumab Plus Pembrolizumab in Participants With Gastric or GEJ Adenocarcinoma, NSCLC or Transitional Cell Carcinoma of the Urothelium. Available from: https://clinicaltrials.gov/ct2/show/NCT02443324

[165] Clinical trials.gov. A Combination Clinical Study of PLX3397 and Pembrolizumab to Treat Advanced Melanoma and Other Solid Tumors. Available from: https://clinicaltrials.gov/ct2/show/NCT02452424

[166] Lutzky J, Antonia SJ, Blake-Haskins A, Li X, Robbins PB, Shalabi AM, Vasselli J, Ibrahim RA, Khleif S, Segal NH. A phase 1 study of MEDI4736, an anti-PD-L1 antibody, in patients with advanced solid tumors. J Clin Oncol. 2014;**32**:abstr 3001

[167] Clinical trials.gov. Durvalumab and Tremelimumab in Combination With First-Line Chemotherapy in Advanced Solid Tumors. Available from: https://clinicaltrials.gov/ct2/show/NCT02658214

[168] Clinical trials.gov. A Phase 1b/2 Study of MEDI4736 With Tremelimumab, MEDI4736 or Tremelimumab Monotherapy in Gastric or GEJ Adenocarcinoma. Available from: https://clinicaltrials.gov/ct2/show/NCT02340975

[169] Clinical trials.gov. Phase 1 Study of MLN0264 in Adult Patients With Advanced Gastrointestinal Malignancies Expressing Guanylyl Cyclase C. Available from: https://clinicaltrials.gov/show/NCT01577758

[170] Messersmith W, Almhanna K, Rodon J, Cruz C, Ryan D, Jung JA, Fasanmade A, Wyant T, Kalebic T. PD-0032MLN0264, an investigational, first-in-class antibody drug conjugate targeting guanylyl cyclase C (GCC): First in-human study in patients with advanced gastrointestinal malignancies. Annals of Oncology. 2013;**24**:piv36

[171] Clinical trials.gov. A Study of MLN0264 in Patients with Cancer of the Stomach or Gastroesophageal Junction. Available from: https://clinicaltrials.gov/ct2/show/NCT02202759

[172] Clinical trials.gov. MLN0264 in Previously Treated Asian Patients with Advanced Gastrointestinal Carcinoma or Metastatic or Recurrent Gastric or Gastroesophageal Junction Adenocarcinoma Expressing Guanylyl Cyclase C. Available from:https://clinicaltrials.gov/ct2/show/NCT02391038

[173] Lim S, Kaldis P. Cdks, cyclins and CKIs: Roles beyond cell cycle regulation. Development. 2013;**140**:3079-3093. PMID: 23861057 DOI: 10.1242/dev.091744

[174] Schwartz GK, Ilson D, Saltz L, O'Reilly E, Tong W, Maslak P, Werner J, Perkins P, Stoltz M, Kelsen D. Phase II study of the cyclin-dependent kinase inhibitor flavopiridol administered to patients with advanced gastric carcinoma. Journal of Clinical Oncology. 2001;**19**:1985-1992. PMID: 11283131

[175] Fujita T, Doihara H, Washio K, Ino H, Murakami M, Naito M, Shimizu N. Antitumor effects and drug interactions of the proteasome inhibitor bortezomib (PS341) in gastric cancer cells. Anti-Cancer Drugs. 2007;**18**:677-686. PMID: 17762396

[176] Bae SH, Ryoo HM, Kim MK, Lee KH, Sin JI, Hyun MS. Effects of the proteasome inhibitor bortezomib alone and in combination with chemotherapeutic agents in gastric cancer cell lines. Oncology Reports. 2008;**19**:1027-1032. PMID: 18357392 DOI: 10.3892/or.19.4.1027

[177] Ocean AJ, Christos P, Sparano JA, Shah MA, Yantiss RK, Cheng J, Lin J, Papetti M, Matulich D, Schnoll-Sussman F, BesanceneyWebler C, Xiang J, Ward M, Dilts KT, Keresztes R, Holloway S, Chen EX, Wright JJ, Lane ME. Phase II trial of bortezomib alone or in combination with irinotecan in patients with adenocarcinoma of the gastroesophageal junction or stomach. Investigational New Drugs. 2014;**32**:542-548. PMID: 24526575 DOI: 10.1007/s10637-014-0070-0

[178] Jatoi A, Dakhil SR, Foster NR, Ma C, Rowland KM, Moore DF, Jaslowski AJ, Thomas SP, Hauge MD, Flynn PJ, Stella PJ, Alberts SR. Bortezomib, paclitaxel, and carboplatin as a firstline regimen for patients with metastatic esophageal, gastric, and gastroesophageal cancer: Phase II results from the North Central Cancer Treatment Group (N044B). Journal of Thoracic Oncology. 2008;**3**:516-520. PMID: 18449005 DOI: 10.1097/JTO.0b013e31816de276

[179] Shah MA, Power DG, Kindler HL, Holen KD, Kemeny MM, Ilson DH, Tang L, Capanu M, Wright JJ, Kelsen DP. A multicenter, phase II study of bortezomib (PS-341) in patients with unresectable or metastatic gastric and gastroesophageal junction adenocarcinoma. Investigational New Drugs. 2011;**29**:1475-1481. PMID: 20574790

[180] Zhang QW, Liu L, Chen R, Wei YQ, Li P, Shi HS, Zhao YW. Matrix metalloproteinase-9 as a prognostic factor in gastric cancer: A meta-analysis. Asian Pacific Journal of Cancer Prevention. 2012;**13**:2903-2908. PMID: 22938481

[181] He L, Chu D, Li X, Zheng J, Liu S, Li J, Zhao Q, Ji G. Matrix metalloproteinase-14 is a negative prognostic marker for patients with gastric cancer. Digestive Diseases and Sciences. 2013;**58**:1264-1270. PMID: 23314917 DOI: 10.1007/s10620-012-2513-9

[182] Bramhall SR, Hallissey MT, Whiting J, Scholefield J, Tierney G, Stuart RC, Hawkins RE, McCulloch P, Maughan T, Brown PD, Baillet M, Fielding JW. Marimastat as maintenance therapy for patients with advanced gastric cancer: A randomised trial. British Journal of Cancer. 2002;**86**:1864-1870. PMID: 12085177

Chapter 8

Systemic Inflammatory Reaction in Gastric Cancer: Biology and Practical Implications of Neutrophil to Lymphocyte Ratio, Glasgow Prognostic Score and Related Parameters

Ilze Strumfa, Tatjana Bogdanova, Arturs Kalva, Boriss Strumfs, Roberts Rumba, Andrejs Vanags, Inese Drike, Dzeina Mezale, Arnis Abolins, Arvids Jakovlevs, Dainis Balodis and Janis Gardovskis

Additional information is available at the end of the chapter

http://dx.doi.org/10.5772/intechopen.69723

Abstract

Gastric cancer induces systemic inflammatory reaction (SIR) manifesting with changes in counts of white blood cell fractions and concentrations of acute phase proteins, clotting factors and albumins. Thus, protein-based scores or blood cell ratios (neutrophil to lymphocyte ratio (NLR); platelet to lymphocyte ratio (PLR)) are used to evaluate SIR. SIR tests are biologically justified by multiple clinically important and fascinating events including bone marrow activation, development of immune-suppressing immature myeloid cells, generation of pre-metastatic niches and neutrophil extracellular trap formation from externalised DNA network in bidirectional association with platelet activation. Despite biological complexity, clinical SIR assessment is widely available, patient-friendly and economically feasible. Here we present concise review on NLR, PLR, Glasgow prognostic score and fibrinogen – parameters that have prognostic role regarding overall, cancer-free and cancer-specific survival in early and advanced cases. Tumour burden can be predicted helping in preoperative detection of serosal or lymph node involvement. Practical consequences abound, including selection of surgical approach in respect to tumour burden, adjustments in treatment intensity by prognosis or evaluation of chemotherapy response. The chapter also scrutinises main controversies including different cut-off levels. Future developments should include elaboration of complex scores as described here. SIR parameters should be wisely incorporated in patients' treatment.

Keywords: gastric cancer, systemic inflammatory reaction, neutrophil to lymphocyte ratio, NLR, platelet to lymphocyte ratio, PLR, Glasgow prognostic score, fibrinogen

1. Introduction

Gastric cancer remains an important issue in world oncology. In 2013, it ranked fifth by the global incidence and second by mortality [1]. Although the death rates have decreased significantly in the USA and Europe over the previous 70 years, gastric cancer is characterised by poor prognosis and high mortality [2] except for early diagnosed cases. Thus, prognostic and predictive estimates are necessary to guide the intensity of treatment and to predict the efficacy of it. Different directions of prognostic evaluation have been studied, including classic means as tumour-node-metastasis (TNM) stage or patient's Eastern Cooperative Oncology Group (ECOG) performance status [3], or novel approaches as the molecular tests [4].

Many tumours, including gastric cancer, evoke systemic inflammatory reaction (SIR). The systemic effects of cancer include alterations in bone marrow function, especially myelopoiesis. The production and release of leukocytes increases. In addition, immature myeloid cells, including the precursors of granulocytes and monocytes, are retained in early stages of differentiation. Immature myeloid cells can act as immune suppressors and generate pre-metastatic niches, among other pathogenetic processes. Thus, it has even been stated that cancer is an inflammatory disease [5]. SIR shows complex associations with the local immune and inflammatory infiltrate in the tumour [6].

Cancer-related SIR involves cells of innate and adaptive immunity as well as soluble factors. Macrophages are recruited in tumour by hypoxia and tumour-released molecular agents including growth factors and cytokines [7]. Macrophage phenotype switch from tumour-suppressing classical M1 to tumour-promoting M2 subtype promotes angiogenesis and immunosuppression. Platelets undergo activation that contributes to cancer progression and patient mortality [8]. Neutrophil activation can stimulate angiogenesis and metastatic spread. Neutrophil extracellular traps formed from externalised DNA network are bidirectionally associated with platelet activation and can contribute to cancer progression via several mechanisms therefore neutrophil extracellular traps represent also an attractive treatment target [8]. Neutrophils are locally recruited in the cancer as well via chemokine signalling; they contribute to angiogenesis and increased blood vessel permeability. These molecular events highlight also the association between infection or surgery-induced inflammation [9, 10] and cancer relapse or metastatic spread. While innate immunity is generally thought to act as tumour enhancers, high numbers of infiltrating neutrophils [11] and macrophages [12] are shown to be protective in gastric cancer.

In contrast, lymphocytes representing the adaptive immunity are considered to have tumour suppressing effects [7] although contrary effects have been ascribed to certain subpopulations [13, 14].

There is increasing body of evidence that patients' survival can vary despite equal TNM parameters. In turn, cancer can cause systemic inflammatory response that might be associated with prognosis and/or response to treatment. SIR can be evaluated by number or ratio of serum neutrophils, lymphocytes, monocytes and platelets as well as by concentrations of acute phase proteins. These blood tests represent patient-friendly, widely available, globally standardised and cheap information that should be wisely incorporated in patients' treatment [15]. Regarding the diagnostics of gastric cancer, several SIR parameters have been found to differ between gastric cancer patients and healthy controls. Such indicators include neutrophil to lymphocyte ratio [16–18], platelet to lymphocyte ratio, platelet count [18], mean platelet volume [18, 19] and red blood cell distribution width [18]. While these changes clearly indicate activation of systemic inflammatory reaction in gastric cancer, additional research is necessary to identify the diagnostic value of SIR parameters in the differential diagnosis between gastric cancer and other gastric pathologies, including precancerous, inflammatory and ulcerative changes.

The correlation between neutrophil to lymphocyte ratio (NLR) and poor survival of gastric cancer patients is the best-known finding regarding SIR in gastric cancer [16, 17, 20]. High NLR is associated not only with shorter overall survival but also with worse progression-free survival [21]. In addition to the general association with survival, the prognostic value of NLR has been tested in specific clinical groups. Thus, NLR predicts post-operative survival of surgically treated patients with resectable cancer [22] and retains independent prognostic role in elderly patients—an expanding group in Western population showing multiple ageing-related changes that could affect the immune and inflammatory processes [23]. For patients undergoing chemotherapy because of unresectable and recurrent advanced gastric cancer, NLR also shows independent prognostic significance [24]. NLR is an independent prognostic factor in metastatic gastric cancer [25] and in metastatic gastric cancer treated with chemotherapy [26]. The predictive value is limited in patients receiving palliative treatment for disseminated gastric cancer [21]. Some authors consider low NLR as an indicator for good prognosis and thus beneficial effect of surgical treatment in stage IV gastric cancer [27, 28].

Some research groups have found that complex assessment of SIR-related parameters has superior prognostic value. For instance, joint analysis of platelet count and NLR was found to predict post-operative survival more exactly [29]. Combined scoring of albumin and neutrophil to lymphocyte ratio was independently associated with overall survival and was especially accurate for patients with stage I–II gastric cancer [30]. Combined evaluation of pre-operative NLR and platelet to lymphocyte ratio (PLR) was independent predictor of survival after curative surgical resection of stage I–II gastric cancer [31].

SIR can highlight wider scope of clinical traits, including manifestations that are not directly related to surgery or oncologic treatment. For example, pre-operative anxiety and depression are significantly associated with NLR [32].

SIR assessment is more comprehensive than NLR analysis. Thus, pre-operative plasma fibrinogen increases with gastric cancer stage and predicts worse recurrence-free and overall survival [33]. Similarly, levels of plasma albumin or the characteristics of platelets can provide significant data. Levels of C-reactive protein, original or modified Glasgow prognostic score can be used for analysis [3, 15].

The systemic inflammatory reaction itself can be an adverse pathogenetic event, facilitating tumour angiogenesis or adhesion of circulating tumour cells to endothelium that would lead to the growth of metastasis. In addition, NLR correlates with other factors known to have adverse prognostic role. Among such parameters, presence of vascular and lymphatic invasion as well as positive resection lines have been reported [22]. In several studies, NLR has been found to correlate with the stage of gastric cancer [16, 20–22]. NLR negatively correlates with mismatch repair protein deficiency [34]. NLR is associated with post-operative infectious complications. Both factors show an independent significant association with poorer survival after gastrectomy [9].

The evaluation of SIR in gastric cancer patients is highly attractive. By increasing awareness of SIR parameters, simple and widely available blood tests can provide information that is helpful in shaping the care of gastric cancer patients from early stages to metastatic spread or locally advanced tumour.

However, unresolved issues remain. Except the prognostic value to NLR, many aspects as the correlation with tumour morphology, type by Lauren classification, invasive properties of cancer, grade, intensity of angiogenesis and microvascular density have been targeted by low number of studies. Only few meta-analyses have been conducted [21, 35–37]. Few data are available on SIR parameters after treatment although it is known that post-chemotherapy NLR correlates with the response in patients with unresectable gastric cancer [38].

The practical unsolved questions include the comparison between NLR and other indicators of systemic inflammatory response, e.g., platelet to lymphocyte ratio [39], the significance of post-treatment NLR as well as cut-off values for practical use. The ultimate goal would be to create and validate an algorithm for fine-tuning of the treatment strategy in gastric cancer from early to advanced stages. Inflammatory markers other than NLR should be included; complex assessment hypothetically could be advised.

Thus, considering the high incidence and mortality of gastric cancer and the need for prognostic and predictive data, the present chapter will be devoted to the assessment of SIR in gastric cancer in order to develop practical recommendations how to adjust gastric cancer treatment by easily available and economically feasible simple blood tests for SIR parameters. Increased awareness of SIR characteristics is important to reach this aim.

2. Neutrophil to lymphocyte ratio in gastric cancer

Neutrophil to lymphocyte ratio is calculated as the ratio between the count of neutrophilic leukocytes and lymphocytes in peripheral blood. Thus, the parameter is easily available, especially in carefully examined cancer patients, and economically non-demanding. In fact, sufficient awareness and algorithm for interpretation are the only prerequisites to obtain an additional piece of information from routine blood tests.

Since the early reports [40, 41], NLR has been studied in relation to the prognosis of gastric cancer patients. Thus, Aliustaoglu et al. reported that high NLR was statistically significantly associated with shorter median survival. In the same study, similar association was found regarding high platelet to lymphocyte ratio and high absolute number of lymphocytes but no difference was found for neutrophil count, platelet count and mean platelet volume [41]. In another early study devoted to the prognostic significance of host- and tumour-related factors in patients with gastric cancer, white blood cell count, NLR, C-reactive protein (CRP) and albumin was found to have prognostic impact, along with age, haemoglobin level, tumour size as well as T and N characteristics. By multivariate analysis, NLR was an independent prognostic factor along with tumour size and T parameter [42].

At present, the association between NLR and different aspects of survival (overall, cancer-specific, cancer-free or progression-free survival) remains one of the best substantiated aspects in the SIR research in gastric cancer.

2.1. NLR and survival: prognostic implications

The prognostic importance of NLR is shown over the whole course of gastric cancer, and is applicable to wide treatment spectrum—from surgically resectable cases, including early gastric cancer, to advanced, recurrent or metastatic tumours subjected to non-surgical treatment. Most researchers have demonstrated that NLR is an independent prognostic factor, based on multivariate analysis [17]. However, in few studies, the association with survival is confirmed by univariate but not multivariate analysis [43–45]. Some of the reports are on better scores, e.g. Glasgow prognostic score had higher informativity in a large and homogeneous group of 324 patients with stage III gastric cancer undergoing resection [43].

The prognostic value of NLR has been reported in different cancers, including lung, colorectal and breast carcinoma, among others [46]. Gastric cancer also follows the same mechanisms. In unselected cohort of patients diagnosed with gastric adenocarcinoma, high NLR (compared with the cut-off value 3) was a significant ($p = 0.016$), independent risk factor for poor survival [17].

Surgery is the mainstay of gastric cancer treatment, if the local and/or systemic tumour spread, or the general condition of the patient does not limit the possibilities of surgical intervention. In patients who have had curative surgery for gastric cancer, high NLR is significantly associated with poor prognosis [39], including overall survival [16, 47–49], cancer-specific survival [47], cancer-free survival [16, 47] and progression-free survival [25, 38, 50].

Thus, in a recent study of 162 patients with resectable gastric cancer, high pre-operative NLR (reaching or exceeding the median of 4.02) was associated with decreased overall and cancer-free survival, confirmed by Kaplan-Meier analysis [16]. In a significantly larger group of 1986 consecutive patients subjected to curative surgical treatment for gastric cancer, NLR was confirmed as an independent prognostic factor for overall survival, associated with hazard ratio of 1.4 [39]. Similarly, in 601 surgically treated gastric cancer patients, high NLR (reaching or exceeding 1.7) was a significant prognostic parameter for overall survival, confirmed as an independent factor by multivariate analysis. The hazard ratio was 2.12 [48]. Analogous observations were reported by Hsu et al. They assessed a large cohort of 1030 gastric cancer patients subjected to complex treatment. In accordance with clinical indications, subtotal or total gastrectomy along with spleen- and pancreas-sparing D2 lymphadenectomy was performed, aiming to accomplish clear resection margins. Metastasectomy was considered depending on clinical symptoms and possibility of radical resections, and adjuvant or palliative chemotherapy was offered for stage II–IV patients. In such a large group, showing the routine clinical diversity of gastric cancer presentation, high NLR (exceeding 3.44) was an independent prognostic factor for overall survival, associated with hazard ratio of 1.57 [22].

In addition to significant statistical findings, the biological differences between groups also are remarkable. The 3- and 5-year survival rates in low versus (vs.) high NLR groups were 71.0% vs. 55.1% and 64.1% vs. 47.2%, respectively [22]. Even more, the 5-year survival was 29.9% in the high NLR group (reaching or exceeding 5.0) contrasting with statistically significantly different value of 85.6% in patients who had low NLR [51].

The overall survival was 86.1 months in patients presenting with low NLR vs. 64.0 months in high NLR (reaching or exceeding 2.3) group [30]. Evaluating 156 surgically treated gastric cancer patients, the median survival in high vs. low NLR groups was 36 vs. 60 months while the five-year survival was 35% and 60%, and the median cancer-free survival was 12 and 20 months, respectively. The survival differences retained significance in N0 patients: 5-year survival was 60% vs. 90%, $p < 0.05$. In this cohort, NLR was also recognised as an independent prognostic factor for overall survival [52].

In advanced gastric cancer (stage III–IV) patients subjected to gastrectomy with curative intent, high NLR was an independent predictor of overall survival at cut-off 2.0 corresponding to median while cut-off value 3.0 (the 75th percentile) was an independent predictor of cancer-free survival. The median overall survival in high vs. low NLR was 21.4 and 45.3 months while the progression-free survival in the redefined high and low NLR groups was 12.8 vs. 27.9 months [53].

NLR retains prognostic significance for surgically treated gastric cancer patients in specific subgroups. For instance, in elderly gastric cancer patients (aged 75 years or older) treated by gastrectomy, high NLR (reaching or exceeding 1.83) was associated with worse survival. Again, NLR was confirmed as an independent risk factor by multivariate analysis. The biological differences were remarkable: the median survival associated with low vs. high NLR was 1209 vs. 587 days, respectively [16]. High NLR is associated with older age in some studies [9, 20, 44, 47, 54, 55] while others report no association [22, 38].

It is very important to identify high risk of cancer progression in early diagnosed cases. Some promising reports have been published. Combined score including NLR and albumin level was shown to have independent prognostic value exceeding the informativity of NLR as justified by higher area under curve (AUC). This score, further described in detail, retained the prognostic ability in stage I–II gastric cancer [30]. A complex score comprising NLR and PLR is another prognostic option, successfully tested in a stage I–II gastric cancer. NLR-PLR score showed a clear trend to improve the prognostic value of TNM staging [31].

Mohri et al. has reported very interesting findings regarding NLR in surgically treatable gastric cancer cases. In 404 patients undergoing curative gastrectomy for gastric cancer, high NLR was an independent risk factor of post-operative infectious complications while it was not predictive of non-infectious complications. In turn, both high NLR and post-operative infectious complications were independent risk factors of worse overall and cancer-specific survival [9]. The preceding NLR increase in patients later developing post-operative infectious complications but not in case of all complications was justified by Japanese scientists [10].

In contrast with the previously described findings, NLR was not informative regarding survival of gastric cancer patients having only local disease while it was significantly associated with survival in advanced cases [56]. Some negative findings, including the cited one, can be explained by small study group comprising only 53 patients with local disease and 50 with advanced cancer [56]. Evaluating Glasgow prognostic score, NLR and PLR in patients with resected stage III gastric adenocarcinoma, only Glasgow prognostic score along with TNM stage was independently associated with cancer-free and overall survival [43]. If the study design includes several SIR parameters, multivariate analysis could highlight only one of those.

Advanced or metastatic cancer represents a situation with continuously significant tumour burden, associated with ongoing inflammation, angiogenesis, antigenic stimulation and thus sustained SIR. The NLR has been evaluated in these situations as well. In 174 advanced gastric cancer patients treated with oxaliplatin/5-fluorouracil (FOLFOX), NLR was associated with overall survival but not with progression-free survival. NLR was also an independent predictor of overall survival. Normalisation of NLR after one cycle of chemotherapy was significant and independent predictor of overall and progression-free survival [57]. Similar findings are reported by Jin et al. [58].

In unresectable and recurrent advanced gastric cancer patients treated by chemotherapy, high NLR (exceeding 4) was associated with significantly lower median survival [24]. Similarly, in another cohort comprising 143 cases of metastatic gastric cancer, high NLR was an independent prognostic factor. The overall and progression-free survival was 11.6 and 7.9 months in low NLR (less than 3.34) group contrasting with 8.3 and 6.2 months in patients having high NLR [25]. In 120 unresectable metastatic and advanced gastric cancer cases, treated by chemoradiotherapy, baseline NLR predicted survival. The median overall and progression-free survival in high vs. low NLR group was 10 and 3 months vs. 18 and 6 months. Treatment-induced changes in NLR also predicted survival. Both baseline NLR and changes upon initiation of treatment predicted treatment outcomes [38]. This finding is in accordance with Cho et al., who also reported significantly higher chemotherapeutic disease control rate in metastatic advanced gastric cancer patients having low NLR, defined as less or equal to 3.0 [50]. Combined scores have been generated to evaluate the prognosis of metastatic gastric cancer as well [26].

Occasionally NLR shows association with survival by univariate but not multivariate analysis. Thus, in a small group of 70 patients affected by locally advanced gastric cancer (stage III–IV) and treated by neoadjuvant chemotherapy, NLR was an independent predictor of overall survival. It was significantly associated with progression-free survival but was not an independent factor [59]. In a large group of 439 patients affected by metastatic or recurrent gastric cancer, NLR was significantly associated with overall survival in univariate but not multivariate analysis. Complex score was favoured by authors [60].

The prognostic findings regarding NLR in gastric cancer have been summarised in **Table 1**.

Study group		Survival				References
Characteristics	**Size**	**Overall**	**Cancer-specific**	**Cancer-free**	**Progression-free**	
Unselected gastric adenocarcinoma	706	X Multivariate				[17]
GC	245	X Kaplan-Meier analysis of multicentre study data				[61]
Gastric adenocarcinoma	236	X Multivariate				[62]
Surgically treated GC						
Consecutive GC patients undergoing curative gastrectomy	404	X Multivariate	X Multivariate			[9]
Curative surgery for GC	288	X Multivariate				[49]
Resectable GC	162	X Kaplan-Meier analysis		X Kaplan-Meier analysis		[16]
GC, subjected to curative surgery	1986	X Multivariate				[39]
Surgically treated GC (R0)	601	X Multivariate				[48]
GC patients undergoing gastrectomy	389	X Multivariate	X Multivariate	X Multivariate		[47]
Surgically treated GC patients	207		X Multivariate	X Multivariate		[63]
GC subjected to radical surgery	291	X Multivariate				[20]

Study group		Survival				References
Characteristics	Size	Overall	Cancer-specific	Cancer-free	Progression-free	
GC subjected to gastrectomy	632	X Univariate (significant) Multivariate (NS)				[45]
GC subjected to potentially curative gastrectomy	156	X Multivariate				[52]
Patients with resectable GC, including advanced cases	377	X Multivariate				[64]
Surgically treated (total or subtotal gastrectomy) GC patients	220	X Univariate (significant) Multivariate (NS)				[44]
Gastrectomy with curative intent for stage III–IV GC	293	X Multivariate		X Multivariate		[53]
Curative gastrectomy	157		X Multivariate			[65]
GC patients, undergoing gastrectomy	1028	X Multivariate				[66]
Elderly patients (at least 75 years old) undergoing gastrectomy	160	X Multivariate				[23]
Curative resection, D2 lymphadenectomy, adjuvant chemotherapy in stage II–III	873	X Kaplan-Meier analysis				[30]
Resectable GC subjected to combined treatment	1030	X Multivariate				[22]

Study group		Survival				References
Characteristics	Size	Overall	Cancer-specific	Cancer-free	Progression-free	
Advanced, unresectable and/or metastatic GC						
Unresectable and recurrent advanced GC, treated by chemotherapy	224	X Multivariate				[24]
Metastatic GC treated by chemotherapy	256	X Multivariate				[26]
Metastatic GC	143	X Multivariate			X Multivariate	[25]
Unresectable, advanced GC, treated by chemotherapy	120	X Kaplan-Meier analysis			X Kaplan-Meier analysis	[38]
Metastatic GC treated by chemotherapy	109	X Kaplan-Meier analysis			X Kaplan-Meier analysis	[67]
GC, stage IV with synchronous distant MTS	123	X Multivariate				[27]
Metastatic advanced GC treated by palliative chemotherapy	268	X Multivariate			X Multivariate	[50]
Locally advanced GC treated by neoadjuvant chemotherapy	70	X Multivariate			X Univariate (significant) Multivariate (NS)	[59]
Metastatic or recurrent GC	439	X Univariate (significant) Multivariate (NS)				[60]

Study group		Survival				References
Characteristics	Size	Overall	Cancer-specific	Cancer-free	Progression-free	
Inoperable advanced or metastatic GC patients receiving chemotherapy	384	X Univariate (significant) Multivariate (NS)				[68]
Advanced GC patients treated by chemotherapy	174	X Multivariate			X (dynamics, not baseline) Multivariate	[57]
Advanced GC treated with neoadjuvant chemotherapy	46	X (baseline and dynamics) X Univariate (significant) Multivariate (NS)			X (baseline and dynamics) Multivariate	[58]
Metastatic unresectable advanced GC patients treated with palliative chemotherapy	104	X Multivariate				[69]

Abbreviations: GC, gastric cancer; R0, resection line free of cancer; NS, not significant; MTS, metastasis.

Table 1. The prognostic value of NLR in gastric cancer patients.

The cut-off levels vary widely among the studies. Most frequently, either the median value is selected as the cut-off [16, 70], or the relevant level is found by receiver operating characteristic curve (ROC) analysis [30, 39]. Youden Index has been successfully employed to detect the optimal cut-off during ROC analysis [30]. This index is defined as the cut-off value showing the highest sum of specifity and sensitivity at the considered value; minus 1 [71]. Less frequently, the 75th percentile is used as the cut-off [44, 53]. Some research groups have applied more complex approach, e.g. combining the patients groups with similar survival [17, 20]. The reported cut-off levels for NLR in gastric cancer patients are summarized in **Table 2**.

Interestingly, different cut-off values can reveal different information. Thus, Jung et al. has reported that cut-off 2.0 based on the median value was valuable in order to show that higher NLR is an independent risk factor for worse overall survival. However, when studying cancer-free survival, NLR was an independent risk factor by cut-off 3.0 corresponding to the 75th percentile [53]. The necessity for different cut-offs in regard to the question of interest is indirectly demonstrated by mean NLR in different patient groups: 4.02 in T1–2; 6.54 in T3–4; 4.81 in N0; 6.41 in N+; 5.00 in M0; 7.82 in M1; 4.74 in stage I–II cancers and 7.07 in stage III–IV cancers [47]. Jung et al. also observed statistically significant differences in median NLR by gastric cancer stage: 1.88 in stage III and 2.17 in stage IV [53].

2.2. Association with tumour features

2.2.1. Local tumour spread: T

Significant association between NLR and the invasion depth of gastric cancer is recognised since the early studies [65] and confirmed by more recent research [20]. The applied cut-off levels again vary widely. Thus, the association with increased depth of invasion has been demonstrated in patients whose high preoperative NLR level was defined as higher than or equal to 4.02 [16] or as exceeding the ROC-set cut-off value of 1.59 [55]. Significant difference in T1–2 vs. T3–4 distribution was reported by Deng et al. The mean NLR was 4.02 in T1–2 cases and 6.54 in T3–4 cases [47].

Many studies have highlighted the association between NLR and serosal invasion that is classified as T4a. Such invasion represents a potential limit to surgical treatment if followed by extensive peritoneal spread. NLR studies in regard to the tumour spread have led to the development of complex predictive scores to forecast serosal invasion. Hence, high NLR can be used as an independent predictive factor for T4 using cut-off 3.2 [73]. The high NLR (exceeding 3.44) group had significantly higher proportion of T4 when 1030 patients with resectable gastric cancer were assessed [22]. Serosal invasion was significantly more frequent in elderly patients having high NLR: 75.5% vs. 57.4% [23]. Finally, in a large prospective study enrolling 1131 surgically treated patients, high NLR (exceeding the median 3.5) was associated with deeper invasion: T3–T4 tumours. The mean NLR was 2.51 in T3–T4 tumours vs. 2.19 in T1–T2 tumours. Within the frames of a complex score, NLR can be used to predict inappropriateness of gastrectomy [54].

The capacity of NLR to predict such tumour spread that would limit surgical treatment has been explored in combined model searching for either peritoneal or metastatic spread due to either gastric or oesophageal adenocarcinoma. Authors concluded that NLR reaching or exceeding

http://dx.doi.org/10.5772/intechopen.69723

Study group		Cut-off		Study target	Level of justification	Main conclusions	References
Characteristics	Size	Value	Approach				
Unselected gastric adenocarcinoma	706	3	Complex	OS	Multivariate	Higher NLR is associated with worse OS	[17]
GC	245	2.56	Ref. [40]	OS	Kaplan-Meier analysis Multicentre study	High NLR is significantly associated with worse OS, presence of N+ and higher stage	[61]
Surgically treated GC							
Operable GC	231	2.97	ROC analysis	N	Multivariate	High NLR shows significant association with N+ in early GC but is not an independent factor	[72]
Stage I–II GC, subjected to radical (R0) surgery including D2 lymphadenectomy	305	2.1	ROC analysis	OS	Multivariate	Within the frames of complex NLR-PLR score is an independent predictor of OS in stage I–II GC	[31]
Stage I–II GC, subjected to radical (R0) surgery including D2 lymphadenectomy	305	3	Ref. [29]	OS	Multivariate	Within the frames of complex score, including platelet count and NLR, is not the most informative predictor of OS by AUC assessment	[31]
Surgically treated T2 GC	230	2.18	Median	N	Multivariate	Higher NLR is associated with higher number of LN MTS and higher N	[70]

Study group		Cut-off		Study target	Level of justification	Main conclusions	References
Characteristics	Size	Value	Approach				
Consecutive patients undergoing curative gastrectomy	404	3.0	ROC analysis	OS CSS Post-operative complications	Multivariate	Higher NLR is an independent risk factor for worse OS, CSS and post-operative infectious complications	[9]
Curative surgery for gastric cancer	288	2.7	ROC analysis for survival	OS Immune cell density within cancer	Multivariate	Higher NLR is an independent risk factor for worse OS Density of CD4 Ly is decreased in high NLR group while CD3 and CD8 + Ly density shows no differences	[49]
Operable GC	492	1.59	ROC analysis	N	Multivariate	High NLR is an independent factor, associated with N+	[55]
Curative resection, D2 lymphadenectomy, adjuvant chemotherapy in high-risk stage II–III	873	2.3	ROC analysis	OS	Kaplan-Meier analysis Multivariate	Although NLR is associated with OS, a complex score including NLR and albumin is more potent predictor of OS based on higher AUC in ROC analysis	[30]
Elderly patients (at least 75 years old) undergoing gastrectomy	160	1.83	ROC analysis	OS	Multivariate	Higher NLR is an independent risk factor for worse OS	[23]
Surgically treated GC	601	1.7	ROC analysis	OS	Multivariate	Higher NLR is an independent risk factor for worse OS	[48]

Study group		Cut-off		Study target	Level of justification	Main conclusions	References
Characteristics	Size	Value	Approach				
Total or subtotal gastrectomy with lymphadenectomy	389	2.36	ROC analysis	OS, CFS, CSS	Multivariate	Higher NLR is a significant risk factor for worse OS, CFS, CSS	[47]
Resectable GC	162	4.02	Median	OS, CFS	Kaplan-Meier analysis	Higher NLR is an associated with worse OS and CFS	[16]
Resectable gastric cancer subjected to combined treatment	1030	3.44	Survival tree assessment by R software	3 and 5-year OS rate	Multivariate	Higher NLR is an independent risk factor for worse OS	[22]
Surgically treated GC	207	5/4	ROC analysis	OS CFS	Multivariate	Higher NLR is an independent risk factor for worse OS. However, GPS has higher prognostic value	[63]
GC subjected to radical surgery	291	3.5	Complex assessment of survival by NLR intervals	OS Tumour and patients characteristics	Multivariate	High NLR is an independent prognostic factor for overall survival and is significantly associated with, age, tumour size, T and TNM stage	[20]
GC subjected to gastrectomy	632	1.83	ROC analysis	OS	Multivariate	High NLR shows significant association with OS but is not an independent factor. Complex score preferred	[45]
GC subjected to potentially curative gastrectomy	156	2.34	Median	OS	Multivariate	Higher NLR is an independent risk factor for worse OS	[52]

Study group		Cut-off		Study target	Level of justification	Main conclusions	References
Characteristics	Size	Value	Approach				
Surgically treated GC, including non-radical cases	1131	3.5	Median	Resection line status Tumour characteristics	Mann Whitney test Fisher test Univariate analysis	High NLR is associated with T3-4, G3-4, larger tumours, higher N and TNM stage Within frames of complex score NLR can be used to predict inappropriateness of gastrectomy	[54]
Surgically treated GC patients	220	2.15	75th percentile	OS	Multivariate	Higher NLR is a significant risk factor for OS by univariate but not multivariate analysis	[44]
Surgically treated GC, T2–4	262	3.2	ROC analysis	T4	Multivariate	High NLR is an independent factor, associated with T4	[73]
Gastrectomy with curative intent for stage III–IV GC	293	2.0	Median	OS	Multivariate	Higher NLR is an independent risk factor for worse OS	[53]
Gastrectomy with curative intent for stage III–IV GC	293	3.0	75th percentile	CFS	Multivariate	Higher NLR is an independent risk factor for worse CFS	[53]
Curative gastrectomy	157	5.0	Refs. [74, 75]	CSS	Multivariate	Higher NLR is an independent risk factor for worse CSS	[65]
Advanced, unresectable and/or metastatic GC							
Metastatic gastric adenocarcinoma treated by chemotherapy	256	3	Refs. [53, 66]	OS	Multivariate	NLR is an independent risk factor	[26]

Study group		Cut-off		Study target	Level of justification	Main conclusions	References
Characteristics	Size	Value	Approach				
Metastatic GC	143	3.34	Median	OS	Multivariate	Higher NLR is an independent risk factor for worse OS	[25]
Metastatic GC treated by chemotherapy	109	2.5	Refs. [40, 58]	OS PFS	Kaplan-Meier analysis	High NLR is significantly associated with worse OS and PFS	[67]
Unresectable, advanced GC, treated by chemotherapy	120	4.62	Median	OS PFS	Kaplan-Meier analysis	Higher baseline NLR or increase of NLR after first-line chemotherapy is associated with worse OS and CFS	[38]
Unresectable, advanced GC, treated by chemotherapy	120	4.62	Median	Response to chemotherapy	χ^2 test	Lower baseline NLR or lower NLR after first-line chemotherapy was associated with improved response to chemotherapy	[38]
Advanced GC treated by chemotherapy//Local GC treated by surgery and adjuvant chemoradiotherapy	50//53	2.75	Median	OS	Kaplan-Meier analysis	High NLR is significantly associated with worse OS in advanced but not local GC	[56]
GC (stage IV) with synchronous distant MTS	123	3.1	Median	OS	Multivariate	Higher NLR is a significant risk factor for worse OS in the whole group and in surgically treated patients	[27]

Study group		Cut-off		Study target	Level of justification	Main conclusions	References
Characteristics	Size	Value	Approach				
Metastatic advanced GC treated by palliative chemotherapy	268	3.0	Median	OS, PFS Response to chemotherapy	Multivariate	Higher NLR is an independent risk factor for worse response to chemotherapy, OS and PFS	[50]
Inoperable advanced and metastatic GC patients receiving palliative chemotherapy	384	2.75	Median	OS	Multivariate	High NLR shows significant association with OS but is not an independent factor	[68]
Advanced GC patients treated with chemotherapy	174	3	OS curve analysis	OS PFS	Multivariate	Low baseline NLR and normalisation of NLR were independent predictors of better OS. Normalisation of NLR was an independent predictor of better PFS.	[57]
Advanced GC treated by neoadjuvant chemotherapy	46	2.5	Ref. [40]	OS PFS	Multivariate		[58]

Abbreviations: OS, overall survival; NLR, neutrophil to lymphocyte ratio; GC, gastric cancer; Ref., reference; N+, presence of metastases in regional lymph nodes; ROC, receiver operating characteristic curve; N, regional lymph node status in respect to metastases by tumour-nodes-metastasis (TNM) classification; R0, resection line free of tumour; PLR, platelet to lymphocyte ratio; AUC, area under the curve; T, local spread of primary gastric cancer by TNM classification; LN, lymph node; MTS, metastasis; CSS, cancer-specific survival; CD, cluster of differentiation; Ly, lymphocyte; CFS, cancer-free survival; GPS, Glasgow prognostic score; TNM, tumour-nodes-metastasis classification; G, grade; PFS, progression-free survival.

Table 2. Cut-offs of NLR in gastric cancer studies.

the cut-off value of 3.28 is an independent predictor of undesirable tumour spread. The median NLR in operable patients vs. those having peritoneal or metastatic disease was 2.2 vs. 3.3 [76].

Negative findings have been published. Some of them could be easily explained by small group size, e.g. only 61 gastric cancer patients were enrolled in the study of Pietrzyk et al. [18]. However, no differences in T distribution by NLR were found by Kim et al. who analysed a large group of 601 patients [48]. No association between invasion depth and NLR was found in a multicentre study [61].

Large tumour size has shown association with high NLR [20, 22, 38, 53–55, 65, 77]. As T in gastric cancer is not defined by size, tumour size could become a confounding factor.

2.2.2. *Metastases in regional lymph nodes: N*

Metastatic involvement of regional lymph nodes is associated with worse prognosis, being especially important in the early stages of gastric cancer. Presence of lymph node metastases also limits and changes the treatment options as endoscopic resection is not feasible anymore but D2 lymphadenectomy becomes more appropriate than D1 lymphadenectomy. In addition, neoadjuvant treatment can be offered now to gastric cancer patients affected by lymph node metastases [55]. NLR can be used to predict lymph node metastasis. In a retrospective study of 230 surgically treated patients, affected by T2 gastric cancer, NLR exceeding the median value of 2.18 was associated with higher number of lymph node metastases and higher N characteristics. The findings were confirmed by multivariate analysis. The relative risk was as high as 4.15 and 7.09 in regard to high number of metastases and N stage, respectively [70]. NLR at the cut-off level 1.59 (detected by ROC) was an independent factor associated with lymph node metastasis; however, higher informativity reflected by higher AUC was achieved by complex score (see further) including NLR, PLR and tumour-related factors [55]. The conclusions are justified by other researchers reporting correlation between NLR and N parameter since the early reports [65] until recent studies [77]. Thus, high NLR (exceeding the ROC-set cut-off value of 1.59) was associated with high N [55] while low preoperative NLR level (less than 4.02) was associated with lower number of lymph node metastases [16]. The variability of applied cut-off values is evident.

Lymph node metastases were significantly more frequent in elderly patients having high NLR: 83.0% vs. 55.6% [23]. In a large cohort of 1030 patients with resectable gastric cancer, high ratio of metastatic to examined lymph nodes defined as exceeding 0.18 was more frequent in those who had high NLR (greater than 3.44). Interestingly, in the same study N distribution showed only a trend to differences [22]. Significant difference in N0 vs. N+ distribution was reported by Deng et al. In addition, the mean NLR was 4.81 in N0 patients and 6.41 in N+ cases [47]. Statistically significant correlation between presence of lymph node metastasis, high NLR was confirmed in a multicentre study [61]. In a prospective study of 1131 surgically treated cases, high NLR (exceeding the median 3.5) was associated with higher N. The mean NLR was 2.31 in N0; 2.32 in N1; 2.43 in N2 and 2.75 in N3 cases [54].

Negative findings have been published as well. Some of them could be easily explained by small group size, e.g. only 61 gastric cancer patients were enrolled in the study of Pietrzyk et al. [18]. No differences in N distribution by NLR were found by Kim et al. who analysed a large group of 601 patients [48] and Yu et al. who assessed another significant cohort of 291 patients. In the same study, association with T and TNM stage was significant [20]. There was no correlation between NLR and N in a reasonable group of 262 surgically treated patients affected by T2–T4 gastric cancer while correlation with T in the same study was meaningful. The cut-off in this study was detected by ROC and was 3.2 [73].

Some reports have re-evaluated the meaning of NLR in predicting N status, arriving to less positive conclusions. In early gastric cancer (T1a–T1b), NLR was significantly associated with presence of lymph node metastases. The mean NLR was 2.07 in N0 group while it increased to 2.60 in N+ group. However, by multivariate analysis NLR was not an independent prognostic factor. Complex score not including NLR was more informative for preoperative estimation of lymph node metastases [72].

2.2.3. Presence of distant metastases: M

Presence of distant metastasis has also been associated with higher NLR [38, 77]. Metastatic tumours were significantly more frequent in patients who had high NLR (exceeding 3.44) assessing 1030 patients with resectable gastric cancer [22]. Significant difference in M0 vs. M1 frequencies by NLR groups was reported by Deng et al. In addition, the mean NLR was 5.00 in M0 cases and 7.82 in M1 cases [47].

In a large study of 491 gastric cancer patients, NLR was significantly associated with peritoneal metastasis. However, it was not an independent predictive factor for peritoneal spread, while tumour morphology, serum level of carbohydrate antigen CA19-9 and lymphocyte count retained independent predictive value [78]. In contrast, evaluating CRP, activated partial thromboplastin time, NLR and hypoalbuminemia, NLR was identified as an independent risk factor of the presence of peritoneal metastasis. The cut-off level was set at 2.37 [79].

2.2.4. TNM stage

Considering the previously discussed links between NLR and TNM parameters, correlation with TNM stage could be expected as well. Indeed, advanced TNM stage was significantly associated with high NLR [9, 20, 44, 47, 65, 77]. High NLR (exceeding the ROC-set cut-off value of 1.59) was associated with high TNM stage [55]. The mean NLR was 4.73 in stage I–II and 7.07 in stage III–IV [47]. In advanced gastric cancer (stage III–IV) patients, there still was difference between stage III and IV [53].

Statistically significant correlation between cancer stage and high NLR was confirmed also by multicentre [61] and prospective study design [54]. In a prospective study of 1131 surgically treated patients, high NLR (exceeding the median 3.5) was associated with higher TNM stage. The mean NLR was 2.13 in stage I, 2.40 in stage II, 2.53 in stage III and 2.60 in stage IV [54].

Regarding negative reports, no NLR differences by TNM stage were found by Kim et al. who analysed a large group of 601 patients [48].

2.2.5. Histological type and grade (G)

The association between NLR and cancer grade is more controversial. The cancer grade was not different between high and low NLR groups in a cohort of 143 metastatic gastric cancer cases as well as in 389 patients who underwent gastrectomy or in 293 gastric cancer patients diagnosed in stage III–IV [22, 25, 47, 53]. No difference by differentiation degree (G1–2 vs. G3) was found by Yu et al. [20].

In contrast, high NLR was associated with differentiated (vs. undifferentiated) gastric cancer [9]. High differentiation degree (vs. moderate and poorly differentiated cases) was associated with low NLR. In the same study, no differences were observed regarding proliferation fraction by Ki-67 [38]. High NLR (exceeding the ROC-set cut-off value of 1.59) was associated with high grade [55]. In a prospective study of 1131 surgically treated patients, high NLR (exceeding the median 3.5) was associated with poor differentiation or undifferentiated tumours while low NLR—with high and moderate differentiation. The relevant mean NLR values were 2.46 in G3–G4 vs. 2.31 in G1–G2 cancers [54].

There was no correlation between NLR and histological differentiation in a large group of 262 surgically treated patients affected by T2–T4 gastric cancer while correlation with T in the same study was meaningful. The cut-off in this study was detected by ROC and was 3.2 [73]. No correlation between histological type of cancer and NLR was observed in a prospective study of 1131 surgically treated patients [54]. No differences in histology distribution by NLR were found by Kim et al. who analysed a large group of 601 patients [48]. Histological types (papillary, tubular, poorly differentiated, mucinous, signet ring cell carcinoma) were scrutinized by Deng et al., also finding no association with NLR level [47].

No NLR differences were observed between Lauren types: intestinal vs. diffuse [38, 53, 65] that might explain the lack of association with HER-2 protein expression [38].

Low NLR shows significant correlations with mismatch repair deficiency [34]. In cancer tissues, the density of CD4-positive lymphocytes was significantly decreased in high NLR group while the density of CD3 and CD8-positive lymphocytes was not associated with NLR [49]. Although NLR correlated with survival, it did not correlate with tumour-infiltrating lymphocytes [62]. Regarding cytokines and angiogenic factors, serum levels of osteopontin and interleukin 6 were significantly associated with NLR in gastric cancer patients [80]. NLR is significantly associated with helper T lymphocyte Th1/Th2 ratio in blood [65].

2.2.6. Manifestations of invasive growth

Only few scientists have assessed the relations between NLR and such manifestations of invasive growth as perineural, lymphatic and vascular invasion. Theoretically, such association could be hypothesised on the basis of prognostic value of NLR and the correlations between NLR and metastatic cancer spread. However, at present, negative reports predominate although are not unequivocal.

The frequency of perineural growth was not different between high and low NLR groups [22]. The frequency of lymphovascular invasion also was not different between high and low NLR groups in a cohort of 143 metastatic gastric cancer cases [25]. In contrast, vascular or lymphatic invasion was significantly more frequent in patients who had high NLR (exceeding 3.44) assessing 1030 cases of resectable gastric cancer. Hypothetically, the higher capacity for invasive growth could be the reason of more frequent occurrence of R1 in patients presenting with high NLR. However, association between NLR and resection line status (R0 vs. R1 vs. R2) was found by Jung et al., who observed no differences in the frequency of lymphatic, vascular and perineural growth regarding NLR level [53].

2.3. The diagnostic role of NLR and confounding factors

Several haematological parameters, including NLR, are significantly higher in gastric cancer patients than in healthy individuals [18]. A number of studies have confirmed that patients affected by gastric carcinoma have significantly higher NLR than healthy controls [16, 17]. NLR was also higher in gastric cancer patients if compared with persons having adenoma or benign gastrointestinal stromal tumour: 2.17 vs. 1.62. Excluding the confounding factors, NLR was an independent predictor of gastric cancer, associated with the odds ratio of 1.446, $p = 0.005$ [77].

NLR is influenced by smoking [81]. Such differences are reported in gastric cancer patients as well [25] while other researchers have found no difference [47]. Non-oncological diseases, including both inflammations and such frequent non-inflammatory pathologies as diabetes mellitus and atrial fibrillation, among others, can also influence NLR [82]. Thus, SIR should be assessed within the frames of complex patient evaluation.

2.4. Meta-analyses of NLR in gastric cancer

Several meta-analyses of NLR in gastric cancer have been carried out. Sun et al. have assessed 19 studies of NLR in gastric cancer. They confirmed the association between high NLR and worse overall, progression- or cancer-free survival, and higher stage. The predictive role was lost for stage IV patients who received palliative surgery only [21]. Nineteen studies were subjected to meta-analysis by Xin-Ji et al. [37]. Elevated NLR was associated with shorter overall (odds ratio (OR) 1.65; 95% CI = 1.47–1.83) and shorter cancer-free survival (OR 1.61; 95% CI = 1.28–1.94). Regarding the tumour characteristics, NLR was associated with presence of lymph node metastasis, and high T (T3 + T4) and high stage (III–IV). The odds ratio for lymph node metastasis, 1.70 (95% CI = 1.05–2.75), for T3 or T4 cancer 2.93 (95% CI = 2.27–3.78) and for stage III–IV: 1.87 (95% CI = 1.48–2.35) as reported by Xin-Ji et al. [37]. By meta-analysis performed by Chen et al. [36], high NLR was associated with poor overall survival (hazard ratio (HR) 2.16; 95% CI = 1.86–2.51) and progression-free survival (HR 2.78; 95% CI = 1.95–3.96). In a meta-analysis of 10 studies, higher NLR was associated with worse overall (HR 1.83; 95% CI = 1.62–2.07), progression-free (HR 1.54; 95% CI = 1.22–1.95) and cancer-free (HR 1.58; 95% CI = 1.12–2.21) survival [35].

3. Platelet to lymphocyte ratio in gastric cancer

3.1. PLR and survival: prognostic implications

Similarly to NLR, platelet to lymphocyte ratio (PLR) has been evaluated as a prognostic and diagnostic marker of gastric cancer. Although the prognostic role has been shown both in surgically treatable and advanced gastric cancer cases, the data are controversial.

Some research groups have demonstrated that PLR could help to predict overall and cancer-free survival of surgically treated gastric cancer patients. Thus, in 377 patients who underwent curative resection for gastric cancer, high PLR was an independent predictive factor for worse overall survival [64]. In 162 patients diagnosed with resectable gastric cancer, high PLR correlated with decreased both overall and cancer-free survival [16].

Later, evaluating several blood test parameters (PLR, NLR, absolute count and relative proportion of neutrophils and lymphocytes, counts of platelets, white and red blood cells as well as mean platelet volume) in 451 surgically treated gastric cancer patients, high PLR was the only independent prognostic marker for poor overall survival, associated with hazard ratio of 1.4 (95% CI = 1.0–1.9). Hence, in this study preoperative PLR was more informative than NLR [83].

PLR has been successfully implemented in complex prognostic score (along with NLR, see also the further description) in order to assess the prognosis in stage I–II gastric cancer. The created score was an independent predictor of overall survival and retained prognostic significance both in stage I and stage II [31].

In contrast, several studies either preferred the NLR as more informative SIR marker, or failed to identify the independent prognostic role of PLR although significant association with survival parameters was found by univariate analysis. In 389 gastric cancer patients who have undergone gastrectomy, elevated PLR was significantly associated with worse overall, cancer-specific and cancer-free survival. The cut-off was estimated by ROC analysis and was 132. However, as a prognostic factor for overall survival, cancer-specific survival and cancer-free survival, PLR was not superior to NLR [47]. PLR was not an independent prognostic factor for overall survival in large Chinese cohort of 591 gastric cancer patients although it was significantly associated with survival by univariate analysis. In the same study, NLR along with age and TNM stage was shown to be an independent prognostic factor [84]. Assessing 207 gastric cancer patients treated by resection, univariate analysis disclosed significant association of PLR (along with serum CRP, albumin, Glasgow prognostic score (GPS), NLR, cancer grade and TNM stage) with overall survival and cancer-specific survival. However, by multivariate analysis, PLR was not an independent predictor of survival, contrasting with NLR, GPS, TNM stage and cancer grade. Glasgow prognostic score and TNM stage were the most robust of the assessed prognostic parameters [63]. Evaluating different SIR markers, namely, GPS, NLR and PLR, as prognostic variables in 324 patients with resected stage III gastric adenocarcinoma, only Glasgow prognostic score along with TNM stage was independently associated with cancer-free and overall survival while PLR was associated with GPS [43]. By univariate analysis, both NLR and PLR were associated with overall survival of gastric cancer patients after gastrectomy. However, none of these parameters was identified as an independent factor by multivariate analysis in this study [45]. A study of 1986 consecutive gastric cancer patients was directly targeting the issue if PLR of NLR is better as a prognostic factor of gastric cancer. Although high PLR was significantly associated with poor prognosis it was not an independent risk factor for decreased overall survival in contrast to NLR. Thus, NLR was preferred [39].

Finally, negative results are reported. In a multicentre study of 245 gastric cancer patients, PLR was not associated with survival [61].

In advanced gastric cancer, many studies have revealed significant and independent association between PLR and survival. However, controversial findings still are reported.

High PLR (exceeding 160) along with high NLR (reaching or exceeding 2.57) and high absolute number of lymphocytes (reaching or exceeding 1500/mm^3) were significantly associated with shorter median overall survival of 168 locally advanced gastric cancer patients. The median survival in high vs. low PLR groups was 27 vs. 45 months [41].

In advanced unresectable gastric cancer, low PLR (less than 235) correlated with less metastasis and improved response to chemotherapy, longer overall survival and progression-free survival. Changes in PLR after first-line chemotherapy also were indicative of prognosis: survival and response to treatment was better in cases that retained low PLR or switched to low PLR group during treatment [38].

In a cohort of 109 metastatic gastric cancer patients treated by chemotherapy, high PLR (exceeding the cut-off 160) was associated with significantly shorter progression-free and overall survival [67].

In 174 advanced gastric cancer cases treated by chemotherapy, low PLR and normalisation of PLR after one cycle of chemotherapy were independent prognostic markers for better overall survival. Normalisation of PLR was also associated with longer progression-free survival: 5.6 months vs. 3.4 months [57].

In a relatively small study group, PLR lacked prognostic role in 53 patients affected by local gastric cancer and treated with surgery and adjuvant chemotherapy while it had significant prognostic meaning in 50 advanced cases treated by chemotherapy. Interestingly, high platelet count was associated with better overall survival in patients having local disease [56].

Again, many studies have identified significant but not independent association between PLR and survival. In 439 patients affected by metastatic or recurrent gastric cancer, PLR (along with NLR, modified Glasgow prognostic score, previous histology with neural and vascular invasion, albumin, CRP and haemoglobin level) was significantly associated with overall survival, but it was not an independent prognostic factor. In this study design, modified Glasgow prognostic score was the only inflammation-related parameter that was independently associated with survival by multivariate analysis [60]. In 384 patients affected by inoperable advanced or metastatic gastric cancer and treated by palliative chemotherapy, PLR (as well as NLR, leucocytosis, elevated number of neutrophils or platelets, decreased lymphocyte count, hypoalbuminemia, high CRP and Glasgow prognostic score) showed association with overall survival by univariate analysis. By multivariate assessment, PLR had no independent meaning. Only elevated count of neutrophils and Glasgow prognostic score were independent survival predictors by multivariate analysis [68].

As the prognostic role of PLR in gastric cancer is controversial, meta-analyses also have brought contrary opinions. Thus, in a meta-analysis of 8 studies comprising 4513 patients with gastric cancer, there was no association between elevated PLR and overall survival: the hazard ratio was 0.99 (95% CI = 0.9–1.1) as described by Xu et al. [85]. In another meta-analysis comprising 14 cohorts and 6280 cases, PLR was associated with poor overall survival (HR 1.3; 95% CI 1.1–1.5) but not with worse cancer-free survival (HR 1.6; 95% = CI 0.9–2.9). High PLR predicted poor survival in Caucasians, patients receiving chemotherapy and patients at advanced stage [86].

In parallel with NLR research, diversity of cut-off levels have been applied in PLR studies (**Table 3**).

In 377 patients who underwent curative resection for gastric cancer, PLR was independently associated with the development of post-operative complications [64].

3.2. Association with tumour features

3.2.1. Local tumour spread: T

PLR has been evaluated for the association with tumour features, mainly—TNM parameters, representing the oncological mainstay. The association between high PLR and deeper invasion has been confirmed in 162 patients diagnosed with resectable gastric cancer [16], in a larger cohort of 451 surgically treated gastric cancer patients [83] and in a multicentre study of 245 gastric cancer patients [61]. In a meta-analysis of 8 studies comprising 4513 patients with gastric cancer, elevated PLR also showed association with deeper invasion (T3–T4). The relevant odds ratios was 2.01 (95% CI 1.49–2.73) as reported by Xu et al. [85]. In addition, in a large cohort of 451 surgically treated gastric cancer patients, high PLR was associated with larger tumour size [83].

3.2.2. Metastases in regional lymph nodes: N

In patients diagnosed with resectable gastric cancer, high PLR correlated with higher number of lymph node metastases [16]. The association between high PLR and presence of lymph node metastasis was re-confirmed by a meta-analysis of 8 studies comprising 4513 patients with gastric cancer. Elevated PLR showed association with lymph node metastasis with the relevant odds ratio of 1.50 (OR 1.24–1.82) as reported by Xu et al. [85]. In another meta-analysis comprising 14 cohorts and 6280 cases, elevated PLR also was significantly associated with lymph node metastases [86]. However, in a multicentre study of 245 gastric cancer patients, PLR was not associated with N [61].

PLR has been investigated as predictive factor for lymph node metastases in a cohort of surgically treatable gastric cancer comprising 492 patients. PLR was identified as an independent predictive factor for lymph node metastasis and along with other independent prognostic factors that can be determined preoperatively was included in scoring system. This complex

Study group		Cut-off		Study target	Level of justification	Main conclusions	References
Characteristics	Size	Value	Approach				
Patients with confirmed GC diagnosis	103	170	Median	OS	Kaplan-Meier analysis	PLR is associated with worse OS in advanced but not local GC	[56]
Patients with confirmed GC diagnosis	245	160	Ref. [87]	OS	Kaplan-Meier analysis Multicentre study	PLR correlated with T and stage but not survival	[61]
Surgically treated GC							
GC patients subjected to curative resection	873	117	ROC analysis	OS	Kaplan-Meier analysis	Higher PLR is associated with worse OS	[30]
Operable GC patients	492	155.67	ROC analysis	N	Multivariate	PLR was an independent factor predicting N+ and was incorporated in complex score	[55]
Operable patients with early GC	312	106	ROC analysis	N	Multivariate	PLR was an independent factor predicting N+ and was incorporated in complex score	[72]
Surgically treated GC	207	3-tiered complex scoring	ND	OS CFS	Multivariate	PLR was associated with OS and CFS by univariate but not multivariate analysis	[63]
GC patients undergoing gastrectomy	632	140	ROC analysis	OS	Multivariate	PLR was associated with OS by univariate but not multivariate analysis	[45]

Study group		Cut-off		Study target	Level of justification	Main conclusions	References
Characteristics	Size	Value	Approach				
Resectable GC	162	208	Median	OS, CFS	Kaplan-Meier analysis	Higher PLR is associated with worse OS and CFS	[16]
GC treated by total or subtotal gastrectomy with lymphadenectomy	389	132	ROC analysis	OS, CFS, CSS	Multivariate	Higher PLR is significantly associated with worse OS, CFS, CSS	[47]
Advanced, unresectable and/or metastatic GC							
Unresectable, advanced GC, treated by chemotherapy	120	235	Median	OS PFS	Kaplan-Meier analysis Multivariate	Higher baseline PLR or increase of PLR after first-line chemotherapy is associated with worse OS and CFS	[38]
Unresectable, advanced GC, treated by chemotherapy	120	235	Median	Response to chemotherapy	χ^2 test	Lower baseline PLR or lower PLR after first-line chemotherapy was associated with improved response to chemotherapy	[38]
Metastatic GC treated by chemotherapy	109	160	Refs. [40, 58]	OS PFS	Kaplan-Meier analysis	High PLR is significantly associated with worse OS and PFS	[67]

Abbreviations: GC, gastric cancer; OS, overall survival; PLR, platelet to lymphocyte ratio; Ref, reference; T, local spread of primary gastric cancer by tumour-nodes-metastasis (TNM) classification; ROC, receiver operating characteristic curve; N, regional lymph node status in respect to metastases by (TNM) classification; N+, presence of metastases in regional lymph nodes; ND, no data available; CFS, cancer-free survival; CSS, cancer-specific survival.

Table 3. Cut-offs of PLR in gastric cancer studies.

score consisted of NLR (cut-off 1.59), PLR (cut-off 155.67), T/depth of invasion, macroscopic type according to Bormann and tumour size [55].

As previously outlined, lymph node status is crucial to select the most appropriate treatment in early gastric cancer. PLR has been analysed in this context. In a retrospective assessment of 312 early gastric cancer cases subjected to surgical treatment, high PLR along with high NLR was significantly associated with lymph node metastases. Although both PLR and NLR showed this association by univariate analysis, only PLR was identified as an independent risk factor by multivariate analysis. Thus PLR, but not NLR was included in a complex score. The scoring system was based on the identified independent risk factors: PLR (cut-off 106, based on ROC analysis), age, tumour size, grade and depth of invasion and successfully validated in a prospective training set [72].

3.2.3. TNM stage

In patients diagnosed with resectable gastric cancer, high PLR correlated with higher stage [16]. The association between high PLR and higher stage was confirmed in a multicentre study of 245 gastric cancer patients [61]. When a meta-analysis of 8 studies was performed comprising data on 4513 patients with gastric cancer, elevated PLR showed association with advanced cancer stage (III–IV). The relevant odds ratios was 1.99 (95% CI 1.60–2.46) as reported by Xu et al. [85].

Generally, PLR can accurately reflect tumour burden. In the study carried out by Cetinkunar et al., the 228 cases were classified as early vs. advanced and non-metastatic vs. metastatic ones. PLR could discriminate the groups in both models. The mean PLR values were 160.3 in early and 231.6 in advanced gastric cancer; 192.7 in non-metastatic and 251.0 in metastatic cases [88].

3.3. The diagnostic role of PLR

The diagnostic role of PLR has been explored as well. Thus, the mean values of PLR were significantly higher in gastric cancer patients than in healthy controls [16, 18]. The parameter might seem promising as it is not affected by smoking in contrast to NLR [81].

3.4. Meta-analyses of PLR in gastric cancer

Several meta-analyses of PLR have been devoted to PLR in gastric cancer, yielding partially conflicting results. In a meta-analysis of 8 studies comprising 4513 cases of gastric carcinoma, elevated PLR correlated with lymph node metastasis, deeper invasion (T3–T4) and advanced cancer stage (III–IV) but it was not predictor of overall survival. The relevant odds ratios were 1.50 (95% CI = 1.24–1.82) for N+, 2.01 (95% CI = 1.49–2.73) for T3–T4 and 1.99 (95% CI = 1.60–2.46) for stage III–IV [85].

Fourteen cohorts and 6280 cases were re-evaluated within the frames of another meta-analysis. Authors found out that PLR was associated with poor overall survival but not with cancer-free survival. High PLR predicted poor survival in Caucasians, patients receiving chemotherapy and patients at advanced stage. Despite the controversies regarding survival, the association with lymph node metastases was reconfirmed [86].

Zhou et al. carried out a general meta-analysis devoted to the prognostic value of PLR in different cancers [89]. There was significant association between elevated PLR and worse overall survival (hazard ratio 1.60; 95% CI = 1.35–1.90). In the subgroup of gastric cancer, the HR was 1.35 (95% CI 0.80–2.25).

4. Peripheral blood monocytes in gastric cancer assessment

Although macrophages are a significant component of tumour microenvironment, quite few studies have been devoted to the prognostic role of monocytes in relation with other cells in peripheral blood of gastric cancer patients.

However, in a recent large study enrolling 3243 gastric cancer patients, high monocyte to white cell ratio (MWR) was identified as an independent prognostic factor of poor survival. In the same study, high NLR, high PLR, high monocyte to lymphocyte ratio, high neutrophil to white cell ratio, low lymphocyte to white cell ratio (LWR) were associated with survival in univariate analysis, but only low LWR and high MWR were independent prognostic factors for poor survival [90].

In gastric cancer patients who have undergone gastrectomy, decreased lymphocyte to monocyte ratio (LMR) was significantly associated with worse overall survival, cancer-specific survival and cancer-free survival. The cut-off was estimated by ROC analysis and was 4.95. However, as a prognostic factor for overall survival, cancer-specific survival and cancer-free survival, LMR was not superior to NLR [47].

5. Glasgow prognostic score in gastric cancer

Glasgow prognostic score is considered the prognostic milestone of SIR assessment in malignant tumours [91]. It is detected on the basis of the prototypic acute phase protein, C-reactive protein and albumin levels in blood serum. CRP is a non-specific, but sensitive marker of systemic inflammatory response, produced as a response to pro-inflammatory cytokines including interleukins IL-1 and IL-6 as well as tumour necrosis factor TNF. Hypoalbuminemia can be caused by malnutrition and cancer cachexia or by systemic inflammation [68]. GPS includes both estimates of elevated acute phase response and malnutrition, resulting in considerable sensitivity [68]. Later, two alterations of Glasgow prognostic score have been developed—the modified GPS and high-sensitivity GPS. In the modified GPS, albumin level influences the score only if CRP is increased [31]. However, the definitions also show variability between authors [92]. High-sensitivity GPS differs from the original GPS by lower cut-off level for CRP [93]. The definitions of GPS and its modifications are summarised in **Table 4**.

5.1. Glasgow prognostic score and survival

Glasgow prognostic score has high informativity both in surgically treatable and advanced, unresectable and/or metastatic gastric cancer. Thus, evaluating Glasgow prognostic score, NLR and PLR in 324 patients with resected stage III gastric adenocarcinoma, only Glasgow prognostic score along with TNM stage was independently associated with overall and cancer-free survival [43]. In 207 gastric cancer patients who underwent surgery, GPS along with NLR, PLR, CRP, albumin and TNM stage were significantly associated with overall and cancer-free

Score	Definition	References
Glasgow prognostic score		[68]
0	CRP < 10 mg/L AND albumin ≥ 35 g/L	
1	One high-risk finding: CRP ≥ 10 mg/L OR albumin < 35 g/L	
2	Both high-risk findings: CRP ≥ 10 mg/L AND albumin < 35 g/L	
Modified Glasgow prognostic score		[31] [94]
0	CRP ≤ 10 mg/L irrespective of albumin level	
1	Increased CRP on the background of normal albumin level: CRP > 10 mg/L AND albumin ≥ 35 g/L	
2	Increased CRP and hypoalbuminemia: CRP > 10 mg/L AND albumin < 35 g/L	
Modified Glasgow prognostic score by Hirashima et al.		[92]
0	CRP ≤ 5 mg/L AND albumin ≥ 38 g/L	
1	One high-risk finding: CRP > 5 mg/L OR albumin < 38 g/L	
2	Both high-risk findings: CRP > 5 mg/L AND albumin < 38 g/L	
High-sensitivity Glasgow prognostic score		[93]
0	CRP ≤ 3 mg/L AND albumin ≥ 35 g/L	
1	One high-risk finding: CRP > 3 mg/L OR albumin < 35 g/L	
2	Both high-risk findings: CRP > 3 mg/L AND albumin < 35 g/L	

Abbreviations: CRP, C-reactive protein.

Table 4. Glasgow prognostic score and its modifications.

survival. However, only GPS and TNM were independent prognostic factors; therefore in this study, GPS was favoured as the most informative SIR parameter [63]. By multivariate analysis, GPS was independent predictor of overall survival in 425 surgically treated gastric cancer patients who had normal serum levels of carcinoembryonic antigen [91]. In a large cohort of 1017 patients subjected to curative resection of gastric cancer, GPS was an independent prognostic factor for overall survival [95].

In a homogeneous group of 88 gastric cancer patients undergoing only surgical treatment, increasing GPS was an independent predictor of worse overall survival and perioperative mortality. The median survival by GPS 0 vs. 1 vs. 2 was 25.2 vs. 15.3 vs. 5.8 months. The perioperative mortality in the same subgroups was 0.0% vs. 20.0% vs. 80.0% [96]. However, the GPS capacity to predict complications is not straightforward. In contrast with the previous report, assessing 1017 patients subjected to curative resection of gastric cancer, GPS was not associated with the incidence of complications [95].

Variations of GPS have been successfully tested. In a large group of 236 gastric cancer patients who underwent gastrectomy, high-sensitivity GPS after surgery was a significant prognostic factor for overall survival while the pre-operative level was less informative [93]. Modified Glasgow prognostic score was an independent prognostic factor for overall and cancer-free survival in 102 consecutive gastric cancer patients treated with resection [97]. Modified GPS was independent predictor of cancer-specific survival in 120 surgically treated gastric cancer patients [98]. The role of modified GPS in stage IV gastric cancer was confirmed by Mimatsu et al., who evaluated cancer-specific survival in 42 patients at stage IV, treated by palliative gastrectomy and chemotherapy. The modified GPS was associated with cancer-specific survival [99]. Pre-operative modified GPS retained prognostic value in elderly patients [92]. Assessing 1710 surgically treated patients with gastric cancer, modified GPS was associated with post-operative mortality [94]. However, high-sensitivity modified GPS was found to be superior prognostic predictor for overall survival compared to modified GPS having especially high prognostic importance in stage I and IV [100].

By some study designs, the informativity of GPS has been estimated lower. In comparison with NLR-PLR score, modified Glasgow prognostic index was not an independent prognostic factor for survival of stage I–I gastric cancer patients [31]. In 224 patients receiving chemotherapy for advanced gastric cancer, NLR and diffuse type histology were independent prognostic factors for overall survival while GPS was not. However, the median survival still was significantly longer in patients having GPS 0 in contrast to those having GPS 1 or 2 [24].

GPS and its variations retain the prognostic value in advanced cases. In 402 patients with advanced gastric adenocarcinoma treated by palliative chemotherapy, GPS was an independent predictor of overall survival [101]. GPS was an independent predictor of cancer-specific and progression-free survival in 83 patients having advanced gastric cancer and receiving chemotherapy. In low GPS group, favourable response to chemotherapy can be obtained [102]. In patients affected by stage IV gastric cancer and treated by chemotherapy, higher modified Glasgow prognostic score was associated with shorter overall survival (along with lower level of albumin, elevated concentration of C-reactive protein, high absolute number of neutrophilic leukocytes and elevated NLR). In multivariate analysis, modified Glasgow prognostic score was identified as an independent prognostic factor along with NLR, presence of lymph node metastasis and histological subtype [69]. In 68 patients affected by advanced gastric cancer and treated by chemotherapy with or without irradiation, high GPS predicted shorter survival [103]. High GPS was an independent prognostic factor in 384 inoperable advanced or metastatic gastric cancer patients treated with chemotherapy. The value of GPS was higher than that of NLR, PLR or CRP [68]. In 125 patients with recurrent or metastatic gastric cancer placed on single agent chemotherapy because of poor performance status, GPS had independent prognostic value [104]. In 91 metastatic or recurrent gastric cancer patients treated by palliative chemotherapy, GPS was significantly associated with survival. The differences were also biologically remarkable: the median survival was 12.3 months if GPS was 0 but only 2.9 if GPS was 2 [105].

Recently, a meta-analysis was carried out including 14 studies and 5579 gastric cancer patients. High GPS was significantly associated with poor overall survival (hazard ratio 1.51; 95% CI 1.37–1.66), and disease-free survival (HR 1.45; 95% CI = 1.26–1.68) as reported by Zhang et al. [106].

Glasgow prognostic score has been further developed into different complex scores. Thus, complex predictive score regarding survival was elaborated, based on NLR and modified Glasgow prognostic score in patients with metastatic gastric adenocarcinoma treated by chemotherapy, after independent prognostic value of both parameters was justified in a group of 256 patients [26]. The design of studies devoted to GPS in gastric carcinoma is summarised in **Table 5**.

5.2. Association with tumour features

5.2.1. Local tumour spread: T

In 88 patients undergoing only surgical treatment, increasing GPS was associated with higher T and resection line status [96]. In a recent meta-analysis, association between high GPS and high TNM stage was found. Although the association with lymph node metastases (OR 4.60; 95% CI = 3.23–6.56) was significant, there was no association with T [106].

5.2.2. Metastases in regional lymph nodes: N

In a recent meta-analysis including 14 studies and 5579 gastric cancer patients, high GPS was significantly associated with presence of lymph node metastases (OR 4.60; 95% CI = 3.23–6.56) as well as with lymphatic (OR 3.04; 95% CI = 2.00–4.62) invasion [106].

5.2.3. Presence of distant metastases: M

In a homogeneous group of 88 gastric cancer patients undergoing only surgical treatment, increasing GPS was associated with presence of synchronous distant metastases and venous invasion [96].

Group		Score	Target	References
Characteristics	Size			
Meta-analysis	14 studies 5579 patients	GPS	OS, CFS TNM stage, N Lymphatic invasion Venous invasion	[106]
Meta-analysis	7 studies 3206 patients	mGPS	OS Lymphatic invasion Venous invasion	[109]
Original studies of surgically treated GC				
Stage I–II GC, treated by curative resection	305	mGPS	OS	[31]
GC undergoing surgical treatment only	88	GPS	T, M, R; Venous invasion Perioperative mortality OS	[96]
GC patients subjected to surgical treatment	207	GPS	OS	[63]
Surgically treated GC patients with normal CEA level	425	GPS	OS	[91]
GC patients subjected to gastrectomy	236	HS-GPS	Clinical and pathological parameters OS	[93]
GC patients subjected to gastrectomy	552	GPS HS-GPS	Clinical and pathological parameters OS	[100]
Consecutive GC patients undergoing surgical treatment	102	mGPS	OS CFS	[97]
GC patients subjected to gastrectomy	294	mGPS	OS	[92]
Surgically treated GC patients	1017	GPS	OS Post-operative complications	[95]
Surgically treated GC patients	1710	mGPS	OS	[94]
Surgically treated GC patients	120	mGPS	CSS	[98]
Surgically treated GC patients, stage III	324	GPS	CFS OS	[43]

Group		Score	Target	References
Characteristics	Size			
Original studies of advanced GC				
Chemotherapy for advanced GC	224	GPS	OS	[24]
Advanced GC treated with chemo- or chemoradiotherapy	68	GPS	OS	[103]
Metastatic GC treated by chemotherapy	256	mGPS	OS	[26]
GC patients at stage IV, treated by palliative gastrectomy	42	mGPS	CSS	[99]
Metastatic or recurrent GC patients considered for palliative chemotherapy	91	GPS	OS	[105]
Inoperable advanced or metastatic GC patients receiving first-line chemotherapy	384	GPS	OS	[68]
Advanced GC patients treated by single agent palliative chemotherapy due to poor performance	125	GPS	OS	[104]
Metastatic GC treated by palliative chemotherapy	104	mGPS	OS	[69]
Advanced GC treated by chemotherapy	83	GPS	CSS, PFS	[102]
Advanced recurrent or metastatic GC patients receiving first-line palliative chemotherapy	402	GPS	PFS OS	[101]
GC patients with vs. without cachexia vs. controls	90 (30 vs. 30 vs. 30)	GPS	Cachexia, adipokines	[107]
Inoperable GC subjected to chemotherapy	71	GPS	Predicting metastasis	[108]

Abbreviations: GC, gastric cancer; mGPS, modified Glasgow prognostic score; OS, overall survival; GPS, Glasgow prognostic score; T, local tumour spread by tumour-nodes-metastasis (TNM) classification; M, presence of distant metastasis by TNM classification; R, resection line status; CEA, carcinoembryonic protein; HS-GPS, high sensitivity Glasgow prognostic score; CFS, cancer-free survival; CSS; cancer-free survival; PFS, progression-free survival; TNM, tumour-nodes-metastasis classification; vs, versus; N, regional lymph node status by TNM classification.

Table 5. The design of studies devoted to Glasgow prognostic score in gastric cancer.

5.2.4. TNM stage

Assessing 1710 patients with gastric cancer, modified GPS was associated with advanced stage [94]. Elevated GPS has been reported in gastric cancer patients having cachexia; higher stage was also observed in cachectic patients [107]. However, GPS did not differ between metastatic and non-metastatic gastric cancer cases. Although the study group was small consisting of only 43 metastatic and 28 non-metastatic cases, a novel score based on pre-albumin and CRP, showed significant differences [108]. In a recent meta-analysis including 14 studies and 5579 gastric cancer patients, elevated GPS was significantly associated with high TNM stage (odds ratio 3.09; 95% CI = 2.11–4.53) as reported by Zhang et al. [106].

5.2.5. Manifestations of invasive growth

In a homogeneous group of 88 gastric cancer patients undergoing only surgical treatment, increasing GPS was associated with presence of venous invasion [96]. In a recent meta-analysis including 14 studies and 5579 gastric cancer patients, high GPS was significantly associated with lymphatic (OR 3.04; 95% CI = 2.00–4.62) and venous (OR 3.56; 95% CI = 1.81–6.99) invasion [106]. In a meta-analysis devoted to the modified Glasgow prognostic score, higher rates of lymphatic (OR 2.51; 95% CI = 1.80–3.51) and venous (OR 2.63; 95% CI = 1.35–5.11) invasion were found in patients in whom the score was at least 1 [109].

5.3. Meta-analyses of Glasgow prognostic score and its modifications in gastric cancer

Recently, a meta-analysis was carried including 14 studies and 5579 gastric cancer patients. High GPS was significantly associated with poor overall survival (hazard ratio 1.51; 95% CI 1.37–1.66), and disease-free survival (HR 1.45; 95% CI = 1.26–1.68) as well as with high TNM stage (odds ratio 3.09; 95% CI = 2.11–4.53), N+ (OR 4.60; 95% CI = 3.23–6.56), lymphatic (OR 3.04; 95% CI = 2.00–4.62) and venous (OR 3.56; 95% CI = 1.81–6.99) invasion [106].

In a meta-analysis devoted to the modified Glasgow prognostic score, worse overall survival (odds ratio OR 2.54; 95% CI = 1.62–3.98 for mGPS = 1 and OR 12.02; 95% CI 6.79–21.28 for mGPS = 2), higher rates of lymphatic (OR 2.51; 95% CI = 1.80–3.51) and venous (OR 2.63; 95% CI = 1.35–5.11) invasion were found in patients in whom the score was not zero [109].

6. Fibrinogen in gastric cancer evaluation

The association between malignant solid tumours and disturbances of blood clotting is well-known. In addition, fibrinogen is an acute phase reactant glycoprotein [110]. Consequently, the presence of hyperfibrinogenaemia in gastric cancer patients can be almost expected. Indeed, increased levels of fibrinogen have been identified and explored regarding the prognostic value or the association with tumour parameters. The studies range from historical to up-to-dated and cover aspects of patient's survival, tumour progression, diagnostic value, estimates of tumour burden and insights into novel treatment options.

Elevated concentration of fibrinogen in the serum of gastric carcinoma patients has negative prognostic value regarding several aspects of survival—overall and cancer-free survival. The independent prognostic value of increased fibrinogen level has been demonstrated in 351 surgically treated gastric cancer patients. The hazard ratio was 2.61 (95% CI = 1.18–5.76) as reported by Suzuki et al. [111]. The independent prognostic role was confirmed in another large surgically treated cohort of 1196 gastric cancer patients [112]. Applying ROC-identified cut-off (3.9 g/L), high fibrinogen level was significantly associated with overall survival in multivariate analysis [113]. In patients who underwent curative gastrectomy, hyperfibrinogenaemia (reaching or exceeding 350 mg/dL) was associated not only with overall but also cancer-free survival. By multivariate analysis, fibrinogen level again was an independent prognostic factor along with pTN [33].

Classic studies have explored the diagnostic meaning of hyperfibrinogenaemia resulting in conclusion that fibrinogen level is significantly elevated in gastric cancer patients but not in individuals having gastric or duodenal peptic ulcer. Such reports stem back as far as to 1975 [114]. Later, it was repeatedly confirmed that fibrinogen levels in gastric cancer are higher than in controls, even if the tumour was non-metastatic. The mean levels in cancer patients vs. control individuals were 505 vs. 336 mg/dL [115]. Nowadays, the ongoing research has identified fibrinogen fragments that could potentially serve as serum markers of gastric cancer. Fibrinogen fragments, e.g., carboxyl terminal fraction of fibrinogen alpha, have been tested as a serum marker of gastric cancer in comparison with healthy controls and individuals affected by chronic gastritis [116, 117].

A 15-amino acid peptide of the fibrinogen alpha chain, fibrinostatin, has anti-angiogenic properties; thus therapeutic applications have been hypothesised [118].

Regarding the local events within the tumour, fibrinogen has been identified in tumour stroma as early as 1984 [119, 120] while fibrin and D-dimers are found in the invasive front [120].

Fibrinogen level parallels the tumour burden, correlates with advanced TNM stage [112] and is associated with adjacent organ involvement [121]. In a recent considerable cohort of 1090 gastric cancer patients treated by gastrectomy, high fibrinogen level (exceeding the ROC-identified cut-off at 3.9 g/L) was significantly associated with tumour size, T, N and TNM stage [113]. Fibrinogen shows statistically significant associations with the invasion depth of gastric cancer confirmed by several other studies focusing on T [122–124]. Several studies have identified meaningful association with presence of metastasis in lymph nodes [122–124]. The association with tumour spread has also been confirmed, regarding the presence of distant metastases [122].

The logical next step is incorporation of fibrinogen measurements into combined scores that could be used to assess the prognosis or tumour spread. A complex score comprising evaluation of hyperfibrinogenemia (exceeding 400 mg/dL) and elevated NLR (exceeding 3.0) was associated with shorter survival. The combined score showed significantly different results in patients developing progressive disease despite chemotherapy or chemoradiotherapy [103]. Similar score comprising evaluation of hyperfibrinogenemia (reaching or exceeding 305 mg/dL) and elevated NLR (reaching or exceeding 2.34) was significantly associated with invasion depth, lymph node metastasis, lymphovascular invasion and stage [110]. Coagulation score based on the assessment of fibrinogen and D-dimer levels, was significantly associated with overall and cancer-free survival as well as with recurrence and development of liver metastases [125].

Other blood clotting parameters show similar associations with patient's prognosis and tumour burden. Thus, D-dimers [126, 127] and thrombocytosis [128] have prognostic role in gastric cancer. In turn, D-dimers and prothrombin time are associated with lymph node involvement [129].

7. Application of SIR in complex scoring systems for gastric cancer

SIR parameters have been incorporated in diverse complex scores that allow reaching higher diagnostic value (see also **Tables 6–7**).

A complex score, based on fibrinogen (cut-off 400 mg/dL) and NLR (cut-off 3.0) levels, was applied to predict the effect of chemotherapy or chemoradiotherapy in advanced gastric cancer. The created score indeed was significantly higher in patients having cancer progression during treatment; it also was an independent prognostic factor by multivariate analysis [103]. The same authors have elaborated similar combined score, based on the same parameters which by different cut-off levels are adjusted for another research target. The fibrinogen-NLR score at cut-off 305 mg/dL and 2.34, respectively, was significantly associated with depth of tumour invasion, lymph node metastasis, lymphatic and venous invasion and tumour stage. The 5-year survival rates by score categories 0 vs. 1 vs. 2 were 92.9, 84.1 and 66.5%; the differences being statistically significant [110].

The coagulation score, recently proposed by Kanda et al., distinguished high-risk patients having low overall and cancer-free survival. High coagulation score was also an independent prognostic factor for recurrence and was associated with liver metastasis as the initial recurrence [125]. It is in accordance with the observation that D-dimer is associated with metastatic tumour spread both in murine gastric carcinoma models and in patients having visceral metastasis [130].

The score developed by Ishizuka et al. was based on platelet count and NLR to predict post-operative survival. The score classified patients into 3 groups: 0 vs. 1 vs. 2 had post-operative survival of 1676 vs. 1310 vs. 1050 days. The differences were statistically significant. The cancer-specific survival also was significantly different by the score levels. The sensitivity and accuracy of the presented score in regard to survival was higher than the informativity of clinical and pathological parameters—carcinoembryonic antigen CEA, CA19-9, venous and lymphatic invasion and lymph node metastasis [29].

NLR-PLR score can be used to assess overall survival in gastric cancer patients diagnosed at stage I–II. This score was an independent prognostic factor while mGPS, the prognostic nutritional index and combination of platelet count and NLR were not. The score had the highest area under ROC curve in comparison with the listed other scores. The hazard ratio associated with NLR-PLR score was 1.51 (95% CI = 1.02–2.24). Interestingly, there was a trend to shorter mean OS in stage I patients having NLR-PLR score of 2 than in stage II patients scored 0: 89 months vs. 127 months. The score retained prognostic value in stage I and II [31].

Target	Score description	References
Lymph node metastases in early gastric cancer	PLR (cut-off 106, based on ROC analysis), age, grade, depth of invasion and tumour size	[72]
Survival of early gastric cancer patients	NLR (cut-off 2.1), PLR (cut-off 120)	[31]
Lymph node metastases	Independent predictive factors (for lymph node metastasis) that can be determined preoperatively: NLR (cut-off 1.59), PLR (cut-off 155.67), T/depth of invasion, macroscopic type (Bormann), tumour size	[55]
Overall survival	Albumin (cut-off 35 g/L), NLR (cut-off 2.3)	[30]
Cancer-specific survival (CSS) and cancer-free survival (CFS)	Nomogram including independent predicting factors: (1) for CSS: NLR, age, tumour stage, presence of lymph node metastases, presence of distant metastases; (2) for CFS: NLR, tumour stage, presence of distant metastases, family history of gastric cancer; CA 19-9 level.	[47]
Overall survival and chemotherapy response	NLR (cut-off 3.0) and fibrinogen (cut-off 400 mg/dL)	[103]
Prognosis and cancer characteristics	NLR (cut-off 2.34) and fibrinogen (cut-off 305 mg/dL)	[110]
Overall survival	Canton score: [1]prognostic nutritional index (PNI; cut-off 48), platelet count (cut-off 3×10^{11}/L) and NLR (cut-off 1.83)	[45]
Overall and cancer-specific survival	Platelet count and NLR	[29]
Overall and cancer-free survival Recurrence Metachronous liver metastases	Coagulation score: increased level of fibrinogen and D-dimers	[125]
Overall survival	NLR, mGPS and patient-generated subjective global assessment score	[26]

Abbreviations: PLR, platelet to lymphocyte ratio; ROC, receiver operating characteristic curve; NLR, neutrophil to lymphocyte ratio; T, local spread of primary gastric cancer by tumour-nodes-metastasis (TNM) classification; CSS, cancer-specific survival; CFS, cancer-free survival; mGPS, modified Glasgow prognostic score.

[1]PNI = albumin (g/L) + 5 × total lymphocyte count ($\times 10^9$/L).

Table 6. Application of SIR in complex scoring systems for gastric cancer.

The score based on albumin and NLR was elaborated to improve the evaluation of overall survival. The resulting score was independently associated with overall survival. It had higher diagnostic value than NLR, PLR and GPS, as shown by higher area under ROC curve. The overall survival by score values 0 vs. 1 vs. 2 was 44.9% vs. 29.8% vs. 20.3%, respectively [30].

Modified Glasgow prognostic score [31]	
0	CRP ≤ 10 mg/L irrespectively of albumin level
1	Albumin ≥ 35 g/L AND CRP > 10 mg/L
2	Albumin < 35 g/L AND CRP > 10 mg/L
Albumin—NLR score [30]	
0	Albumin ≥ 35 g/L AND NLR < 2.3
1	Albumin ≥ 35 g/L AND NLR ≥ 2.3 OR Albumin < 35 g/L AND NLR < 2.3
2	Albumin < 35 g/L AND NLR ≥ 2.3
NLR—PLR score [31]	
0	Both values are low: NLR < 2.1 AND PLR < 120
1	Only one elevated value: NLR ≥ 2.1 AND PLR < 120 OR NLR < 2.1 AND PLR ≥ 120
2	Both values are elevated: NLR ≥ 2.1 AND PLR ≥ 120
Inflammation and nutrition based score [26]	
0–2	Favourable group
3–4	Intermediate risk
5–6	High risk
	Definitions of the score components: NLR > 3 equals 1, otherwise scored 0 mGPS > 1 equals 3, otherwise scored 0 Patient-Generated Subjective Global Assessment C equals 2, otherwise (A or B) scored 0
Hyperfibrinogenemia—NLR score [103]	
0	NLR ≤ 3.0 AND fibrinogen ≤ 400 mg/dL
1	NLR >3.0 OR fibrinogen > 400 mg/dL
2	NLR >3.0 AND fibrinogen > 400 mg/dL
Hyperfibrinogenemia—NLR score II [110]	
0	NLR < 2.34 AND fibrinogen > 305 mg/dL
1	NLR ≥ 2.34 OR fibrinogen ≥ 305 mg/dL
2	NLR ≥ 2.34 AND fibrinogen ≥ 305 mg/dL
Combined score to predict lymph node metastases [55]	
0–155	Low risk
>156	High risk
	Definitions of the score components: Tumour size ≥ 3 cm scored 39, otherwise scored 0 Macroscopic type: early vs. Borrmann I–II vs. Borrmann III–IV scored 0 vs. 32 vs. 59 PLR > 155.67 scored 28, otherwise scored 0 NLR > 1.59 scored 28, otherwise scored 0 Depth of invasion: T3—4 scored 60, otherwise scored 0
Combined score to predict lymph node metastases [72]	
0–11	Low risk

12–20	High risk
	Definitions of the score components: Age ≥ 65 scored 3, otherwise scored 0 Tumour size ≥ 1.8 cm scored 4, otherwise scored 0 Grade: G3 scored 5, otherwise scored 0 Depth of invasion: submucosa scored 3, while mucosa scored 0 PLR > 106 scored 3, otherwise scored 0
Canton score [45]	
0	No high-risk parameters: [1]PNI ≥ 48 AND NLR ≤ 1.83 AND PLT ≤ 3 × 10^{11}/L
1	One high-risk parameter: PNI < 48 AND NLR ≤ 1.83 AND PLT ≤ 3 × 10^{11}/L PNI ≥ 48 AND NLR > 1.83 AND PLT ≤ 3 × 10^{11}/L PNI ≥ 48 AND NLR ≤ 1.83 AND PLT > 3 × 10^{11}/L
2	Two high-risk parameters: PNI < 48 AND NLR > 1.83 AND PLT ≤ 3 × 10^{11}/L PNI < 48 AND NLR ≤ 1.83 AND PLT > 3 × 10^{11}/L PNI ≥ 48 AND NLR > 1.83 AND PLT > 3 × 10^{11}/L
3	Three high-risk parameters: PNI < 48 AND NLR > 1.83 AND PLT > 3 × 10^{11}/L
Platelet count and NLR score [29]	
0	No elevated parameters: PLT ≤ 300 × 10^3/mkL AND NLR ≤ 3
1	One elevated parameter: PLT > 300 × 10^3/mkL OR NLR >3
2	Two elevated parameters: PLT > 300 × 10^3/mkL AND NLR >3
Coagulation score [125]	
0	Normal level of D-dimer AND fibrinogen
1	Increased level of either D-dimer OR fibrinogen
2	Increased level of both D-dimer AND fibrinogen

Abbreviations: CRP, C-reactive protein; NLR, neutrophil to lymphocyte ratio; PLR, platelet to lymphocyte ratio; mGPS, modified Glasgow prognostic score; T, local spread of primary gastric cancer by tumour-nodes-metastasis (TNM classification), G, grade; PNI, prognostic nutritional index; PLT, platelet count.

[1]PNI = albumin (g/L) + 5 × total lymphocyte count (×10^9/L).

Table 7. The definitions of complex scores.

The inflammation and nutrition-based score was elaborated to predict overall survival in patients diagnosed with metastatic gastric cancer. According to this score, patients were classified into favourable, intermediate and high-risk groups exhibiting the median overall survival of 27.6 vs. 13.2 vs. 8.2 months. The respective two-year survival rates were 52% vs. 16% vs. 3%. The ROC curve analysis confirmed that the novel score has higher informativity than any of its components [26].

Deng et al. elaborated complex nomograms to predict cancer-specific and cancer-free survival in surgically treated gastric cancer patients [47].

Pang et al. developed complex system to predict lymph node metastases based on those tumour and systemic parameters that were independently associated with N+ and could be detected preoperatively. The point system was based on hazard ratios detected by logistic regression analysis. Youden Index was applied to detect the cut-off of the novel combined system. Finally, the developed score had specifity of 72.4%, sensitivity 82.7%, positive predictive value 88.7% and negative predictive value 61.5%. Besides the informative value of the score itself, the mathematical model of score design is flawless [55].

Lou et al. developed score to predict lymph node metastases in early gastric cancer. The scoring system reached reasonable accuracy of 0.817 when evaluating prospective cases [72].

The Canton score was created to predict overall survival after gastrectomy. The novel score possessed higher AUC than the classic parameters. The HR for Canton score values 1 vs. 2 vs. 3 (in comparison to 0) were 1.08 (95% CI = 0.80–1.45) vs. 1.55 (95% CI = 1.15–2.10) vs. 1.64 (95% CI = 1.14–2.36) as reported by Sun et al. [45].

8. Conclusions

Gastric cancer induces systemic inflammatory reaction. The biological background is complex, involving bone marrow activation, development of immune-suppressing immature myeloid cells, generation of pre-metastatic niches and neutrophil extracellular trap formation from externalised DNA network in bidirectional association with platelet activation. These mechanisms have been demonstrated in general studies of carcinogenesis as well as in animal models and human studies of gastric cancer.

Systemic inflammatory reaction can be easily evaluated by simple, patient friendly and economically non-demanding blood tests practically lacking complications. These tests could be broadly classified as cellular and protein-based. Among cellular tests, neutrophil to lymphocyte ratio is the most widely explored followed by platelet to lymphocyte ratio. Glasgow prognostic score is the prototype of protein-based test.

Although controversies still exist, most researchers have recognised the independent prognostic value of NLR, encompassing overall, cancer-specific, cancer-free or progression-free survival both in early and advanced gastric cancer. NLR can bring significant prognostic information in surgically treated individuals, in case of combined treatment and in patients receiving only chemotherapy.

NLR shows associations with TNM parameters. Thus, it can be incorporated in patient's evaluation for tumour burden. The possibility to predict serosal invasion, peritoneal and/or metastatic spread can be an adjunct to avoid inappropriate attempts of technically impossible gastrectomy. Lymph node status can be predicted as well.

PLR and GPS also possess diagnostic and prognostic information in gastric cancer patients, as well as show correlations with tumour parameters.

The cut-offs for NLR and PLR show significant variability. Mostly, the cut-off levels are identified either based on ROC analysis and Youden Index, or the median is selected for cut-off. Less frequently, the 75th percentile is applied.

Combined scores appear, based on SIR data in complex with patient's characteristics as well as tumour features. The informativity of such scores is generally higher than that of separate components; therefore, wider testing of these scores in different populations should be necessary to bring the promising novel scores to clinical application.

Abbreviations

AUC	Area under curve
CD	Cluster of differentiation
CEA	Carcinoembryonic antigen
CI	Confidence interval
CRP	C-reactive protein
DNA	Deoxyribonucleic acid
ECOG	Eastern Cooperative Oncology Group
G	Grade
GPS	Glasgow prognostic score
HR	Hazard ratio
IL	Interleukin
LMR	Lymphocyte to monocyte ratio
LWR	Lymphocyte to white cell ratio
M	Presence or absence of distant metastases in accordance with TNM classification
mGPS	Modified Glasgow prognostic score
MWR	Monocyte to white cell ratio
N	Status of regional lymph nodes regarding metastases in accordance with TNM classification
NLR	Neutrophil to lymphocyte ratio
OR	Odds ratio
PLR	Platelet to lymphocyte ratio

R	Resection line status regarding presence or absence of tumour
ROC	Receiver operating characteristics
SIR	Systemic inflammatory reaction
T	Local tumour spread in accordance with TNM classification
TNF	Tumour necrosis factor
TNM	Tumour-node-metastasis classification to reflect the extent of tumour growth and spread
USA	The United States of America
vs.	versus

Author details

Ilze Strumfa[1]*, Tatjana Bogdanova[1], Arturs Kalva[1], Boriss Strumfs[2], Roberts Rumba[3], Andrejs Vanags[3], Inese Drike[1], Dzeina Mezale[1], Arnis Abolins[1], Arvids Jakovlevs[1], Dainis Balodis[1] and Janis Gardovskis[3]

*Address all correspondence to: ilze.strumfa@rsu.lv

1 Department of Pathology, Riga Stradins University, Riga, Latvia

2 Latvian Institute of Organic Synthesis, Riga, Latvia

3 Department of Surgery, Riga Stradins University, Riga, Latvia

References

[1] Global Burden of Disease Cancer Collaboration, Fitzmaurice C, Allen C, Barber RM, Barregard L, Bhutta ZA, Brenner H, Dicker DJ, Chimed-Orchir O, Dandona R, Dandona L, Fleming T, Forouzanfar MH, Hancock J, Hay RJ, Hunter-Merrill R, Huynh C, Hosgood HD, Johnson CO, Jonas JB, Khubchandani J, Kumar GA, Kutz M, Lan Q, Larson HJ, Liang X, Lim SS, Lopez AD, MacIntyre MF, Marczak L, Marquez N, Mokdad AH, Pinho C, Pourmalek F, Salomon JA, Sanabria JR, Sandar L, Sartorius B, Schwartz SM, Shackelford KA, Shibuya K, Stanaway J, Steiner C, Sun J, Takahashi K, Vollset SE, Vos T, Wagner JA, Wang H, Westerman R, Zeeb H, Zoeckler L, Abd-Allah F, Ahmed MB, Alabed S, Alam NK, Aldhahri SF, Alem G, Alemayohu MA, Ali R, Al-Raddadi R, Amare A, Amoako Y, Artaman A, Asayesh H, Atnafu N, Awasthi A, Saleem HB, Barac A, Bedi N, Bensenor I, Berhane A, Bernabé E, Betsu B, Binagwaho A, Boneya D, Campos-Nonato I, Castañeda-Orjuela C, Catalá-López F, Chiang P, Chibueze C, Chitheer A, Choi JY, Cowie B, Damtew S, das Neves J, Dey S, Dharmaratne S, Dhillon P, Ding E, Driscoll T, Ekwueme D, Endries AY, Farvid M, Farzadfar F, Fernandes J, Fischer F, G/Hiwot TT, Gebru A, Gopalani S,

Hailu A, Horino M, Horita N, Husseini A, Huybrechts I, Inoue M, Islami F, Jakovljevic M, James S, Javanbakht M, Jee SH, Kasaeian A, Kedir MS, Khader YS, Khang YH, Kim D, Leigh J, Linn S, Lunevicius R, El Razek HM, Malekzadeh R, Malta DC, Marcenes W, Markos D, Melaku YA, Meles KG, Mendoza W, Mengiste DT, Meretoja TJ, Miller TR, Mohammad KA, Mohammadi A, Mohammed S, Moradi-Lakeh M, Nagel G, Nand D, Le Nguyen Q, Nolte S, Ogbo FA, Oladimeji KE, Oren E, Pa M, Park EK, Pereira DM, Plass D, Qorbani M, Radfar A, Rafay A, Rahman M, Rana SM, Søreide K, Satpathy M, Sawhney M, Sepanlou SG, Shaikh MA, She J, Shiue I, Shore HR, Shrime MG, So S, Soneji S, Stathopoulou V, Stroumpoulis K, Sufiyan MB, Sykes BL, Tabarés-Seisdedos R, Tadese F, Tedla BA, Tessema GA, Thakur JS, Tran BX, Ukwaja KN, Uzochukwu BS, Vlassov VV, Weiderpass E, Wubshet Terefe M, Yebyo HG, Yimam HH, Yonemoto N, Younis MZ, Yu C, Zaidi Z, Zaki ME, Zenebe ZM, Murray CJ, Naghavi M. Global, regional, and national cancer incidence, mortality, years of life lost, years lived with disability, and disability-adjusted life-years for 32 cancer groups, 1990 to 2015: A systematic analysis for the global burden of disease study. JAMA Oncology. 2016 Dec 3;**3**:DOI: 10.1001/jamaoncol.2016.5688

[2] Crew KD, Neugut AI. Epidemiology of gastric cancer. World Journal of Gastroenterology. 2006;**12**(3):354-362

[3] Gao Y, Huang D. The value of the systematic inflammation-based Glasgow Prognostic Score in patients with gastric cancer: a literature review. Journal of Cancer Research and Therapeutics. 2014;**10**(4):799-804

[4] Riquelme I, Saavedra K, Espinoza JA, Weber H, Garcia P, Nervi B, Garrido M, Corvalan AH, Roa JC, Bizama C. Molecular classification of gastric cancer: Towards a pathway-driven targeted therapy. Oncotarget. 2015;**6**(28):24750-24779

[5] Rutkowski MR, Svoronos N, Perales-Puchalt A, Conejo-Garcia JR. The tumor macroenvironment: Cancer promoting networks beyond tumor beds. Advances in Cancer Research. 2015;**128**:235-262

[6] Diakos CI, Charles KA, McMillan DC, Clarke SJ. Cancer-related inflammation and treatment effectiveness. The Lancet Oncology. 2014;**15**(11):e493-e503

[7] Cederval J, Dimberg A, Olsson AK. Tumor-induced local and systemic impact on blood vessel function. Mediators of Inflammation. 2015;**2015**:418290

[8] Olsson AK, Cederval J. NETosis in cancer—Platelet-neutrophil crosstalk promotes tumor-associated pathology. Frontiers in Immunology. 2016;**7**:373

[9] Mohri Y, Tanaka K, Toiyama Y, Ohi M, Yasuda H, Inoue Y, Kusunoki M. Impact of preoperative neutrophil to lymphocyte ratio and postoperative infectious complications on survival after curative gastrectomy for gastric cancer: A single institutional cohort study. Medicine (Baltimore). 2016;**95**(11):e3125. DOI: 10.1097/MD0000000000003125

[10] Sagawa M, Yagawa H, Konno S, Usuda A, Maeda H, Kim K, Watanabe T, Yamaya E, Usui T, Yokomizo H, Yoshimatsu K, Shimakawa T, Katsube T, Naritaka Y. Significance

of perioperative neutrophil lymphocyte ratio (NLR) in gastric cancer and colon cancer. [Article in Japanese] Gan to Kagaku Ryoho. 2016;**43**(10):1243-1245

[11] Caruso RA, Muda AO, Bersiga A, Rigoli L, Inferrera C. Morphological evidence of neutrophil-tumor cell phagocytosis (cannibalism) in human gastric adenocarcinomas. Ultrastructural Pathology. 2002;**26**(5):315-321

[12] Ohno S, Inagawa H, Dhar DK, Fujii T, Ueda S, Tachibana M, Suzuki N, Inoue M, Soma G, Nagasue N. The degree of macrophage infiltration into the cancer cell nest is a significant predictor of survival in gastric cancer patients. Anticancer Research. 2003;**23**(6D):5015-5022

[13] De Visser KE, Coussens LM. The interplay between innate and adaptive immunity regulates cancer development. Cancer Immunology, Immunotherapy. 2005;**54**(11):1143-1152

[14] Nishikawa H, Sakaguchi S. Regulatory T cells in cancer immunotherapy. Current Opinion in Immunology. 2014;**27**:1-7

[15] Maeda K, Shibutani M, Otani H, Nagahara H, Ikeya T, Iseki Y, Tanaka H, Muguruma K, Hirakawa K. Inflammation-based factors and prognosis in patients with colorectal cancer. World Journal of Gastrointestinal Oncology. 2015;**7**(8):111-117

[16] Lian L, Xia YY, Zhou C, Shen XM, Li XL, Han SG, Zheng Y, Mao ZQ, Gong FR, Wu MY, Chen K, Tao M, Li W. Application of platelet/lymphocyte and neutrophil/lymphocyte ratios in early diagnosis and prognostic prediction in patients with resectable gastric cancer. Cancer Biomarkers. 2015;**15**(6):899-907

[17] Qiu M, Zhou Y, Jin Y, Wei XL, Wang DS, Ren C, Bai L, Yang DJ, Xu RH. Prognostic effect of high pretreatment neutrophil to lymphocyte ratio on survival of patients with gastric adenocarcinoma in China. The International Journal of Biological Markers. 2015;**30**(1): e96-e103

[18] Pietrzyk L, Plewa Z, Denisow-Pietrzyk M, Zebrowski R, Torres K. Diagnostic power of blood parameters as screening markers in gastric cancer patients. Asian Pacific Journal of Cancer Prevention. .2016;**17**(9):4433-4437

[19] Shen XM, Xia YY, Lian L, Zhou C, Li XL, Han SG, Zheng Y, Gong FR, Tao M, Mao ZQ, Li W. Mean platelet volume provides beneficial diagnostic and prognostic information for patients with resectable gastric cancer. Oncology Letters. 2016;**12**(4):2501-2506

[20] Yu L, Lv CY, Yuan AH, Chen W, Wu AW. Significance of the preoperative neutrophil-to-lymphocyte ratio in the prognosis of patients with gastric cancer. World Journal of Gastroenterology. 2015;**21**(20):6280-6286

[21] Sun J, Chen X, Gao P, Song Y, Huang X, Yang Y, Zhao J, Ma B, Gao X, Wang Z. Can the neutrophil to lymphocyte ratio be used to determine gastric cancer treatment outcomes? A systematic review and meta-analysis. Dis Markers. 2016;**2016**:7862469. DOI: 10.1155/2016/7862469

[22] Hsu JT, Liao CK, Le PH, Chen TH, Lin CJ, Chen JS, Chiang KC, Yeh TS. Prognostic value of the preoperative neutrophil to lymphocyte ratio in resectable gastric cancer. Medicine (Baltimore). 2015;**94**(39):e1589. DOI: 10.1097/MD.000 0000000001589

[23] Zhang X, Li S, Guo Z, Xue Y. Prognostic value of preoperative neutrophil-to-lymphocyte ratio in the elderly patients over 75 years old with gastric cancer. [Article in Chinese] Zhonghua Wei Chang Wai Ke Za Zhi. 2016;**19**(5):526-529

[24] Namikawa T, Munekage E, Munekage M, Maeda H, Yatabe T, Kitagawa H, Kobayashi M, Hanazaki K. Evaluation of systemic inflammatory response biomarkers in patients receiving chemotherapy for unresectable and recurrent advanced gastric cancer. Oncology. 2016;**90**(6):321-326

[25] Musri FY, Mutlu H, Eryilmaz MK, Salim DK, Gunduz S, Coskun HS. The neutrophil to lymphocyte ratio is an independent prognostic factor in patients with metastatic gastric cancer. Asian Pacific Journal of Cancer Prevention. 2016;**17**(3):1309-1312

[26] Hsieh MC, Wang SH, Chuah SK, Lin YH, Lan J, Rau KM. A prognostic model using inflammation- and nutrition-based scores in patients with metastatic gastric adenocarcinoma treated with chemotherapy. Medicine (Baltimore). 2016;**95**(17):e3504. DOI:10.1097/MD.0000000000003504

[27] Mohri Y, Tanaka K, Ohi M, Saigusa S, Yasuda H, Toiyama Y, Araki T, Inoue Y, Kusunoki M. Identification of prognostic factors and surgical indications for metastatic gastric cancer. BMC Cancer. 2014;**14**:409. DOI: 10.1186/1471-2407-14-409

[28] Tanaka H, Muguruma K, Toyokawa T, Kubo N, Ohira M, Hirakawa K. Differential impact of the neutrophil-lymphocyte ratio on the survival of patients with stage IV gastric cancer. Digestive Surgery. 2014;**31**(4-5):327-333

[29] Ishizuka M, Oyama Y, Abe A, Kubota K. Combination of platelet count and neutrophil to lymphocyte ratio is a useful predictor of postoperative survival in patients undergoing surgery for gastric cancer. Journal of Surgical Oncology. 2014;**110**(8):935-941

[30] Sun X, Wang J, Liu J, Chen S, Liu X. Albumin concentrations plus neutrophil lymphocyte ratios for predicting overall survival after curative resection for gastric cancer. Onco Targets and Therapy. 2016;**9**:4661-4669

[31] Sun X, Liu X, Liu J, Chen S, Xu D, Li W, Zhan Y, Li Y, Chen Y, Zhou Z. Preoperative neutrophil-to-lymphocyte ratio plus platelet-to-lymphocyte ratio in predicting survival for patients with stage I-II gastric cancer. Chinese Journal of Cancer. 2016;**35**(1):57. DOI: 10.1186/s40880-016-0122-2

[32] Xu L, Pan Q, Lin R. Prevalence rate and influencing factors of preoperative anxiety and depression in gastric cancer patients in China: Preliminary study. The Journal of International Medical Research. 2016;**44**(2):377-388

[33] Yamamoto M, Kurokawa Y, Miyazaki Y, Makino T, Takahashi T, Yamasaki M, Nakajima K, Takiguchi S, Mori M, Doki Y. Usefulness of preoperative plasma fibrinogen versus

other prognostic markers for predicting gastric cancer recurrence. World Journal of Surgery. 2016;**40**(8):1904-1909

[34] Giampieri R, Maccaroni E, Mandolesi A, Del Prete M, Andrikou K, Faloppi L, Bittoni A, Bianconi M, Scarpelli M, Bracci R, Scartozzi M, Cascinu S. Mismatch repair deficiency can affect clinical outcome through immune response activation in metastatic gastric cancer patients receiving first-line chemotherapy. Gastric Cancer. 2016;**20**. DOI: 10.1007/s10120-016-0594-4

[35] Zhang X, Zhang W, Feng LJ. Prognostic significance of neutrophil lymphocyte ratio in patients with gastric cancer: A meta analysis. PloS One. 2014;**9**(11):e111906. DOI: 10.1371/journal.pone.0111906

[36] Chen J, Hong D, Zhai Y, Shen P. Meta-analysis of associations between neutrophil-to-lymphocyte ratio and prognosis of gastric cancer. World Journal of Surgical Oncology. 2015;**13**:122. DOI: 10.1186/s12957-015-0530-9

[37] Xin-Ji Z, Yong-Gang L, Xiao-Jun S, Xiao-Wu C, Dong Z, Da-Jian Z. The prognostic role of neutrophils to lymphocytes ratio and platelet count in gastric cancer: A meta-analysis. International Journal of Surgery. 2015;**21**:84-91

[38] Wang F, Liu ZY, Xia YY, Zhou C, Shen XM, Li XL, Han SG, Zheng Y, Mao ZQ, Gong FR, Tao M, Lian L, Li W. Changes in neutrophil/lymphocyte and platelet/lymphocyte ratios after chemotherapy correlate with chemotherapy response and prediction of prognosis in patients with unresectable gastric cancer. Oncology Letters. 2015;**10**(6):3411-3418

[39] Kim EY, Lee+ JW, Yoo HM, Park CH, Song KY. The platelet-to-lymphocyte ratio versus neutrophil-to-lymphocyte ratio: Which is better as a prognostic factor in gastric cancer? Annals of Surgical Oncology. 2015;**22**(13):4363-4370

[40] Yamanaka T, Matsumoto S, Teramukai S, Ishiwata R, Nagai Y, Fukushima M. The baseline ratio of neutrophils to lymphocytes is associated with patient prognosis in advanced gastric cancer. Oncology. 2007;**73**(3-4):251-20

[41] Aliustaoglu M, Bilici A, Ustaalioglu BB, Konya V, Gucun M, Seker M, Gumus M. The effect of peripheral blood values on prognosis of patients with locally advanced gastric cancer before treatment. Medical Oncology. 2010;**27**(4):1060-1065

[42] Mohri Y, Tanaka K, Ohi M, Yokoe T, Miki C, Kusunoki M. Prognostic significance of host- and tumor-related factors in patients with gastric cancer. World Journal of Surgery. 2010;**34**(2):285-290

[43] Wang DS, Ren C, Qiu MZ, Luo HY, Wang ZQ, Zhang DS, Wang FH, Li YH, Xu Rh. Comparison of the prognostic value of various preoperative inflammation-based factors in patients with stage III gastric cancer. Tumour Biology. 2012;**33**(3):749-756

[44] Lee DY, Hong SW, Chang YG, Lee WY, Lee B. Clinical significance of preoperative inflammatory parameters in gastric cancer patients. Journal of Gastric Cancer. 2013;**13**(2):111-116

[45] Sun KY, Xu JB, Chen SL, Yuan YJ, Wu H, Peng JJ, Chen CQ, Guo P, Hao YT, He YL. Novel immunological and nutritional-based prognostic index for gastric cancer. World Journal of Gastroenterology. 2015;**21**(19):5961-5971

[46] Proctor MJ, Morrison DS, Talwar D, Balmer SM, Fletcher CD, O'Reilly DS, Foulis AK, Horgan PG, McMillan DC. A comparison of inflammation-based prognostic scores in patients with cancer. A Glasgow Inflammation Outcome Study. European Journal of Cancer. 2011;**47**(17):2633-2641

[47] Deng Q, He B, Liu X, Yue J, Ying H, Pan Y, Sun H, Chen J, Wang F, Gao T, Zhang L, Wang S. Prognostic value of pre-operative inflammatory response biomarkers in gastric cancer patients and the construction of a predictive model. Journal of Translational Medicine. 2015;**13**:66. DOI: 10.1186/s12967-015-0409-0

[48] Kim JH, Han DS, Bang HY, Kim PS, Lee KY. Preoperative neutrophil-to-lymphocyte ratio is a prognostic factor for overall survival in patients with gastric cancer. Annals of Surgical Treatment and Researh. 2015;**89**(2):81-86

[49] Choi Y, Kim JW, Nam KH, Han SH, Kim JW, Ahn SH, Park DJ, Lee KW, Lee HS, Kim HH. Systemic inflammation is associated with the density of immune cells in the tumor microenvironment of gastric cancer. Gastric Cancer. 2016 [Epub ahead of print; accessed 21.06.2017.]; DOI: 10.1007/s10120-016-0642-0

[50] Cho IR, Park JC, Park CH, Jo JH, Lee HJ, Kim S, Shim CN, Lee H, Shin SK, Lee SK, Lee YC. Pre-treatment neutrophil to lymphocyte ratio as a prognostic marker to predict chemotherapeutic response and survival outcomes in metastatic advanced gastric cancer. Gastric Cancer. 2014;**17**(4):703-710

[51] Ubukata H, Konishi S, Nakachi T, Motohashi G, Goto Y, Watanabe Y, Nakada I, Tabuchi T. Characteristics of the serum pepsinogen (Pg) test, and the relationship between Pg test results and gastric cancer outcomes. Scandinavian Journal of Surgery. 2010;**99**(4):201-207

[52] Graziosi L, Marino E, De Angelis V, Rebonato A, Cavazzoni E, Donini A. Prognostic value of preoperative neutrophils to lymphocytes ratio in patients resected for gastric cancer. American Journal of Surgery. 2015;**209**(2):333-337

[53] Jung MR, Park YK, Jeong O, Seon JW, Ryu SY, Kim DY, Kim YJ. Elevated preoperative neutrophil to lymphocyte ratio predicts poor survival following resection in late stage gastric cancer. Journal of Surgical Oncology. 2011;**104**(5):504-510

[54] Xu AM, Huang L, Zhu L, Wei ZJ. Significance of peripheral neutrophil-lymphocyte ratio among gastric cancer patients and construction of a treatment-predictive model: A study based on 1131 cases. American Journal of Cancer Research. 2014;**4**(2):189-195

[55] Pang W, Lou N, Jin C, Hu C, Arvine C, Zhu G, Shen X. Combination of preoperative platelet/lymphocyte and neutrophil/lymphocyte rates and tumor-related factors to predict lymph node metastasis in patients with gastric cancer. European Journal of Gastroenterology & Hepatology. 2016;**28**(5):493-502

[56] Aldemir MN, Turkeli M, Simsek M, Yildirim N, Bilen Y, Yetimoglu H, Bilici M, Tekin SB. Prognostic value of baseline neutrophil-lymphocyte and platelet-lymphocyte ratios in local and advanced gastric cancer patients. Asian Pacific Journal of Cancer Prevention. 2015;**16**(14):5933-5937

[57] Lee S, Oh SY, Kim SH, Lee JH, Kim MC, Kim KH, Kim HJ. Prognostic significance of neutrophil lymphocyte ratio and platelet lymphocyte ratio in advanced gastric cancer patients treated with FOLFOX chemotherapy. BMC Cancer. 2013;**13**:350. DOI: 10.1186/1471-2407-13-350

[58] Jin H, Zhang G, Liu X, Liu X, Chen C, Yu H, Huang X, Zhang Q, Yu J. Blood neutrophil-lymphocyte ratio predicts survival for stages III-IV gastric cancer treated with neoadjuvant chemotherapy. World Journal of Surgical Oncology. 2013;**11**:112. DOI: 10.1186/1477-7819-11-112

[59] El Aziz LM. Blood neutrophil-lymphocyte ratio predicts survival in locally advanced cancer stomach treated with neoadjuvant chemotherapy FOLFOX 4. Medical Oncology. 2014;**31**(12):311. DOI: 10.1007/s12032-014-0311-2

[60] Wang Q, Yang Y, Zhang YP, Zou Z, Qian X, Liu B, Wei J. Prognostic value of carbohydrate tumor markers and inflammation-based markers in metastatic or recurrent gastric cancer. Medical Oncology. 2014;**31**(12):289. DOI: 10.1007/s12032-014-0289-9

[61] Gunaldi M, Goksu S, Erdem D, Gunduz S, Okuturlar Y, Tiken E, Kahraman S, Inan YO, Genc TB, Yildirim M. Prognostic impact of platelet/lymphocyte and neutrophil/lymphocyte ratios in patients with gastric cancer: A multicenter study. International Journal of Clinical and Experimental Medicine. 2015;**8**(4):5937-5942

[62] Dirican A, Ekinci N, Avci A, Akyol M, Alacacioglu A, Kucukzeybek Y, Somali I, Erten C, Demir L, Can A, Bayoglu IV, Koyuncu B, Ulger E, Tarhan MO. The effects of hematological parameters and tumor-infiltrating lymphocytes on prognosis in patients with gastric cancer. Cancer Biomarkers. 2013;**13**(1):11-20

[63] Pan QX, Su ZJ, Zhang JH, Wang CR, Ke SY. A comparison of the prognostic value of preoperative inflammation-based scores and TNM stage in patients with gastric cancer. Onco Targets and Therapy. 2015;**8**:1375-1385

[64] Jiang N, Deng JY, Liu Y, Ke B, Liu HG, Liang H. The role of preoperative neutrophil-lymphocyte and platelet-lymphocyte ratio in patients after radical resection for gastric cancer. Biomarkers. 2014;**19**(6):444-451

[65] Ubukata H, Motohashi G, Tabuchi T, Nagata H, Konishi S, Tabuchi T. Evaluations of interferon-gamma/interleukin-4 ratio and neutrophil/lymphocyte ratio as prognostic indicators in gastric cancer patients. Journal of Surgical Oncology. 2010;**102**(7):742-747

[66] Shimada H, Takiguchi N, Kainuma O, Soda H, Ikeda A, Cho A, Miyazaki A, Gunji H, Yamamoto H, Nagata M. High preoperative neutrophil-lymphocyte ratio predicts poor survival in patients with gastric cancer. Gastric Cancer. 2010;**13**(3):170-176

[67] Dogan M, Eren T, Ozdemir N, Cigirgan CL, Zengin N. The relationship between platelet-lymphocyte ratio, neutrophil-lymphocyte ratio, and survival in metastatic gastric cancer on firstline modified docetaxel and cisplatinum plus 5 fluorurasil regimen: A single institute experience. Saudi Journal of Gastroenterology. 2015;**21**(5):320-324

[68] Li QQ, Lu ZH, Yang L, Lu M, Zhang XT, Li J, Zhou J, Wang XC, Gong JF, Gao J, Li J, Li Y, Shen L. Neutrophil count and the inflammation-based glasgow prognostic score predict survival in patients with advanced gastric cancer receiving first-line chemotherapy. Asian Pacific Journal of Cancer Prevention. 2014;**15**(2):945-950

[69] Jeong JH, Lim SM, Yun JY, Rhee GW, Lim JY, Cho JY, Kim YR. Comparison of two inflammation-based prognostic scores in patients with unresectable advanced gastric cancer. Oncology. 2012;**83**(5):292-299

[70] Zheng D, Lin Y, Yu Y, Wang K, Ouyang X, Dang Y, Huang Q. The value of preoperative neutrophil to lymphocyte ratio in indicating lymph node metastasis in patients with resectable T2 stage gastric adenocarcinoma. Clinical Laboratory. 2016;**62**(4):659-665

[71] Ruopp MD, Perkins NJ, Whitcomb BW, Schisterman EF. Youden Index and optimal cut-point estimated from observations affected by lower limit of detection. Biometrical Journal. 2008;**50**(3):419-430

[72] Lou N, Zhang L, Chen XD, Pang WY, Arvine C, Huang YP, Zhuang CL, Shen X. A novel scoring system associating with preoperative platelet/lymphocyte and clinicopathologic features to predict lymph node metastasis in early gastric cancer. The Journal of Surgical Research 2017;**209**:153-161

[73] Aizawa M, Gotohda N, Takahashi S, Konishi M, Kinoshita T. Predictive value of baseline neutrophil/lymphocyte ratio for T4 disease in wall-penetrating gastric cancer. World Journal of Surgery. 2011;**35**(12):2717-2722

[74] Gomez D, Farid S, Malik HZ, Young AL, Toogood GJ, Lodge JP, Prasad KR. Preoperative neutrophil-to-lymphocyte ratio as a prognostic predictor after curative resection for hepatocellular carcinoma. World Journal of Surgery. 2008;**32**(8):1757-1762

[75] Halazun KJ, Hardy MA, Rana AA, Woodland DC 4th, Luyten EJ, Mahadev S, Witkowski P, Siegel AB, Brown RS Jr, Emond JC. Negative impact of neutrophil-lymphocyte ratio on outcome after liver transplantation for hepatocellular carcinoma. Annals of Surgery. 2009;**250**(1):141-151

[76] Grenader T, Plotkin Y, Mohammadi B, Dawas K, Hashemi M, Mughal M, Bridgewater JA. Predictive value of the neutrophil/lymphocyte ratio in peritoneal and/or metastatic disease at staging laparoscopy for gastric and esophageal adenocarcinoma. Journal of Gastrointestinal Cancer. 2015;**46**(3):267-271

[77] Jiang Y, Xu H, Jiang H, Ding S, Zheng T. Pretreatment neutrophil-lymphocyte count ratio may associate with gastric cancer presence. Cancer Biomarkers. 2016;**16**(4):523-528

[78] Ohi M, Mori K, Toiyama Y, Mohri Y, Okigami M, Yasuda H, Saigusa S, Tanaka K, Inoue Y, Kusunoki M. Preoperative prediction of peritoneal metastasis in gastric cancer as an indicator for neoadjuvant treatment. Anticancer Research. 2015;**35**(6):3511-3518

[79] Nakayama Y, Gotohda N, Shibasaki H, Nomura S, Kinoshita T, Hayashi R. Usefulness of the neutrophil/lymphocyte ratio measured preoperatively as a predictor of peritoneal metastasis in patients with advanced gastric cancer. Surgery Today. 2014;**44**(11):2146-2152

[80] Ock CY, Nam AR, Lee J, Bang JH, Lee KH, Han SW, Kim TY, Im SA, Kim TY, Bang YJ, Oh DY. Prognostic implication of antitumor immunity measured by the neutrophil-lymphocyte ratio and serum cytokines and angiogenic factors in gastric cancer. Gastric Cancer. 2016. DOI: 10.1007/s10120-016-0613-5

[81] Tulgar YK, Cakar S, Tulgar S, Dalkilic O, Cakiroglu B, Uyanik BS. The effects of smoking on neutrophil/lymphocyte and platelet/lymphocyte ratio and platelet indices: A retrospective study. European Review for Medical and Pharmacological Sciences. 2016;**20**:3112-3118

[82] Min K, Kwon S, Cho SY, Choi WJ, Park SU, Jung WS, Moon SK, Park JM, Ko CN, Cho KH. Atrial fibrillation is strongly associated with the neutrophil to lymphocyte ratio in acute ischemic stroke patients: A retrospective study. Journal of Clinical Laboratory Analysis 2016;**31**. DOI: 10.1002/jcla.22041

[83] Zhou X, Xu L, Huang Z, Zhang L, Zhang H, Zhu W, Liu P. The hematologic markers as prognostic factors in patients with resectable gastric cancer. Cancer Biomarkers. 2016;**17**(3):359-367

[84] Li S, Xu X, Liang D, Tian G, Song S, He Y. Prognostic value of blood neutrophil-to-lymphocyte ratio (NLR) and platelet-to-lymphocyte ratio (PLR) in patients with gastric cancer. [Article in Chinese]. Zhonghua Zhong Liu Za Zhi. 2014;**36**(12):910-915

[85] Xu Z, Xu W, Cheng H, Shen W, Ying J, Cheng F, Xu W. The prognostic role of the platelet-lymphocytes ratio in gastric cancer: A meta-analysis. PloS One. 2016;**11**(9):e0163719. DOI: 10.1371/journal.pone.0163719

[86] Gu X, Gao XS, Cui M, Xie M, Peng C, Bai Y, Guo W, Han L, Gu X, Xiong W. Clinicopathological and prognostic significance of platelet to lymphocyte ratio in patients with gastric cancer. Oncotarget. 2016;**7**(31):49878-49887

[87] Smith RA, Ghaneh P, Sutton R, Raraty M, Campbell F, Neoptolemos JP. Prognosis of resected ampullary adenocarcinoma by preoperative serum CA 19-9 levels and platelet –lymphocyte ratio. Journal of Gastrointestinal Surgery. 2008;**12**(8):1422-1428

[88] Cetinkunar S, Guzel H, Emre Gokce I, Erdem H, Gulkan S, Aktimur R, Kucuk B, Imamoglu I, Kargici H. High levels of platelet/lymphocyte ratio are associated with metastatic gastric cancer. Journal of BUON. 2015;**20**(1):78-83

[89] Zhou X, Du Y, Huang Z, Xu J, Qiu T, Wang J, Wang T, Zhu W, Liu P. Prognostic value of PLR in various cancers: A meta-analysis. PloS One. 2014;**9**(6):e101119. DOI: 10.1371/journal.pone.0101119

[90] Feng F, Sun L, Zheng G, Liu S, Liu Z, Xu G, Guo M, Lian X, Fan D, Zhang H. Low lymphocyte-to-white blood cell ratio and high monocyte-to-white blood cell ratio predict poor prognosis in gastric cancer. Oncotarget. 2016. DOI: 10.18632/oncotarget.14136

[91] Ishizuka M, Oyama Y, Abe A, Tago K, Tanaka G, Kubota K. Clinical significance of an inflammation-based prognostic system for gastric cancer patients with a preoperative normal serum level of carcinoembryonic antigen. Anticancer Research. 2014;**34**(12):7219-7226

[92] Hirashima K, Watanabe M, Shigaki H, Imamura Y, Ida S, Iwatsuki M, Ishimoto T, Iwagami S, Baba Y, Baba H. Prognostic significance of the modified Glasgow prognostic score in elderly patients with gastric cancer. Journal of Gastroenterology. 2014;**49**(6):1040-1046

[93] Takeno S, Hashimoto T, Shibata R, Maki K, Shiwaku H, Yamana I, Yamashita R, Yamashita Y. Improvement of high-sensitivity inflammation-based Glasgow prognostic score by gastrectomy is a favorable prognostic factor in patients with gastric cancer. Anticancer Research. 2014;**34**(10):5695-5702

[94] Jiang X, Hiki N, Nunobe S, Kumagai K, Kubota T, Aikou S, Sano T, Yamaguchi T. Prognostic importance of the inflammation-based Glasgow prognostic score in patients with gastric cancer. British Journal of Cancer. 2012;**107**(2):275-279

[95] Kubota T, Hiki N, Nunobe S, Kumagai K, Aikou S, Watanabe R, Sano T, Yamaguchi T. Significance of the inflammation-based Glasgow prognostic score for short- and long-term outcomes after curative resection of gastric cancer. Journal of Gastrointestinal Surgery. 2012;**16**(11):2037-2044

[96] Melling N, Gruning A, Tachezy M, Nentwich M, Reeh M, Uzunoglu FG, Vashist YK, Izbicki JR, Bogoevski D. Glasgow Prognostic Score may be a prognostic index for overall and perioperative survival in gastric cancer without perioperative treatment. Surgery. 2016;**159**(6):1548-1556

[97] Aurello P, Tierno SM, Berardi G, Tomassini F, Magistri P, D'Angelo F, Ramacciato G. Value of preoperative inflammation-based prognostic scores in predicting overall survival and disease-free survival in patients with gastric cancer. Annals of Surgical Oncology. 2014;**21**(6):1998-2004

[98] Dutta S, Crumley AB, Fullarton GM, Horgan PG, McMillan DC. Comparison of the prognostic value of tumour and patient related factors in patients undergoing potentially curative resection of gastric cancer. American Journal of Surgery. 2012;**204**(3):294-299

[99] Mimatsu K, Oida T, Fukino N, Kano H, Kawasaki A, Kida K, Kuboi Y, Amano S. Glasgow prognostic score is a useful predictive factor of outcome after palliative gastrectomy for stage IV gastric cancer. Anticancer Research. 2014;**34**(6):3131-3136

[100] Takeno S, Hashimoto T, Shibata R, Maki K, Shiwaku H, Yamana I, Yamashita R, Yamashita Y. The high-sensitivity modified Glasgow prognostic score is superior to the modified Glasgow prognostic score as a prognostic predictor in patients with resectable gastric cancer. Oncology. 2014;**87**(4):205-214

[101] Hwang JE, Kim HN, Kim DE, Choi HJ, Jung SH, Shim HJ, Bae WK, Hwang EC, Cho SH, Chung IJ. Prognostic significance of a systemic inflammatory response in patients receiving first-line palliative chemotherapy for recurred or metastatic gastric cancer. BMC Cancer. 2011;**11**:489. DOI: 10.1186/1471-2407-11-489

[102] Kunisaki C, Takahashi M, Ono HA, Oshima T, Takagawa R, Kimura J, Kosaka T, Makino H, Akiyama H, Endo I. Inflammation-based prognostic score predicts survival in patients with advanced gastric cancer receiving biweekly docetaxel and s-1 combination chemotherapy. Oncology. 2012;**83**(4):183-191

[103] Arigami T, Uenosono Y, Ishigami S, Okubo K, Kijima T, Yanagita S, Okumura H, Uchikado Y, Kijima Y, Nakajo A, Kurahara H, Kita Y, Mori S, Maemura K, Natsugoe S. A novel scoring system based on fibrinogen and the neutrophil-lymphocyte ratio as a predictor of chemotherapy response and prognosis in patients with advanced gastric cancer. Oncology. 2016;**90**(4):186-192

[104] Hwang JE, Kim HN, Kim DE, Shim HJ, Bae WK, Hwang EC, Cho SH, Chung IJ. First-line single-agent chemotherapy for patients with recurrent or metastatic gastric cancer with poor performance status. Experimental and Therapeutic Medicine. 2012;**4**(4):562-568

[105] Sachlova M, Majek O, Tucek S. Prognostic value of scores based on malnutrition or systemic inflammatory response in patients with metastatic or recurrent gastric cancer. Nutrition and Cancer. 2014;**66**(8):1362-1370

[106] Zhang CX, Wang SY, Chen SQ, Yang SL, Wan L, Xiong B. Association between pretreatment Glasgow prognostic score and gastric cancer survival and clinicopathological features: A meta-analysis. Onco Targets and Therapy. 2016;**9**:3883-3891

[107] Kerem M, Ferahkose Z, Yilmaz UT, Pasaoglu H, Ofluoglu E, Bedirli A, Salman B, Sahin TT, Akin M. Adipokines and ghrelin in gastric cancer cachexia. World Journal of Gastroenterology. 2008;**14**(23):3633-3641

[108] Esfahani A, Makhdami N, Faramarzi E, Asghari Jafarabadi M, Ostadrahimi A, Ghayour Nahand M, Ghoreishi Z. Prealbumin/CRP based prognostic score, a new tool for predicting metastasis in patients with inoperable gastric cancer. Gastroenterology Research and Practice. 2016;**2016**:4686189. DOI: 10.1155/2016/4686189

[109] Zhang X, Chen X, Wu T, Zhang Y, Yan K, Sun X. Modified glasgow prognostic score as a prognostic factor in gastric cancer patients: A systematic review and meta-analysis. International Journal of Clinical and Experimental Medicine. 2015;**8**(9):15222-15229

[110] Arigami T, Uenosono Y, Matsushita D, Yanagita S, Uchikado Y, Kita Y, Mori S, Kijima Y, Okumura H, Maemura K, Ishigami S, Natsugoe S. Combined fibrinogen concentration

and neutrophil-lymphocyte ratio as a prognostic marker of gastric cancer. Oncology Letters. 2016;**11**(2):1537-1544

[111] Suzuki T, Shimada H, Nanami T, Oshima Y, Yajima S, Ito M, Washizawa N, Kaneko H. Hyperfibrinogenemia is associated with inflammatory mediators and poor prognosis in patients with gastric cancer. Surgery Today. 2016;**26**(12):1394-1401

[112] Yu X, Hu F, Yao Q, Li C, Zhang H, Xue Y. Serum fibrinogen levels are positively correlated with advanced tumor stage and poor survival in patients with gastric cancer undergoing gastrectomy: a large cohort retrospective study. BMC Cancer 2016;**16**:480. DOI: 10.1186/s12885-016-2510-z

[113] Yu W, Wang Y, Shen B. An elevated plasma fibrinogen level is associated with poor overall survival in Chinese gastric cancer patients. Cancer Epidemiology 2016;**42**:39-45

[114] Brajerski W, Sikorska K, Bisztyga A, Ilenda M. Blood fibrinogen level in peptic ulcer and gastric carcinoma. Polish Medical Science and History Bulletin. 1975;**15**(5-6):557-560

[115] Di Micco P, Romano M, Niglio A, Nozzolillo P, Federico A, Petronella P, Nunziata L, Di Micco B, Torella R. Alteration of haemostasis in non-metastatic gastric cancer. Digestive and Liver Disease. 2001;**33**(7):546-550

[116] Liu C, Pan C, Liang Y. Screening and identification of serum proteomic biomarkers for gastric adenocarcinoma. Experimental and Therapeutic Medicine. 2012;**3**(6):1005-1009

[117] Wu C, Luo Z, Tang D, Liu L, Yao D, Zhu L, Wang Z. Identification of carboxyl terminal peptide of fibrinogen as a potential serum biomarker for gastric cancer. Tumour Biology. 2016;**37**(5):6963-6970

[118] Zhao C, Su Y, Zhang J, Feng Q, Qu L, Wang L, Liu C, Jiang B, Meng L, Shou C. Fibrinogen-derived fibrinostatin inhibits tumor growth through anti-angiogenesis. Cancer Science. 2015;**106**(11):1596-1606

[119] Maeda M. Distribution of fibronectin and other plasma proteins in gastric cancer tissues: investigation of mechanisms of desmoplasia of the stroma. [Article in Japanese]. Nihon Geka Gakkai Zasshi. 1984;**85**(11):1454-1463

[120] Wojtukiewicz MZ, Sierko E, Zacharski LR, Zimnoch L, Kudryk B, Kisiel W. Tissue factor-dependent coagulation activation and impaired fibrinolysis in situ in gastric cancer. Seminars in Thrombosis and Hemostasis. 2003;**29**(3):291-300

[121] Lee SE, Lee JH, Ryu KW, Nam BH, Cho SJ, Lee JY, Kim CG, Choi IJ, Kook MC, Park SR, Kim YW. Preoperative plasma fibrinogen level is a useful predictor of adjacent organ involvement in patients with advanced gastric cancer. Journal of Gastric Cancer. 2012;**12**(2):81-87

[122] Lee JH, Ryu KW, Kim S, Bae JM. Preoperative plasma fibrinogen levels in gastric cancer patients correlate with extent of tumor. Hepato-Gastroenterology. 2004;**51**(60):1860-1863

[123] Yamashita H, Kitayama J, Nagawa H. Hyperfibrinogenemia is a useful predictor for lymphatic metastasis in human gastric cancer. Japanese Journal of Clinical Oncology. 2005;**35**(10):595-600

[124] Yamashita H, Kitayama J, Kanno N, Yatomi Y, Nagawa H. Hyperfibrinogenemia is associated with lymphatic as well as hematogenous metastasis and worse clinical outcome in T2 gastric cancer. BMC Cancer. 2006;**6**:147. DOI: 10.1186/1471-2407-6-147

[125] Kanda M, Tanaka C, Kobayashi D, Mizuno A, Tanaka Y, Takami H, Iwata N, Hayashi M, Niwa Y, Yamada S, Fujii T, Sugimoto H, Murotani K, Fujiwara M, Kodera Y. Proposal of the coagulation score as a predictor for short-term and long-term outcomes of patients with resectable gastric cancer. Annals of Surgical Oncology. 2017;**24**(2):502-509

[126] Liu L, Zhang X, Yan B, Gu Q, Zhang X, Jiao J, Sun D, Wang N, Yue X. Elevated plasma D-dimer levels correlate with long term survival of gastric cancer patients. PloS One. 2014;**9**(3):e90547. DOI: 10.1371/journal.pone.0090547

[127] Go SI, Lee MJ, Lee WS, Choi HJ, Lee US, Kim RB, Kang MH, Kim HG, Lee GW, Kang JH, Lee JH, Kim SJ. D-dimer can serve as a prognostic and predictive biomarker for metastatic gastric cancer treated by chemotherapy. Medicine (Baltimore). 2015;**94**(30):e951. DOI: 10.1097/MD.0000000000000951

[128] Hu C, Chen R, Chen W, Pang W, Xue X, Zhu G, Shen X. Thrombocytosis is a significant indicator of hypercoagulability, prognosis and recurrence in gastric cancer. Experimental and Therapeutic Medicine. 2014;**8**(1):125-132

[129] Kwon HC, Oh SY, Lee S, Kim SH, Han JY, Koh RY, Kim MC, Kim HJ. Plasma levels of prothrombin fragment F1+2, D-dimer and prothrombin time correlate with clinical stage and lymph node metastasis in operable gastric cancer patients. Japanese Journal of Clinical Oncology. 2008;**38**(1):2-7

[130] Diao D, Wang Z, Cheng Y, Zhang H, Guo Q, Song Y, Zhu K, Li K, Liu D, Dang C. D-dimer: not just an indicator of venous thrombosis but a predictor of asymptomatic hematogenous metastasis in gastric cancer patients. PloS One. 2014;**9**(7):e101125. DOI: 10.1371/journal.pone.0101125

Chapter 9

Surgical Management of Malignant Gastric Tumours: A Practical Guide

Roberts Rumba, Andrejs Vanags, Arturs Kalva,
Tatjana Bogdanova, Inese Drike, Dzeina Mezale,
Marta Vitola, Janis Gardovskis and Ilze Strumfa

Additional information is available at the end of the chapter

http://dx.doi.org/10.5772/intechopen.69825

Abstract

Gastric cancer is one of the most common gastrointestinal malignancies, known also for its dismal prognosis, except early cases. Despite the advances in systemic therapy, surgery remains the cornerstone of treatment. The majority of gastric cancers are carcinomas, while neuroendocrine tumours and gastrointestinal stromal tumours (GISTs) rank next by frequency. Tumour biology, disease course and prognosis differ amongst the aforementioned gastric cancers; thus, surgical treatment has to be adjusted as well. Accumulation of evidence ensures an individualised approach in all aspects of surgical treatment. Specific criteria are set to choose the best surgical treatment while maintaining postoperative function and acceptable life quality. Minimally invasive techniques continue to gain acceptance, while usage is still highly variable. Endoscopic resection is suitable for very early adenocarcinomas, whereas more advanced tumours require standard gastrectomy. Despite the initial concerns, subtotal gastrectomy (SG) is feasible and safe, especially for distal adenocarcinomas. In recent years, D2 lymphadenectomies have become more frequent in Western countries, and evidence supports this tendency. Surgery for gastric neuroendocrine tumours is type-specific and will be discussed in detail. Gastrointestinal stromal tumours are treated by local resection without wide margins or extensive lymph node dissection. Novel targeted therapy can aid surgical treatment by downstaging larger GISTs.

Keywords: gastric cancer, gastric carcinoma, neuroendocrine tumours, GIST, surgery, gastrectomy, lymphadenectomy, laparoscopy

1. Introduction

Despite significant reduction in incidence, important advances in understanding of tumour biology and improvements of complex management of this disease, gastric cancer is still a major and in many aspects poorly resolved oncological problem. Thus, the title 'silent killer' still remains.

Gastric cancer is the fourth most common cancer and second leading cause of cancer death in the world, with nearly a million of new cases in 2012 [1]. There are substantial geographical variations in gastric cancer incidence and survival, with half of all cases diagnosed in East Asia (GLOBOCAN data). This is related to the prevalence of risk factors, mainly *Helicobacter pylori* infection (**Table 1**) [2].

Similarly, stage at diagnosis is also dependent on geographical factors and local screening policies. In most countries, the majority of cases are still diagnosed at an advanced stage (see **Figure 1**).

There are many classifications for gastric cancer. Anatomically, it can be divided in true gastric (noncardia) cancers and gastro-oesophageal (cardia) cancers, which differ in epidemiology and surgical treatment [1]. Histologically, the majority of gastric cancers are malignant epithelial tumours, namely, carcinomas (>90%), while neuroendocrine tumours (NETs) and gastrointestinal stromal tumours (GISTs) rank next by frequency [3].

Surgery is still the only potentially curative treatment of gastric cancer. Despite adequate surgical resection, gastric cancer has a high recurrence rate after operation [4]. Survival parameters have traditionally been higher in Asian countries due to screening and higher proportion of early disease [5]. A 5-year overall survival of 72.3% has been reported in one Korean study, whereas European studies report survival of 28.0–44.3% [2]. To improve these figures, a systematic and evidence-based approach must be used to treat gastric cancer.

Since gastric carcinomas, NETs and GISTs have different characteristics, natural history and prognosis, the cornerstone of treatment, surgical resection, has to be adjusted as well. In this chapter, we discuss the common features and differences in surgical treatment of different gastric cancers according to TNM stage as well as the latest advances in minimally invasive and endoscopic surgical techniques.

Risk factor	Influence and relative risk
H. pylori infection	↑ 3.02
Pernicious anaemia	↑ 6.8
Cigarette smoking	↑ 1.53
Heavy alcohol consumption	↑ 1.20
High dietary salt	↑ 1.07
Dietary fruit and vegetables	↓ 0.81

Table 1. Risk factors of gastric cancer.

http://dx.doi.org/10.5772/intechopen.69825

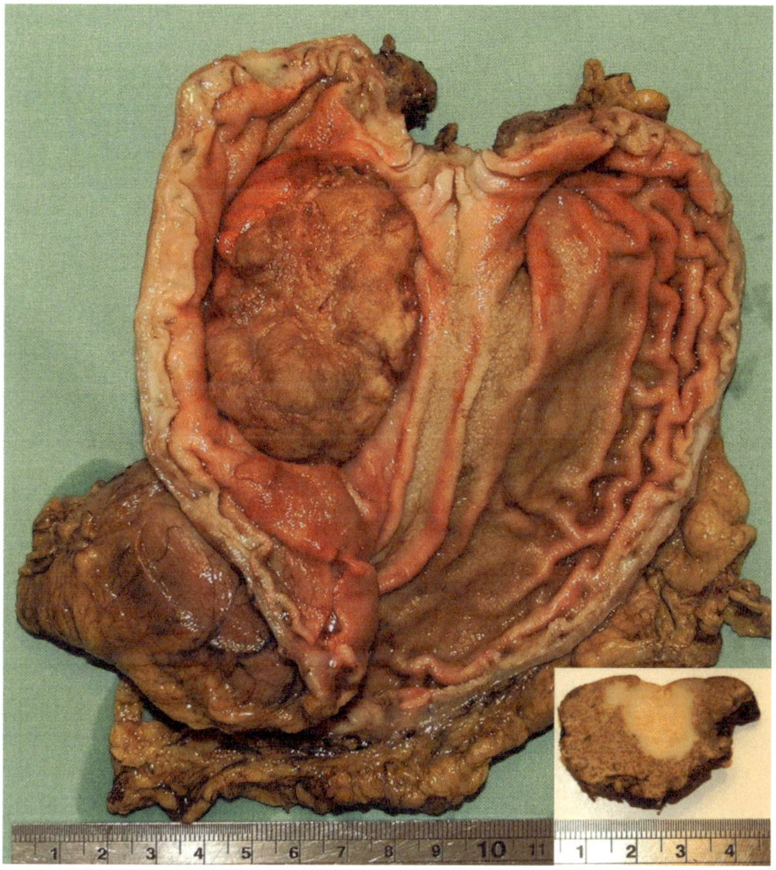

Figure 1. Haematogenous spread of intestinal gastric cancer. Gastrectomy showing a dominant mass lesion. Inset: synchronously resected liver metastasis.

2. Gastric adenocarcinomas

Carcinomas, representing malignant epithelial tumours, arise from epithelial cells in the most superficial, mucosal layer of gastric wall. Traditionally, carcinomas have been divided, according to Lauren classification, in diffuse and intestinal type (**Figure 2**). The former is poorly differentiated, lacks glands, has a more pronounced genetic component, spreads via transmural and lymphatic route and generally has a worse prognosis. Intestinal type is characterised by glandular structures, well or moderately differentiated tumours with haematogenous spread and more pronounced environmental risk factor influence [6]. More recently, the WHO produced a classification that was in concert with histological division of gut tumours—tubular, papillary, mucinous adenocarcinomas, poorly cohesive carcinoma and rare variants [1]. However, there is very little evidence that the aforementioned classifications have additional prognostic value compared to TNM staging [6]. Therefore, for this practical guide, only TNM stage will be taken into consideration.

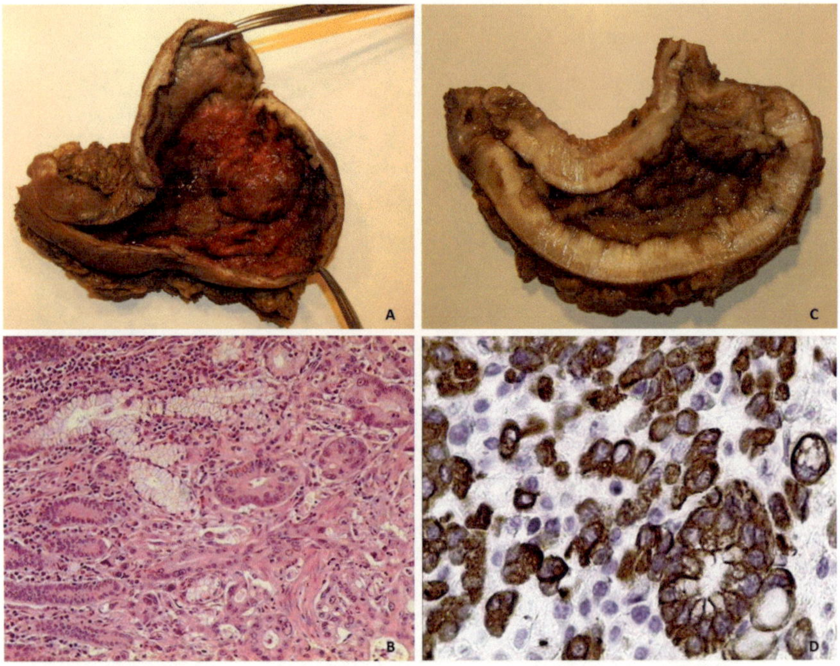

Figure 2. Types of gastric carcinoma by Lauren classification. (A and B) Intestinal type: (A) gross view in gastrectomy and (B) morphological structure showing adenocarcinoma. Haematoxylin-eosin, original magnification (OM) 100×. (C and D) Diffuse type: (C) gross view in gastrectomy and (D) morphological structure showing signet ring cells. Immunoperoxidase, cytokeratin AE1/AE3, OM 400×.

2.1. Early gastric adenocarcinomas

For very early gastric carcinomas (T1a), endoscopic treatment is possible. Precise patient selection is essential to avoid suboptimal treatment. The target is to identify a subgroup of patients for whom the risk of lymph node metastases is virtually zero [5]. Both Japanese and European guidelines have similar criteria for patient selection for endoscopic treatment [5, 7]:

1. Confined to mucosa (T1a)
2. Well differentiated
3. Non-ulcerated
4. Diameter of ≤2 cm

However, in the guidelines, issued by european society for medical oncology (ESMO), these criteria are necessary to consider endoscopic treatment [III, B], whereas Japanese guidelines state them as an absolute indication for endoscopic resection [5, 7]. This underlines the experience of Japanese doctors in endoscopic treatment of very early gastric cancer. The resection is considered curative when a meticulous pathologic examination of specimen reveals an en bloc resection of a tumour with previously mentioned features, negative resection margins and no lymphovascular invasion [7].

http://dx.doi.org/10.5772/intechopen.69825

There are two principal methods for endoscopic removal of gastric cancer. In endoscopic mucosal resection (EMR), a saline injection is used to elevate the tumour and is followed by an excision with a snare device using electrocautery [6] (**Figure 3**). This is generally indicated for lesions smaller than 10–15 mm [5].

In endoscopic submucosal dissection (ESD), electrocautery is used to mark the borders of the tumour followed by hydrodissection with epinephrine and indigo carmine. The lesion is then removed en bloc by dissecting the submucosal layer from the proper muscle layer using insulation-tipped electric knife [6, 7] (**Figure 4**).

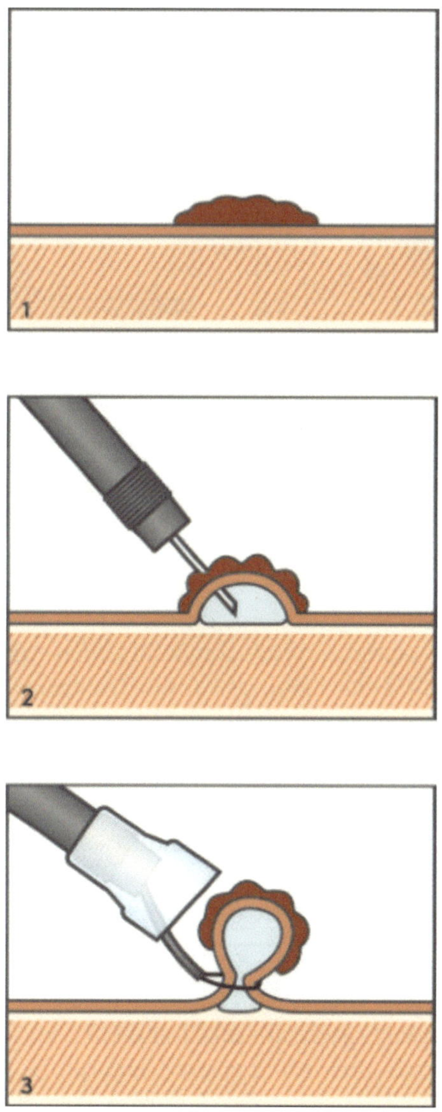

Figure 3. Endoscopic mucosal resection: (1) Localisation of tumour, (2) submucosal injection of saline to elevate the area and (3) electrocautery is applied through snare device to perform resection followed by removal of the lesion.

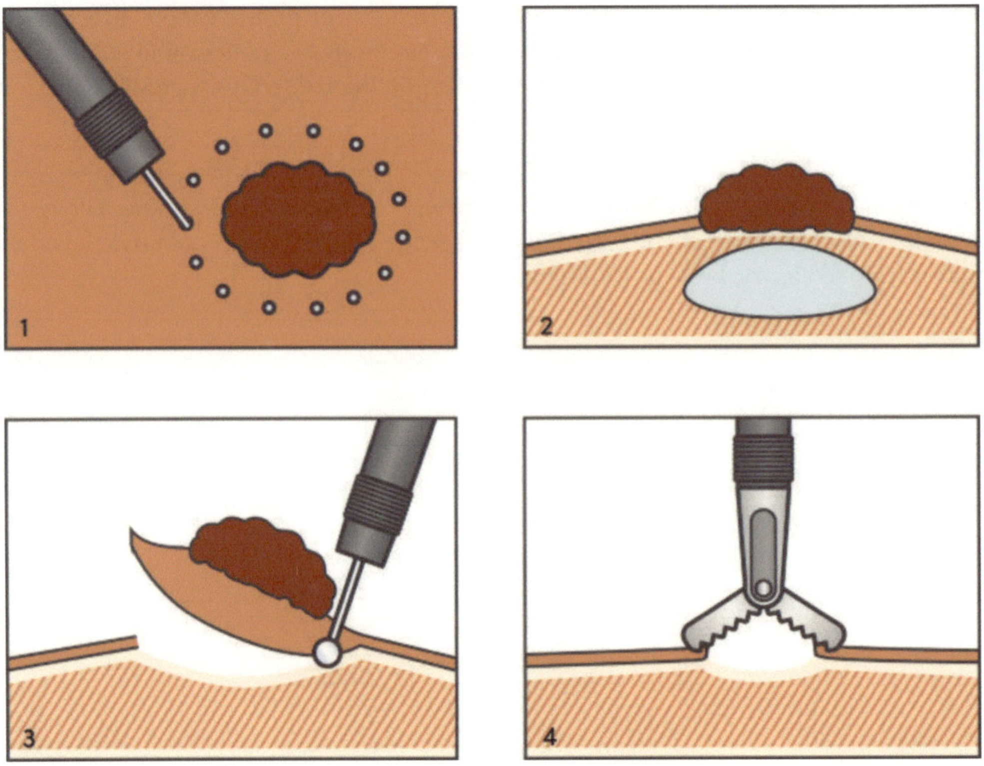

Figure 4. Endoscopic submucosal dissection. (1) Marking borders of the tumour with electrocautery, (2) submucosal injection of a lifting agent, (3) circumferential mucosal incision followed by submucosal dissection with insulation-tipped electric knife and (4) haemostasis.

A meta-analysis comparing both methods was performed, and the results indicated significantly higher en bloc and complete histologic resection rates for ESD (odds ratio, OR = 9.69 vs. OR = 5.66, $p < 0.001$). This increased radicality and also resulted in lower recurrence rate (OR = 0.009, $p < 0.001$). On the other hand, perforation rate was significantly higher for ESD (OR = 4.67, $p < 0.001$) [8]. The European Society of Gastrointestinal Endoscopy Guidelines recommend ESD as the standard procedure for most early gastric tumours [IV, B] [5].

Extended criteria for ESD also are known. One Korean study found no statistically significant differences in recurrence rates between absolute indication and extended indication groups (7.7% vs. 9.3%, $p = 0.524$). However, due to the lack of high-quality evidence, these indications remain investigational and will not be discussed in detail here [7].

Surgical resection is indicated in patients with T1 tumours that do not meet the criteria for endoscopic treatment. However, the extent of resection can be reduced compared to more advanced cancers [5]. For patients with clinical T1 and N0 who require surgical resection for middle gastric cancer, a pylorus-preserving gastrectomy can be offered if the distal extent of tumour is at least 4 cm proximal to pylorus (see **Figure 5**). For early proximal gastric tumours, proximal gastrectomy is an option if more than half of the distal stomach can be preserved (**Figure 6**) [4]. As for segmental gastrectomy and local resection under sentinel navigation, these are still considered investigational [7]. If the above-mentioned criteria are not met, early gastric cancer is treated with a standard gastrectomy. In addition, lymphadenectomy is required because of the risk of lymph node metastases due to submucosal invasion. The extent of lymphadenectomy in early gastric cancer will be discussed in the following chapter.

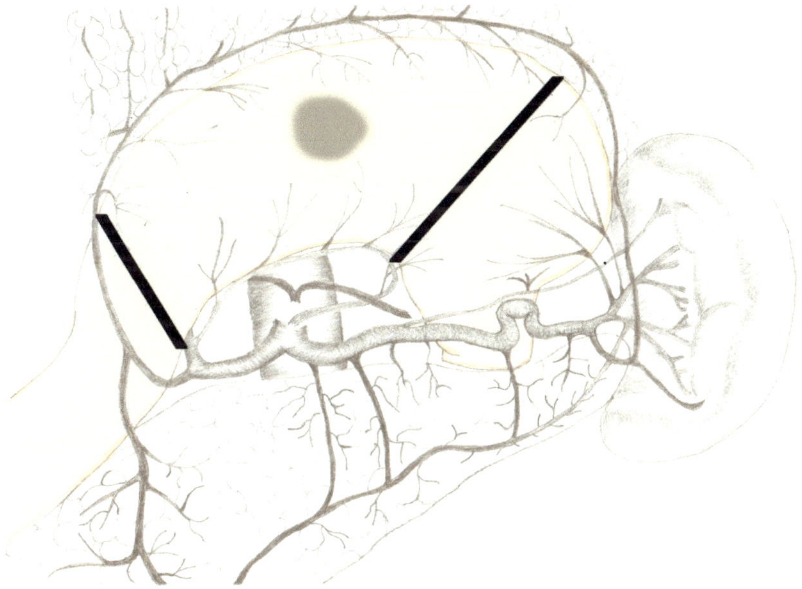

Figure 5. Pylorus-sparing gastrectomy.

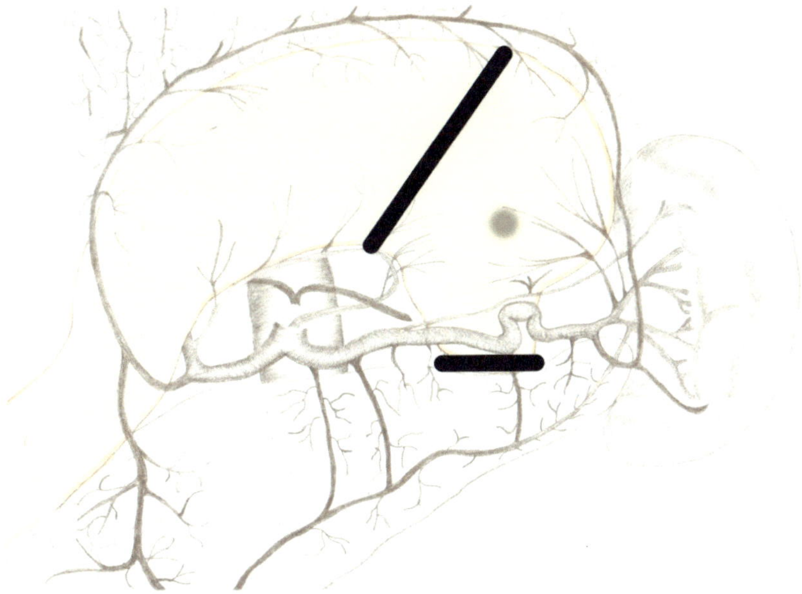

Figure 6. Proximal gastrectomy.

2.1.1. Extent of lymphadenectomy for early gastric tumours

Lymphadenectomy is an essential part of radical gastric cancer surgery. According to the latest UICC/AJCC TNM classification (seventh edition), at least 15 lymph nodes must be harvested to perform adequate staging [5]. However, in a USA-based study comprising more than 3000 patients, it was found that only 23.8% of cases had more than 15 lymph nodes harvested [6].

All of the relevant lymph nodes are divided in 16 stations (see **Figure 7**). The first six stations, perigastric nodes, are grouped together as N1. Stations 7–11, coeliac axis, are grouped as N2 [4]. Depending on the extent of lymph node removal, the term D1 (perigastric nodes) or D2 (perigastric nodes plus clearance of coeliac axis) is used [5]. However, traditionally, the extent of lymphadenectomy was classified relative to the location of tumour [6]. In the latest Japanese gastric cancer treatment guidelines (2014), a more rational approach is suggested. What constitutes D1 or D2 lymphadenectomy is actually dependent on the extent of gastrectomy, regardless of tumour location [7]. For example, in total gastrectomy (TG), D1 means removal of the first seven nodal stations, whereas in distal gastrectomy, D1 constitutes removal of stations 1, 3, 4sb, 4d and 5–7 [7].

For all cT1a tumours which are not amenable to endoscopic treatment as well as cT1b tumours, D1 lymphadenectomy is necessary. If the tumour is well differentiated and does not exceed 1.5 cm in diameter, D1 lymphadenectomy is sufficient. For larger and less differentiated tumours, an extended D1+ lymphadenectomy is required based on the tumour localisation and the extent of gastric resection. Several but not all of the D2 nodes are included in this lymphadenectomy [7].

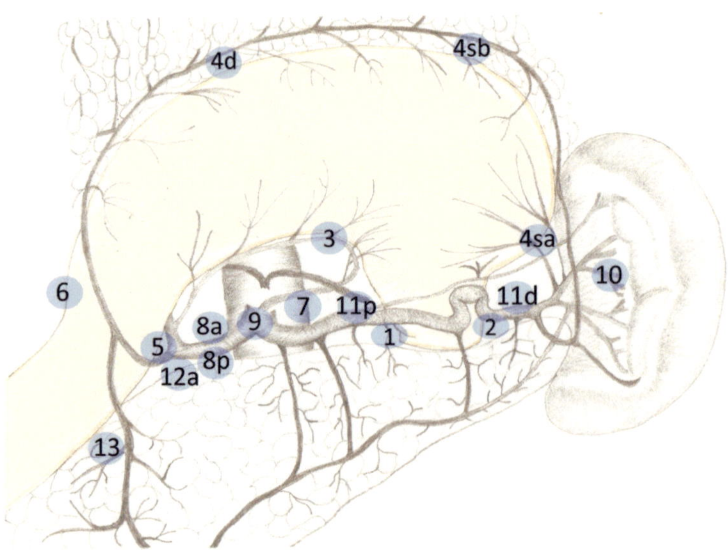

Figure 7. Lymph node stations: (1) right paracardial, (2) left paracardial, (3) lesser curvature, (4sa) short gastric, (4sb) left gastroepiploic, (4d) right gastroepiploic, (5) suprapyloric, (6) infrapyloric, (7) left gastric artery, (8a) anterior common hepatic, (8p) posterior common hepatic, (9) celiac trunk, (10) splenic hilum, (11p) proximal splenic, (11d) distal splenic, (12a) left hepatoduodenal and (13) retropancreatic.

2.2. Gastric carcinoma stage IB–III

There is a consensus amongst specialists and societies that gastric carcinoma invading proper muscular layer or having positive lymph nodes requires a standard gastrectomy [4–7]. A standard gastrectomy means either total gastrectomy (**Figure 8**) or distal subtotal gastrectomy removing at least two-thirds of the stomach (**Figure 9**) [4]. In Japanese guidelines, a D2 lymphadenectomy is an integral part of standard gastrectomy. However, in Western countries this recommendation is not so strict. General recommendation is that a D2 dissection should be performed in high-volume specialised centres with appropriate experience if the patient is medically fit [5].

2.2.1. Extent of lymphadenectomy for stage IB–III gastric carcinoma

There used to be a fierce debate between Asian and Western surgeons about the extent of lymphadenectomy. Asian specialists advocated D2 lymphadenectomy because of superior oncologic outcomes. However, Western surgeons argued that D2 lymphadenectomy only added to perioperative morbidity and mortality with no significant survival benefit [4]. There were three randomised controlled trials (RCTs) that addressed this issue. The Dutch trial randomised 711 patients in D1 and D2 lymphadenectomy groups. It has to be noted that distal pancreatectomy with splenectomy was performed in all cases with D2 dissection but only selectively in D1 dissection. This trial reported a significantly higher morbidity (42% vs. 4%, $p < 0.001$) and mortality (10% vs. 4%, $p < 0.004$) in D2 group. Furthermore, there was no 5-year survival benefit in D2 group (D1 = 34% vs. D2 = 33%). However, this study was criticised because of many shortcomings. One of them was the fact that surgeons participating in this trial had no previous experience in D2 lymphadenectomies and they were trained using video

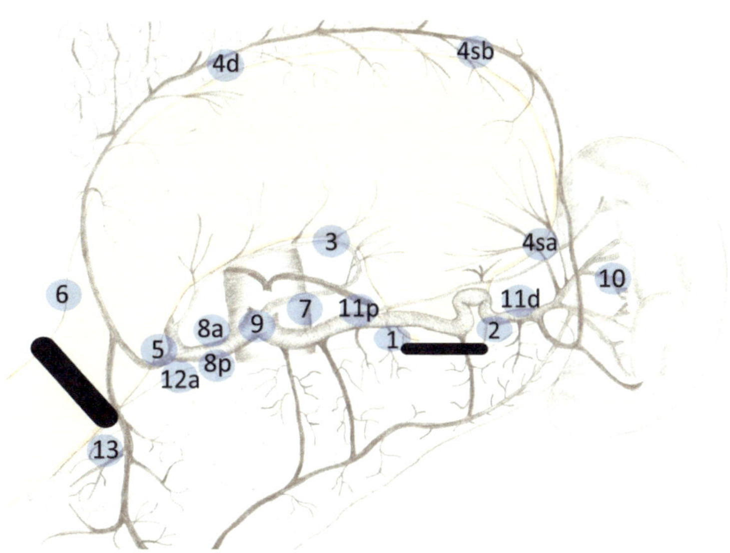

Figure 8. Total gastrectomy. In total gastrectomy, D1 lymphadenectomy constitutes dissection of nodal stations 1–7. D2 lymphadenectomy constitutes dissection of D1 + stations 8a, 9, 10, 11p, 11d and 12a.

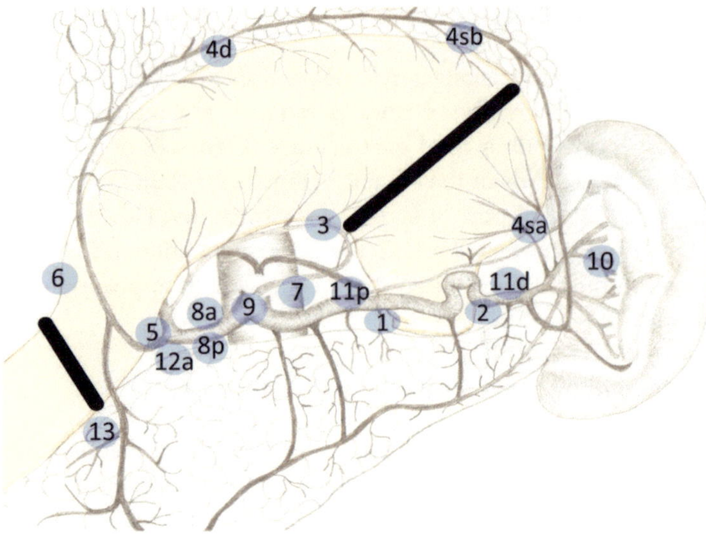

Figure 9. Distal subtotal gastrectomy. In distal subtotal gastrectomy, D1 lymphadenectomy constitutes dissection of nodal stations 1, 3, 4sb, 4d, 5, 6 and 7. D2 lymphadenectomy constitutes dissection of D1 + stations 8a, 9, 11p and 12a.

materials and booklets. It was only after the 15-year survival data were analysed that the evidence showed positive results for D2 dissection. Gastric cancer-related deaths were significantly lower in D2 group (37% vs. 48%). Local (12% vs. 22%) and regional (13% vs. 19%) recurrence rates were also lower in D2 group. The overall 15-year survival was 21% in D1 group and 29% in D2, without statistically significant difference ($p = 0.34$) [4, 9].

Another famous study that questioned the usefulness of D2 dissection was Medical Research Council trial. The results of this study drew similar conclusions – there was no evidence to support routine use of D2 lymphadenectomy. Again, distal pancreatectomy with splenectomy was performed in D2 dissections just as it was in the Dutch study. Significantly, lower survival on subgroup analysis was noted in both studies for patients with distal pancreatectomy and splenectomy. The third landmark RCT on this subject, the Italian study, found comparable overall morbidity (12.0% in D1 vs. 17.9% in D2, $p = 0.178$) and no significant difference in 30-day postoperative mortality rate (3.0% in D1 vs. 2.2% in D2, $p = 0.72$). The essential difference was that only experienced surgeons participated in this trial and that distal pancreatectomy with splenectomy was not routinely performed [4, 9]. The main conclusion is that in Western countries D2 lymphadenectomy can be safely performed in high-volume centres by experienced surgeons. Distal pancreatectomy and splenectomy are no longer considered an integral part of modern D2 lymphadenectomy and are considered beneficial only if the primary tumour or metastatic nodes invade these organs [4, 7, 9].

2.2.2. Extent of resection

Microscopically, negative resection margins are required to qualify any gastric resection as curative. Although not all patients with positive resection margins develop cancer recurrence, this undoubtedly worsens prognosis [10]. There seems to be a lack of agreement about what is an adequate margin from gastric carcinoma with different articles suggesting slightly different numbers. There are studies that have illustrated tumour cell spread as far as 5 cm laterally from the primary tumour. Therefore, a margin of at least 6 cm seems necessary [6]. However, according to other experts, a 4 cm margin is sufficient [1, 4].

Discussion about distal resection margin is simpler. This margin is limited by the papilla of Vater and is generally 2–4 cm from the pylorus. If the tumour invades papilla or further down the duodenum, a metastatic disease is expected, and gastrectomy alone will not suffice [10].

Regarding proximal resection margin, the Japanese guidelines have specific recommendation. For T1 gastric carcinoma, a gross resection margin of 2 cm is recommended. In case the tumour margins are equivocal on preoperative endoscopy, a biopsy-guided marking with clips can be used to aid in intraoperative decision-making [7]. If the cancer is invading proper muscular layer or deeper, a 3 cm margin is needed for expansively growing tumours, and 5 cm are necessary for infiltrating tumours [7]. The idea that optimal proximal margin distance is stage-dependent is highlighted by a multicentre US study reporting on 465 patients who underwent gastric resection due to distal gastric carcinoma. Authors found that in stage I there was no difference in overall survival between 3.1–5.0 cm and >5.0 cm proximal margin [11]. For a diffuse gastric carcinoma, an 8 cm margin is recommended [5]. If the resection margin is negative, the distance from the tumour does not per se influence the prognosis [10]. Therefore, in case the aforementioned criteria regarding proximal margin distance cannot be followed, frozen section examination is highly recommended [7]. In case of positive resection margins on the final histology, the benefits of reoperation must be weighed against the risks of repeated operation. Reoperation is usually warranted in low-stage cases with minimal (N0–N1) nodal involvement [10].

2.2.3. *Total vs. subtotal gastrectomy*

Unlike the debate regarding lymphadenectomy, total gastrectomy (TG) vs. subtotal gastrectomy (SG) is a less polarising topic. Since the 'en principle' total gastrectomy was suggested in the 1970s, several large studies have provided evidence to support the role of distal subtotal gastrectomy [12]. Currently, it is the procedure of choice for early gastric cancer located in the distal and middle third of the stomach if the resection margins are located well within the healthy stomach (distances discussed previously). The advantages of subtotal gastric resection are the following: several studies have reported lower morbidity and mortality, reduced hospital stay and superior nutritional status with better quality of life in long term [12]. Two large randomised trials performed in Europe found no significant difference in long-term survival between TG and SG for distal gastric cancer but lower morbidity, mortality and better quality of life in SG group [12]. A recently performed meta-analysis of six trials also found no significant difference in 5-year survival between TG and SG groups ($p = 0.18$). However, it did not show higher postoperative complication rates ($p = 0.30$) or hospital mortality ($p = 0.12$) in TG group which was in contrast to previously mentioned studies [13].

There are several proposed advantages of TG. It could reduce the risk of inadequate lymph node harvest, thus lowering local recurrence risk. Due to removal of all gastric tissue, it eliminates the risks of multicentric synchronous or metachronous carcinoma [13]. TG is recommended for gastric carcinoma located in the upper third of the stomach, signet ring cell cancers (*linitis plastica*), cancer arising on the background of atrophic gastritis, multicentric cancers, advanced distally located tumours with lymph node metastasis to allow extended lymphadenectomy, invasion of pancreas (which requires pancreaticosplenectomy) and patients with inherited E-cadherin mutation as a prophylactic measure (due to 80% lifetime risk of developing gastric cancer) [1, 6, 7, 12, 13].

2.2.4. Laparoscopic vs. open gastrectomy

Laparoscopic gastric cancer surgery is technically demanding and is currently performed more routinely by Asian surgeons. Nevertheless, more and more specialists around the globe are becoming more confident in laparoscopic surgery, and, with the help of technological advancements, usage of laparoscopy will certainly increase [14]. As discussed previously, very early gastric carcinomas are preferably treated by endoscopic resection. However, criteria for endoscopic treatment are very strict, and these methods are more widely used in high-incidence countries with high proportion of early cases. Therefore, the most solid indication for laparoscopic surgery is gastric carcinoma located in the distal or middle third of the stomach and limited to submucosa without evidence of lymph node involvement or mucosal cancers not amenable to endoscopic treatment [14]. In case of laparoscopic total gastrectomy, the more widely accepted indication is T1N0 tumour of proximal third of the stomach [14]. There is evidence that laparoscopy is a safe and feasible option even for advanced gastric carcinomas if performed in high-volume specialised centres [1]. A systematic review comprising 3411 patients revealed similar lymph node harvest and long-term survival for laparoscopic distal gastrectomy compared to open approach. Hospital stay, analgetic consumption, postoperative complication rate and blood loss in surgery were all reduced in laparoscopic approach group [1]. Surgeons in Eastern Asia have expanded the use of laparoscopy to advanced cancers even with limited involvement of perigastric nodes [14]. There is still a small amount of high-quality evidence to support these expanded indications [4, 14]. However, one large systematic review analysing 23 studies with 7336 patients was recently published. Authors found comparable 5-year overall survival ($p = 0.45$), recurrence ($p = 0.08$) and gastric cancer-related death rates ($p = 0.28$) between laparoscopic and open gastrectomy groups. These results led them to conclude that laparoscopic gastrectomy was comparable to the open approach and did not worsen oncologic results [15]. To evaluate the role of laparoscopy in advanced gastric cancer, a meta-analysis comprising 11 studies and 1904 patients was performed. A D2 dissection was performed in both open and laparoscopic cases. Researchers found reduced blood loss, morbidity, shorter postoperative ileus and length of hospital stay in laparoscopic group, although the operation time was longer by almost 42 min ($p < 0.05$). No significant difference was noted in lymph node harvest, intrahospital mortality, recurrence rate and 3-year overall survival rates. This indicates that laparoscopy has several advantages in short-term results and is equivalent from oncologic standpoint [16].

While many surgeons perform the so-called laparoscopy-assisted gastrectomy which requires mini-laparotomy incision and extracorporeal anastomosis, several options for totally laparoscopic gastrectomy are available. Even single-port laparoscopy is being performed frequently in high-volume centres. A small study comparing 50 single-port laparoscopies with 50 multi-port surgeries indicated superior short-term results for single-port surgery. However, this did not lead to reduced hospital stay. Most specialists use at least five ports for laparoscopic gastrectomy [14].

Despite the aforementioned studies, the present state of laparoscopic gastric surgery is not entirely clear. A lot of the evidence comes from Asian countries, high-volume specialised centres with considerable experience. Current studies have been criticised for bias and heterogeneity, for example, not including the most advanced gastric cancers in studies comparing open with laparoscopic approach. Some authors have found reduced lymph node harvest at specific nodal stations during laparoscopic D2 dissection. This has raised the question of robotic surgery as a valid tool to overcome some of the technical difficulties that comes with laparoscopic surgery. Robotic system has superior manoeuvrability and visualisation, which is essential in performing dissection along the celiac axis, spleen and pancreas. Another advantage is the relatively easier restoration of gastrointestinal continuity using robotic system. As with other procedures, robotic gastrectomy seems to take less time to master than conventional laparoscopic surgery although this could in part be related to previous experience in laparoscopic approach. There is currently not enough high-quality evidence to draw any definitive conclusions on robotic gastric cancer surgery in comparison with conventional laparoscopic and open surgery [17].

3. Gastric neuroendocrine tumours (NETs)

NETs arise from the cells of the diffuse neuroendocrine system that are scattered all around the body and have both neural and endocrine characteristics (**Figure 10**). This is a heterogeneous group of tumours with wide variations in biologic behaviour, clinical picture and optimal management. Despite the fact that these tumours are typically indolent in nature, often

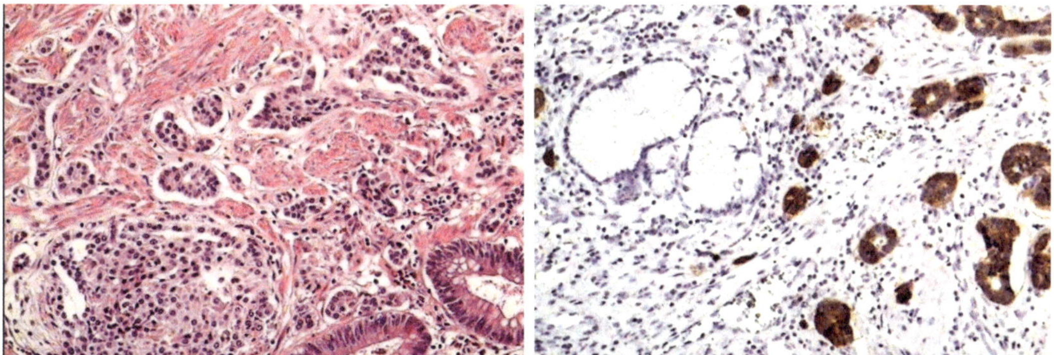

Figure 10. Gastric NET. (A) Haematoxylin-eosin, original magnification (OM) 100×. (B) Synaptophysin expression. Immunoperoxidase, OM 100×.

described as slowly growing, they all have malignant potential. Therefore, surgical resection is the only definitive treatment [18].

Gastric NETs (GNETs) are rare tumours, but their incidence is growing. The proportion of GNETs amongst all gastrointestinal NETs also increases. The current incidence is 1–2 per 100,000 persons per year which accounts for 8.7% of all gastrointestinal NETs. This increase of incidence is at least partly related to more widespread use of gastrointestinal endoscopy [18, 19].

There are three to four types of GNETs which differ significantly in terms of biologic behaviour, malignancy, prognosis and optimal treatment [18–20]. Some discrepancy in literature regarding classification of GNETs is noted. Although the latest European Neuroendocrine Tumour Society (ENETS) guidelines still divide GNETs in three types, a further subclassification of type 3 tumours is considered appropriate [20]. A comparison of different GNET types is depicted in **Table 2**.

Tumour characteristics	Type 1 GNET	Type 2 GNET	Type 3 GNET
Proportion of GNETs (%)	70–80	5–6	10–15
Associated diseases/syndromes	Chronic atrophic gastritis	MEN1-ZES	Sporadic
Typical tumour size (cm)	<1–2 cm	<1–2 cm	>2 cm
Tumour number	Multiple	Multiple	Solitary
Location	Fundus, corpus	Fundus, corpus	Any
Serum gastrin	↑	↑	N
Histology (most common)	NET G1	NET G1/G2	NEC G3
Invasion	Mucosa, submucosa	Mucosa, submucosa	Any
Frequency of metastasis (%)	2–5	10–30	>50
Prognosis	Excellent	Good	Poor

GNET, gastric neuroendocrine tumour; MEN1-ZES, multiple endocrine neoplasia type 1 and Zollinger-Ellison syndrome; N, normal; NET, neuroendocrine tumour; G, grade; NEC, neuroendocrine carcinoma.

Table 2. Features of different gastric NETs.

3.1. Type 1 GNETs

This is the most common type of GNETs (70–80%) and is more frequently seen in female patients. Type 1 GNETs develop from enterochromaffin-like (ECL) cells and are associated with chronic gastric mucosal atrophy caused by *H. pylori* or autoimmune gastritis. These tumours are well differentiated, usually small (<1 cm), multiple, located in the fundus or corpus, limited to mucosa or submucosa and have an excellent prognosis [18–20]. They have a very low mitotic rate and metastatic potential (2–5%) [18, 19]. Pathophysiological mechanism of type 1 GNET development is achlorhydria caused by atrophic gastritis, which stimulates gastrin production, which in turn evokes ECL cell hyperplasia [19].

These tumours are best treated with conservative approach, with surgery reserved for selected cases. In ENETS guidelines, endoscopic surveillance every 1–2 years is recommended for lesions <1 cm without evidence of invasion into the proper muscular layer or metastasis. However, other specialists have recently suggested removal of all visible lesions with biopsy forceps or EMR (>5 mm tumours). This approach has to be compared with the previously mentioned less aggressive management in randomised trials to support its use. Any GNET with size close to 10 mm or threatening proper muscular layer has to be resected to avoid metastatic spread [18–20]. Research has shown superior complete resection rates for ESD compared to EMR in the treatment of GNETs [19].

Surgical resection is recommended for type 1 GNETs that are invading the proper muscular layer (T2), have recurred after endoscopic removal and are poorly differentiated or in case of positive resection margins after endoscopic resection [18–20]. Depending on the location and number of lesions as well as potential involvement of lymph nodes, local excision, partial or total gastrectomy is selected. Antrectomy to reduce hypergastrinemia is questionable and is rarely performed [18, 20].

3.2. Type 2 GNETs

These tumours are less frequently encountered (5–6%) and are associated with multiple endocrine neoplasia type 1 and Zollinger-Ellison syndrome (MEN1-ZES). Just like type 1 GNETs, they are gastrin-dependent, consist of ECL cells, are small, multiple and relatively benign. These are equally distributed amongst genders and in 10–30% of cases are metastatic at presentation. Although type 2 GNETs are asymptomatic per se, they can present with peptic ulcer disease due to hypersecretion of gastric acid caused by ZES [18–20].

According to the National Comprehensive Cancer Network (NCCN) guidelines, the treatment of type 2 GNETs is similar to type 1 tumours. In ENETS guidelines, however, only local surgical excision is recommended. The fact that the patient has multiple tumours does not alter surgical treatment by itself. Local or limited resection of the coexisting gastrinoma is recommended, but decision has to be made in a multidisciplinary setting in high-volume centres [18, 20].

3.3. Type 3 GNETs

Type 3 NETs (10–15%) are sporadic, usually poorly differentiated, single tumours >10 mm in size not associated with gastrin hypersecretion. These tumours have the tendency to invade proper muscular layer and are frequently metastatic (in regional lymph nodes, liver) at the time of diagnosis [18–20].

There are reports that suggest that in selected cases (<2 cm, well differentiated, submucosal, without lymphovascular invasion) type 3 GNETs should be treated with endoscopic or wedge resection. Despite that, ENETS guidelines strictly recommend type 3 GNETs to be treated like gastric carcinomas with distal or total gastrectomy and lymphadenectomy [18, 20].

4. Gastric gastrointestinal stromal tumours (GISTs)

GISTs are mesenchymal tumours that develop from the interstitial cells of Cajal (gastrointestinal pacemakers) anywhere in the GI tract. GISTs are rare constituting only less than 1% of all GI malignancies. Although the annual reported incidence is just 10 cases per million, the actual Incidence is believed to be much higher [22]. The stomach is the most common location for GISTs (70%). The driving force for GIST development is a gain-of-function mutation in tyrosine kinase receptor gene *c-KIT* [21].

Although the discovery of tyrosine kinase inhibitor imatinib has been the most significant change in GIST treatment over recent years, surgery as the only potentially curative method remains the cornerstone of treatment [23].

Gastric GISTs start their growth in deeper layers, mostly in the smooth muscle layer of gastric wall; expand intra- or extraluminally and eventually produce haematogenous metastasis in solid organs or peritoneum. They can also cause sarcomatosis by perforating into peritoneal cavity [21].

Any patient who is medically fit should undergo complete surgical resection of gastric GIST. However, NCCN and ESMO guidelines recommend endoscopic surveillance for small (<1 cm and <2 cm, respectively) gastric lesions if high-risk features are not present by endoscopic ultrasound investigation (ulcerations (see **Figure 11**), cystic spaces, irregular borders, echogenic foci and heterogeneity). All other cases and patients who do not want to undergo endoscopic surveillance should be treated by surgical resection [21, 24].

Unlike for carcinoma, a wide resection margin of healthy tissue is not necessary for GISTs. It is of paramount importance to be meticulous and remove the entire lesion without damaging tumour pseudocapsule or causing tumour spillage or bleeding as this would increase the risk of locoregional recurrence and sarcomatosis. GISTs rarely spread via lymphatics; therefore, lymphadenectomy is not necessary. If noted, enlarged lymph nodes near the tumour can selectively be dissected. Either wedge resection or full-thickness partial gastrectomy is usually sufficient for lesser and greater curvature tumours, whereas a transgastric resection after anterior gastrotomy incision is performed for posterior wall gastric GISTs. Total or subtotal gastrectomy is only required for tumours occupying large portions of the stomach. If the tumour is borderline resectable or a extensive operation

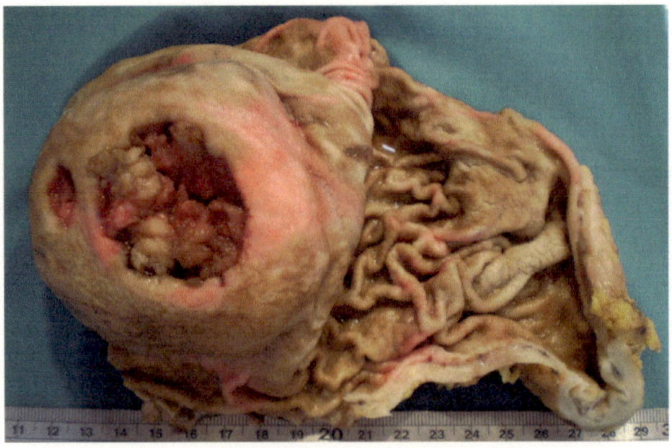

Figure 11. Gastrointestinal stromal tumour. Note the umbilicated ulceration.

(total gastrectomy, en bloc resection of adjacent organs) is predicted, neoadjuvant treatment with imatinib is used to downstage the tumour and perform less extensive surgery in advanced cases [21–24].

Laparoscopic surgery is considered a feasible and safe option for the treatment of small (<5 cm) gastric GISTs as long as the general oncologic principles are followed. This statement is supported by evidence from several retrospective cohort studies [23]. Direct manipulation of the tumour with instruments is contraindicated, and a plastic bag must be used on extraction to reduce the risk of spillage. Both ESMO and NCCN guidelines support the use of laparoscopic technique for small gastric GISTs (<5 cm) [23]. Although there are studies that indicate feasibility for larger tumours [25], more high-quality research is needed to widen this indication. A hybrid procedure, endoscopy-assisted laparoscopic resection, can aid in tumour localisation and preservation of gastric volume. While it is currently performed in a limited amount of centres, it will probably take a more prominent place amongst minimally invasive gastric procedures [21].

5. Conclusions

Gastric cancer at present remains one of the most difficult oncological problems the surgeon has to deal with. Despite extensive research in novel systemic therapeutic options, surgery is still the only potentially curative treatment. Accumulation of evidence has made surgical treatment of gastric cancer more personalised allowing to select the extent of resection and lymphadenectomy according to specific tumour. Increased skills combined with technological advances have further improved the postoperative function by making minimally invasive approach safe and effective. Even complex procedures like D2 lymph node dissection are nowadays performed laparoscopically in specialised centres. Despite being rare, gastric NETs and GISTs need special consideration when it comes to surgical treatment because these tumours differ from adenocarcinomas in biology and best management. Robotic surgery and hybrid endoscopic surgical procedures will probably have a more prominent role in the future because of their potential advantages over conventional laparoscopic surgery.

Author details

Roberts Rumba[1], Andrejs Vanags[1*], Arturs Kalva[2], Tatjana Bogdanova[2], Inese Drike[2], Dzeina Mezale[2], Marta Vitola[3], Janis Gardovskis[1] and Ilze Strumfa[2]

*Address all correspondence to: Andrejs.Vanags@rsu.lv

1 Department of Surgery, Riga Stradins University, Riga, Latvia

2 Department of Pathology, Riga Stradins University, Riga, Latvia

3 Pediatric Dentistry Clinic Villadent, Riga, Latvia

References

[1] Van Cutsem E, Sagaert X, Topal B, Haustermans K, Prenen H. Gastric cancer. Lancet. 2016;388(10060):2654-2664. DOI: 10.1016/S0140-6736(16)30354-3

[2] Thrumurthy SG, Chaudry MA, Hochhauser D, Mughal M. The diagnosis and management of gastric cancer. BMJ. 2013;347:f6367. DOI: 10.1136/bmj.f6367

[3] Karimi P, Islami F, Anandasabapathy S, Freedman ND, Kamangar F. Gastric cancer: Descriptive epidemiology, risk factors, screening, and prevention. Cancer Epidemiol Biomarkers Prev. 2014;23(5):700-713. DOI: 10.1158/1055-9965.EPI-13-1057

[4] Kuo CY, Chao Y, Li CP. Update on treatment of gastric cancer. Journal of the Chinese Medical Association. 2014;77(7):345-353. DOI: 10.1016/j.jcma.2014.04.006

[5] Smyth EC, Verheij M, Allum W, Cunningham D, Cervantes A, Arnold D; ESMO Guidelines Committee. Gastric cancer: ESMO Clinical Practice Guidelines for diagnosis, treatment and follow-up. Ann Oncol. 2016;27(Suppl. 5):v38-v49. DOI: 10.1093/annonc/mdw350

[6] Townsend CM Jr., Beauchamp RD, Evers BM, Mattox KL. Sabiston Textbook of Surgery: the Biological Basis of Modern Surgical Practice. 20th ed. Philadelphia: Elsevier Sounders; 2017. 1213-1231 p.

[7] Japanese Gastric Cancer Association. Japanese gastric cancer treatment guidelines. Gastric Cancer. 2017;20(1):1-19. DOI: 10.1007/s10120-016-0622-4

[8] Facciorusso A, Antonino M, Di Maso M, Muscatiello N. Endoscopic submucosal dissection vs endoscopic mucosal resection for early gastric cancer: A meta-analysis. World J Gastrointest Endosc. 2014;6(11):555-563. DOI: 10.4253/wjge.v6.i11.555

[9] Garg PK, Jakhetiya A, Sharma J, Ray MD, Pandey D. Lymphadenectomy in gastric cancer: Contentious issues. World J Gastrointest Surg. 2016;8(4):294-300. DOI: 10.4240/wjgs.v8.i4.294

[10] Shin D, Park SS. Clinical importance and surgical decision-making regarding proximal resection margin for gastric cancer. World J Gastrointest Oncol. 2013;5(1):4-11. DOI: 10.4251/wjgo.v5.i1.4

[11] Squires MH 3rd, Kooby DA, Poultsides GA, Pawlik TM, Weber SM, Schmidt CR, Votanopoulos KI, Fields RC, Ejaz A, Acher AW, Worhunsky DJ, Saunders N, Levine EA, Jin LX, Cho CS, Bloomston M, Winslow ER, Russell MC, Cardona K, Staley CA, Maithel SK. Is it time to abandon the 5-cm margin rule during resection of distal gastric adenocarcinoma? A multi-institution study of the U.S. Gastric Cancer Collaborative. Ann Surg Oncol. 2015;22(4):1243-1251. DOI: 10.1245/s10434-014-4138-z

[12] Santoro R, Ettorre GM, Santoro E. Subtotal gastrectomy for gastric cancer. World J Gastroenterol. 2014;20(38):13667-13680. DOI: 10.3748/wjg.v20.i38.13667

[13] Kong L, Yang N, Shi L, Zhao G, Wang M, Zhang Y. Total versus subtotal gastrectomy for distal gastric cancer: Meta-analysis of randomized clinical trials. Onco Targets Ther. 2016;9:6795-6800. DOI: 10.2147/OTT.S110828.

[14] Son T, Hyung WJ. Laparoscopic gastric cancer surgery: Current evidence and future perspectives. World J Gastroenterol. 2016;22(2):727-735. DOI: 10.3748/wjg.v22.i2.727

[15] Chen XZ, Wen L, Rui YY, Liu CX, Zhao QC, Zhou ZG, Hu JK. Long-term survival outcomes of laparoscopic versus open gastrectomy for gastric cancer: A systematic review and meta-analysis. Medicine (Baltimore). 2015;94(4):e454. DOI: 10.1097/MD.0000000000000454

[16] Huang YL, Lin HG, Yang JW, Jiang FQ, Zhang T, Yang HM, Li CL, Cui Y. Laparoscopy-assisted versus open gastrectomy with D2 lymph node dissection for advanced gastric cancer: A meta-analysis. Int J Clin Exp Med. 2014;7(6):1490-1499

[17] Caruso S, Patriti A, Roviello F, De Franco L, Franceschini F, Coratti A, Ceccarelli G. Laparoscopic and robot-assisted gastrectomy for gastric cancer: Current considerations. World J Gastroenterol. 2016;22(25):5694-5717. DOI: 10.3748/wjg.v22.i25.5694

[18] Li TT, Qiu F, Qian ZR, Wan J, Qi XK, Wu BY. Classification, clinicopathologic features and treatment of gastric neuroendocrine tumors. World J Gastroenterol. 2014;20(1):118-125. DOI: 10.3748/wjg.v20.i1.118

[19] Sato Y, Hashimoto S, Mizuno K, Takeuchi M, Terai S. Management of gastric and duodenal neuroendocrine tumors. World J Gastroenterol. 2016;22(30):6817-6828. DOI: 10.3748/wjg.v22.i30.6817

[20] Delle Fave G, O"Toole D, Sundin A, Taal B, Ferolla P, Ramage JK, Ferone D, Ito T, Weber W, Zheng-Pei Z, De Herder WW, Pascher A, Ruszniewski P; Vienna Consensus Conference participants. ENETS consensus guidelines update for gastroduodenal neuroendocrine neoplasms. Neuroendocrinology. 2016;103(2):119-124. DOI: 10.1159/000443168

[21] Roggin KK, Posner MC. Modern treatment of gastric gastrointestinal stromal tumors. World J Gastroenterol. 2012;18(46):6720-6728. DOI: 10.3748/wjg.v18.i46.6720.

[22] Kong SH, Yang HK. Surgical treatment of gastric gastrointestinal stromal tumor. J Gastric Cancer. 2013;13(1):3-18. DOI: 10.5230/jgc.2013.13.1.3

[23] Nishida T, Blay JY, Hirota S, Kitagawa Y, Kang YK. The standard diagnosis, treatment, and follow-up of gastrointestinal stromal tumors based on guidelines. Gastric Cancer. 2016;19(1):3-14. DOI: 10.1007/s10120-015-0526-8

[24] ESMO/European Sarcoma Network Working Group. Gastrointestinal stromal tumours: ESMO Clinical Practice Guidelines for diagnosis, treatment and follow-up. Ann Oncol. 2014;25(Suppl. 3):iii21-iii26. DOI: 10.1093/annonc/mdu255

[25] Kasetsermwiriya W, Nagai E, Nakata K, Nagayoshi Y, Shimizu S, Tanaka M. Laparoscopic surgery for gastric gastrointestinal stromal tumor is feasible irrespective of tumor size. J Laparoendosc Adv Surg Tech A. 2014;24(3):123 -129. DOI: 10.1089/lap.2013.0433

Section 5

Treatment Strategies in Patients with Gastric Cancer

Chapter 10

Molecular Targeting Therapy for Gastric Cancer: Current Advances and Obstacles

Shouji Shimoyama

Additional information is available at the end of the chapter

http://dx.doi.org/10.5772/intechopen.69724

Abstract

Although the incidence of gastric cancer (GC) has declined steadily in recent years, GC remains a major cancer burden. Multimodal therapies have been developed and first-line chemotherapy for advanced GC patients, even they have good performance status, could provide only modest efficacy. Furthermore, treatment outcomes after failure of first-line chemotherapy remain poor. In order to provide a solution to this unmet clinical need, since the management of various types of cancer has progressed rapidly into the molecular era, biomarker-targeted therapy for GC has received enormous attention in recent years. This review focuses on the current treatment achievement of molecular targeting agents for GC, such as trastuzumab, pertuzumab, trastuzumab emtansine, lapatinib, cetuximab, panitumumab, nimotuzumab, mammalian target of rapamycin, bevacizumab, ramucirumab, sunitinib, sorafenib, apatinib, rilotumumab, and onartuzumab. However, problems are also emerged with regard to resistance and refractoriness. This chapter also focuses on the current obstacles concerning resistance and refractoriness, as well as provides discussions concerning future directions with regard to molecular categorization to predict response and toxicities leading to select patients most likely to benefit.

Keywords: gastric cancer, molecular targeting therapy, human epidermal growth factor receptors, angiogenesis, resistance

1. Introduction

Although the incidence of gastric cancer (GC) has declined steadily in recent years, GC remains a major cancer burden. GC is still the fifth most common malignancy and third leading cause of cancer death in both sexes worldwide, comprising 8.8% of total cancer deaths [1]. Radical resection is the only potentially curative approach for GC; however, approximately 40–70% of GC recurs even after curative resection [2]. When the disease reaches an advanced state, chemotherapy becomes a mainstay of the treatment [3]. The most frequently used first-line chemotherapy regimens worldwide are platinum derivatives plus fluoropyrimidine doublet or a triplet regimen with the addition of epirubicin or docetaxel. The reality is that chemotherapy has reached a plateau of efficacy for GC with a median overall survival (mOS) of around or less than 12 months [4, 5]. Furthermore, although second-line treatment is recommended for the patients with failure after first-line chemotherapy because it prolongs survival as compared with the best supportive care [6–8], the global standard regimens of second-line chemotherapy have not yet been determined [4].

These somewhat painfully slow rates of advances in treatment have been impetus to develop new concepts of strategies. As an example, receptor tyrosine kinases (RTKs) consist of the ligand binding of extracellular domains, a transmembrane domain, and a tyrosine kinase motif, which is involved in a subsequent downstream signal cascade. Since this cascade leads to cell growth, differentiation, adhesion, migration, and apoptosis [9], each step is theoretically a therapeutic target. This review focuses on advances in molecular targeted therapy for GC in recent years, as well as problems to be resolved.

2. Focus on human epidermal growth factor receptors (HERs)

Membrane-bound human epidermal growth factor receptors (HERs) consist of a ligand-binding domain at the extracellular surface, a single transmembrane segment, and a cytoplasmic portion harboring the protein kinase activity. The HER family includes four structurally related members, namely the epidermal growth factor receptor (EGFR, also known as HER1), HER2, HER3, and HER4. Ligand binding to the extracellular domain triggers conformational changes of receptors that form HER-dimerization, and subsequently, activates downstream a signaling cascade and ultimately stimulates tumor cell proliferation. Therefore, HERs are the most innovative targets for GC treatment.

2.1. Trastuzumab

HER2 is responsible for GC cell growth when overexpressed [10]. A literature review demonstrates that the mean incidence of HER2-positive gastric cancer is 18%, ranging from 4 to 53% [11], and the most recent research confirmed that the HER2 positivity rate to be 21% among Japanese patients [12]. A systematic analysis demonstrated the potential role for HER2 as a negative prognostic factor [11]; thus, it has become a rational therapeutic target. Trastuzumab, a humanized monoclonal antibody that targets the extracellular domain IV of the HER2, was evaluated by the first landmark randomized controlled trial (RCT) (ToGA trial) [M]. The ToGA trial provided evidence of a significant improvement by the addition of trastuzumab to chemotherapy as compared with chemotherapy alone as a first-line setting. In patients with HER2-positive GC, while trastuzumab could achieve longer mOS, a higher response rate (RR), and a longer median progression free survival (mPFS) (**Table 1**), toxicity did not differ between groups. A post-hoc analysis revealed that the survival differences between groups were more evident in patients with immunohistochemistry (IHC) 2+

Reference	Publication year	Design	Phase	Experimental arm		Control arm		RR			mPFS			mOS			Study name
				Agents	*n*	Agents	*n*	Experimental arm	Control arm	*p*	Experimental arm	Control arm	*p*	Experimental arm	Control arm	*p*	
[13]	2010	1st	III	F, Cis, T	294	F, Cis	290	47%	35%	0.0017	6.7	5.5	0.0002	13.8	11.1	0.0046	ToGA
[36]	Ongoing	1st	III	T, F, Cis, Per	NA	T, F, Cis	ND	ND	ND	ND	ND	ND	ND	ND	ND	ND	JACOB (NCT01 774786)
[37]	2016	2nd	II/III	T-DM1	228	TAX	117	21%	20%	ND	2.7	2.9	NS	7.9	8.6	NS	GATSBY (NCT016 41939)
[39]	2015	1st	III	Cape, Ox, L	249	Cape, Ox	238	53%	39%	0.0031	6	5.4	0.04	12.2	10.5	NS	LoGiC
[40]	2014	2nd	III	PTX, L	132	PTX	129	27%	9%	<0.001	5.4	4.4	NS	11	8.9	NS	TyTAN
[41]	2013	1st	III	Cape, Cis, Cet	455	Cape, Cis	449	30%	29%	NS	4.4	5.6	NS	9.4	10.7	NS	EXPAND
[42]	2010	1st	III	EOC, Pani	278	EOC	275	42%	46%	NS	7.4	6	NS	8.8	11.3	0.013	REAL-3
[43]	2015	1st	rII	S1, Cis, Nimo	31	S1, Cis	31	55%	58%	NS	7.2	4.8	0.011	14.2	10.2	0.06	
[44]	2015	2nd	rII	Iri, Nimo	40	Iri	43	18%	10%	NS	73d	85d	NS	251d	232d	NS	
[50]	2013	2nd or further	III	Eve	439	–	217	4	2	ND	1.7	1.4	<0.001	5.3	4.3	NS	GRANITE-1
[56]	2011	1st	III	Cape, Cis, Bev	387	Cape, Cis	387	46%	37%	0.03	6.7	5.3	0.0037	12.1	10.1	NS	AVAGAST
[57]	2015	1st	III	Cape, Cis, Bev	102	Cape, Cis	100	41%	34%	NS	6.3	6	NS	10.5	11.4	NS	AVATAR
[62]	2014	2nd	III	Ram	238	–	117	3%	3%	NS	2.1	1.3	<0.0001	5.2	3.8	0.047	REGARD
[63]	2014	2nd	III	PTX, Ram	330	PTX	335	28%	16%	0.0001	4.4	2.9	<0.0001	9.6	7.4	0.017	RAINBOW

Reference	Publication year	Design	Phase	Experimental arm		Control arm		RR			mPFS			mOS			Study name
				Agents	*n*	Agents	*n*	Experimental arm	Control arm	*p*	Experimental arm	Control arm	*p*	Experimental arm	Control arm	*p*	
[65]	Ongoing	1st	III	F, Cis, Ram	NA	F, Cis	NA	ND	ND	ND	ND	ND	ND	ND	ND	ND	RAINFALL (NCT02 314177)
[66]	2014	1st	rII	FOLFOX, Ram	84	FOLFOX	84	45	46	ND	6.4	6.7	ND	11.7	11.5	ND	
[67]	2014	3rd	III	Apatinib	176	–	91	2.8	0	NS	2.6	1.8	<0.001	6.5	4.7	0.0149	
[73]	2016	2nd or further	rII	FOLFILI, sunitinib	45	FOLFILI	45	20	29	ND	3.5	3.3	NS	10.4	8.9	NS	
[87]	2015	1st	III	E, Cis, Cape, rilotumumab	304	E, Cis, Cape	305	30	39	0.027	5.7	5.7	0.016	9.6	11.5	0.016	RILOMET-1 (NCT016 97072)
[88]	Ongoing	1st	III	Cis, Cape, rilotumumab	NA	Cis, Cape	NA	ND	ND	ND	ND	ND	ND	ND	ND	ND	RILOMET-2 (NCT021 37343)
[92]	2017	1st	III	FOLFOX6, Ona	279	FOLFOX6	283	46	41	NS	6.7	6.8	NS	11	11.3	NS	

RR—response rate; mPFS—median progression free survival; mOS—median overall survival; rII—randomized phase II; NA—not described; NS—not significant; Bev—bevacizumab; Cape—capecitabine; Cet—cetuximab; Cis—cisplatin; E—epirubicin; EOC—epirubicin, oxaliplatin, capecitabine; Eve—everolimus; F—fluoropyrimidines; FOLFIRI—leucovorin + 5-fluorouracil + irinotecan; FOLFOX—leucovorin + 5-fluorouracil + oxaliplatin; Iri—irinotecan; L—lapatinib; Nimo—nimotuzumab; Ona—onartuzumab; Ox—oxaliplatin; Pani—panitumumab; Per—pertuzumab; PTX—paclitaxel; Ram—ramucirumab; T—trastuzumab; T-DM1—trastuzumab emtansine.

Table 1. Results of phase III or randomized phase II trials of molecular targeting therapy for gastric cancer.

and fluorescence *in situ* hybridization (FISH) positive tumors or IHC3+ tumors [13]. The ToGA trial also provided evidence of a prolongation of time to the deterioration of health-related quality of life [14]. Furthermore, the subgroup analyses of the ToGA trial restricted to Japanese patients [15] and a subsequent similar phase III study recruiting only Chinese patients [16] have confirmed again such promising results, suggesting the efficacy of trastuzumab irrespective of country of origin. The results of the ToGA study have changed the treatment paradigm for GC harboring HER2 overexpression. Subsequently, a HELOISE study has been conducted to investigate the efficacy of different doses of trastuzumab with cisplatin and capecitabine [17], resulting in no differences between 6 and 10 mg of trastuzumab in terms of mOS and mPFS.

However, targeting HER2 raises important issues that must be discussed, namely, heterogeneity and resistance. Heterogeneity should be considered because of a different HER2 positivity rate according to cancer histology, the location of GC, and geographic area, making for various prevalence rates of HER2-positive GC from study to study or from country to country. In the ToGA trial discussed above, the HER2 positivity rate was higher in the intestinal type (31.8%) than in the diffuse type (6.1%), in specimens from the gastroesophageal junction (32.2%) than in those from the stomach (21.4%), and in patients from Asia-Pacific (23.9%) or Europe (23.6%) than in patients from Central/South America (16.1%) [18]. In addition, one-third of IHC3+ patients had <30% of stained cells, suggesting staining variability within the same tumor. Furthermore, variations of scoring criteria between studies may be another explanation for heterogeneity [11]. Since these variations may undoubtedly complicate the interpretation of the results of the clinical trials, there is a need for establishing a unique scoring system specific for GC [19], which could help identify and select HER2-positive patients who benefit from trastuzumab. Another important issue is a trastuzumab resistance, which has begun to arise along with the accumulation of experience of trastuzumab use. Not all HER2-positive patients immediately benefit from trastuzumab, and even those who initially respond to trastuzumab will eventually experience progress, suggesting refractories and resistance. In breast cancer, the majority of those who initially responded to trastuzumab ultimately became resistant during prolonged treatment [20, 21]. In looking at the ToGA trial, mPFS was 6.7 months in the trastuzumab arm or the absolute increase in the RR was only 12%, suggesting that half of the GC patients—even though they were HER2 positive—exhibit acquired resistance within 7 months or do not necessarily respond to trastuzumab.

When considering the onset of nonresponsiveness to trastuzumab, two statuses should be distinguished, namely, resistance and refractoriness. Resistance is a condition of disease progression at first evaluation even under trastuzumab use, whereas refractoriness is a condition of disease progression at second or later evaluations after an initial clinical response [22]. The resistance may be ascribed to intrinsic mechanisms, while refractoriness may be related to acquired properties. The precise mechanisms of these phenomena are unclear; several pathways may be involved, including phosphatidylinositol-3-kinase (PI3K) [23], a mammalian target of rapamycin (mTOR) [23], insulin-like growth factor-1 (IGF-1) [24], and a phosphatase and tensin homolog (PTEN) [25]. This encourages the development of second-generation agents of targeting HER2 to overcome HER2 resistance.

2.2. Pertuzumab

Pertuzumab is a humanized monoclonal antibody that binds to the HER2 domain II—the interface of the dimer formation of HER. As discussed earlier, since trastuzumab binds to the HER2 domain IV—a region not involved in receptor dimerization [26, 27], trastuzumab inhibits ligand-independent dimerization of HER2 while it is not effective for the inhibition of ligand-dependent heterodimerization. These biological properties could imply one mechanism of trastuzumab resistance. For example, HER ligands are able to induce the formation of HER2-containing heterodimers such as the ligand-dependent HER2/HER3 heterodimer even in the presence of trastuzumab; thus HER3 plays some roles in trastuzumab resistance. Notably, HER3 is overexpressed in 14–62% of GC [28–30], and HER3 *per se* is associated with poor survival rates. Considering that pertuzumab binds to the HER2 domain II and subsequently blocks the heterodimerization of HER2 with other members of the HER family, pertuzumab is expected to overcome trastuzumab resistance.

In *in vitro* studies and animal models, pertuzumab and trastuzumab showed synergistic antitumor effects [31–33]. Subsequent RCT in HER2-positive metastatic breast cancer demonstrated that pertuzumab, trastuzumab, and docetaxel significantly improved overall survival rates for HER2-positive metastatic breast cancer when compared with placebos, trastuzumab, and docetaxel [34]. Such positive results were maintained when the follow-up period was extended [35]. Motivated by the promising results, a phase III study is ongoing which randomizes HER2-positive advanced GC patients to first-line trastuzumab, cisplatin, and fluoropyrimidine with or without pertuzumab [36].

2.3. T-DM1

T-DM1 is an antibody drug conjugate of trastuzumab and emtansine (DM1), a microtubule inhibitor. TDM-1 is expected to deliver a cytotoxic agent directly to cancer cells. Unfortunately, however, the efficacy of T-DM1 as compared to taxane as a second-line setting failed to meet its primary endpoint (GATSBY trial). The mOS, mPFS, and RR were not different between the two arms [37].

2.4. Lapatinib

Lapatinib is a small molecule inhibitor of the intracellular domain of tyrosine kinase of EGFR and HER2, thus interrupting EGFR- and HER2-associated downstream signaling cascades. Theoretically, lapatinib and trastuzumab synergistically act even on the status of trastuzumab resistance. Indeed, a meta-analysis has revealed [38] the efficacy of lapatinib on HER2-positive breast cancer patients. Accordingly in GC, lapatinib in combination with chemotherapy has been evaluated by two randomized trials as first-line [39] and second-line [40] settings. Unfortunately, the addition of lapatinib to capecitabine plus oxaliplatin (LoGiC trial) [39] or the addition of lapatinib to paclitaxel (TyTAN trial) [40] failed to demonstrate any significant improvement of mOS when compared with chemotherapy without lapatinib.

However, some confusion may exist when considering clinicopathological subsets that receive benefit from agents against HER2. A LoGiC study revealed that Asian or younger (age <60 years old) patients may benefit from lapatinib [39], while a ToGA trial proved trastuzumab efficacy to be more effective in patients from Central/South America or from Europe, or in older patients [13]. In addition, the TyTAN study, which was conducted only in Asia, failed to identify any clear subgroup benefit from lapatinib except for patients from mainland China. Therefore, it is important to clarify biomarkers that may predict which patients may benefit from dual EGFR/HER2 inhibition.

2.5. Cetuximab, panitumumab, and nimotuzumab

Cetuximab is a recombinant human-mouse chimeric anti-EGFR antibody. A randomized EXPAND study as a first-line setting revealed that the addition of cetuximab to capecitabine plus cisplatin provided no additional benefit to chemotherapy [41]. Panitumumab is a fully humanized anti-HER1 antibody. A REAL-3 study randomized advanced GC patients to first-line epirubicin, oxaliplatin, and capecitabine with or without panitumumab [42]. Again, pertuzumab provided no additional survival benefit to chemotherapy or seemed to be even harmful.

Following by the negative results of the two RCTs (EXPAND and REAL-3), another anti-EGFR antibody, nimotuzumab, a recombinant humanized monoclonal antibody against EGFR [43, 44] has been developed. Regrettably, however, a randomized phase II study adding first-line nimotuzumab to S-1 plus cisplatin failed to improve mOS when compared to S-1 plus cisplatin. In this study, even among the EGFR2+/3+ subgroup, adding nimotuzumab did not provide any additional benefit to the S-1 plus cisplatin combination [43]. However, nimotuzumab and irinotecan could improve survival rates in the EGFR2+/3+ subgroup [44]. The exact reasons underlying these different results according to the chemotherapy agents combined with nimotuzumab are unclear, but putative mechanisms responsible for the confusing results may be negative synergistic effects between the anti-EGFR antibody and capecitabine.

Unlike in colorectal cancer, KRAS mutations have not been a negative predictive marker for EGFR-targeting therapy in GC [45], and prespecified KRAS mutations have limited clinical value. Therefore, the significance of KRAS gene mutations, which is a predictive factor for a lack of efficacy in colorectal cancer, may not be extrapolated to GC, and KRAS mutations are not validated at this time. It is possible that alternative mechanisms other than KRAS mutations to escape from cetuximab action may exist. In this regard, attempts to find predictors of the efficacy of EGFR-targeting therapies have been reported in Refs. [46–48]; however, a small number of patients investigated in such biomarker analyses and a retrospective study design may preclude drawing a meaningful conclusion. Furthermore, the very low rate of KRAS mutation in GC (3–9%) [46–48] also hinders further application in clinical practice. The identification of reliable predictive markers is of paramount importance for selecting the most appropriate agents to the patients benefiting most.

2.6. Mammalian target of rapamycin (mTOR)

The mammalian target of rapamycin (mTOR) is one of the key protein kinases that regulate cell growth, proliferation, and angiogenesis [49] and is integrated in the downstream cascade of HER. The inhibition of mTOR is thus an intriguing new therapeutic approach. Everolimus, an oral mTOR inhibitor, did not significantly improve mOS but could reduce the risk of disease progression ($p < 0.001$) when compared with the best supportive care (GRANITE-1 trial) [50].

3. Anti-antigenic

Angiogenesis was postulated 40 years ago as an essential event for tumors to grow beyond a critical size of few millimeters. Except for physiological conditions requiring angiogenesis such as embryogenesis and wound healing, inhibiting neovascularization may contribute to tumor growth arrest with minimal toxicities to normal tissues. Therefore, targeting molecules involved in neovascularization has gained recognition as a rational therapeutic option.

3.1. Bevacizumab

Bevacizumab is a monoclonal antibody targeting vascular endothelial growth factor (VEGF)-A, which is effective in combination with chemotherapy in several kinds of malignancies including the colon [51], breast [52], and lung [53]. Against the background that the overexpression of VEGF was correlated with tumor aggressiveness and poor prognosis in GC [54, 55], a randomized AVAGAST study was conducted to evaluate the efficacy of adding bevacizumab to capecitabine plus cisplatin in the first-line treatment of advanced GC [56]. The results did not meet the primary outcome; however, adding bevacizumab to chemotherapy resulted in a significant prolongation of mPFS and a significant increase in RR. In the subgroup analysis of AVAGAST study, geographical differences in efficacy were suggested, it being effective in Pan-America whereas not so in Asia and Europe. Subsequently, an AVATAR trial in which the trial design is similar with that of AVAGAST has been conducted for 202 Chinese patients with the results recently published [57]. Again, neither mOS nor mPFS were improved by the addition of bevacizumab to chemotherapy. Based on the negative results of the two RCTs, research should be continued to seek the biomarker predictive for bevacizumab efficacy in order to determine the bevacizumab rational position in the treatment of advanced GC [58]. Candidates for potential predictive biomarkers include plasma VEGF-A level and tissue neuropilin-1 expression [58]. However, other cancers had potential other predictive markers for bevacizumab efficacy, being VEGF-A and VEGFR-2 in breast cancer [59] or VEGFR-1 single-nucleotide polymorphism in pancreatic and renal cell cancer [60].

3.2. Ramucirumab

Ramucirumab is a fully humanized monoclonal antibody that blocks the binding of VEGF-A, C, and D to the extracellular domain of VEGF receptor-2 (VEGFR-2); thus, ramucirumab inhibits the ligand activation of a downstream signal transduction of VEGF-R [61]. The REGARD trial is the first RCT demonstrating survival benefits for second-line ramucirumab when compared with the best supportive care [62]. Subsequently, the RAINBOW trial was conducted to evaluate the second-line efficacy of weekly paclitaxel with or without ramucirumab [63]. The subgroup analysis demonstrated that ramucirumab was not effective in Asian patients when compared with those from Europe and the USA; however, this geographical difference was ascribed partly to the high proportion of patients receiving postdiscontinuation therapy—at least for Japanese patients [64]. Currently, ramucirumab has been evaluated as a first-line setting in combination with fluoropyrimidines and cisplatin (RAINFALL trial) [65] or in combination with FOLFOX [66].

3.3. VEGFR tyrosine kinase inhibitors—sunitinib, sorafenib, and apatinib

VEGFR-1, -2, and -3 are RTKs by which a downstream signaling cascade is stimulated to induce angiogenesis when corresponding ligands VEGF-A, -B, -C, and -D bind to the receptors. Several small molecules, which block some steps of this cascade, have been developed. Apatinib is a small molecule of VEGFR-2 tyrosine kinase inhibitor that has been compared with placebos for the second-line treatment of advanced GC. One RCT revealed that apatinib achieved significantly prolonged mOS and mPFS when compared with placebos [67]. These positive findings by inhibiting VEGFR-2 and its related tyrosine kinases have promoted interest in VEGFR inhibition as a therapeutic strategy.

However, pathways of other growth factors, such as platelet-derived growth factor (PDGF), may be responsible for alternative escape mechanisms to the VEGF-VEGFR blockade [68, 69] and may be one reason for resistance to antiangiogenic therapy. These findings have prompted the development of several small molecules targeting multiple RTKs with expectations to overcome an escape from the VEGF-VEGFR blockade. Sorafenib is a multikinase inhibitor that targets multiple RTKs such as VEGFR-2, -3, PDGF-receptor (PDGF-R), c-Kit, and Raf [70, 71]. Sunitinib is another oral multitarget kinase inhibitor of VEGFR, PDGFR, and the Kit receptor [72]. A randomized phase II trial demonstrated a trend toward better mOS in sunitinib plus FORFIRI arm as compared with a FOLFIRI arm, whereas PFS and RR were similar between both arms [73]. Regorafenib is another oral multikinase inhibitor of receptor tyrosine kinases of VEGFR, B-RAF, and PDGFR [74]. A PFS was significantly improved by regorafenib as compared with a placebo in patients with gastrointestinal stromal tumor (GIST) refractory to standard therapy [75]. Encouraged by these results, a phase II INTEGRATE study was conducted and revealed a significant prolongation of mPFS in favor of regorafenib as compared with a placebo [76].

3.4. Resistance to antiangiogenic therapy

In consideration of targeting molecules to suppress angiogenesis, the caveats lie in a paradoxical increase in tumor growth or in a rebound phenomenon that is greater tumor aggressiveness followed by the cessation of antiangiogenic therapy. An animal xenograft model exhibited the worrying observation of a higher incidence of metastasis and/or shorter survival time by antiangiogenic therapy [77], suggesting angiogenesis inhibition as a driving force in tumor progression to stages of greater malignancy. It is plausible for cancer cells exposed to hypoxic conditions to acquire properties that allow them to overcome the lack of energy and oxygen supply. This acquisition means a transformation to a threatening form of tumor adaptation against starving strategy, leading to assume a malignant behavior. In addition, the rebound phenomenon should be mentioned because the withdrawal of antiVEGF TKI resulted in a rapid regrowth of the tumor vasculature that was suppressed during the therapy [78]. For example, renal cell cancer patients showing complete response by sunitinib and sorafenib experienced a relapse on discontinuation of the therapy, but all responded again to a reintroduction of the drug [79]. These findings have confirmed several current limitations to antiangiogenic therapy, posing future challenges for their expanded use.

The precise mechanisms for this phenomenon are unclear. In addition to the multiple pathways to escape from the VEGF-VEGFR blockade as described earlier, it is possible that tumor hypoxia induced by antiangiogenic therapy triggers another angiogenic switch for cancer cells to survive or forces cancer cells to migrate to their nonhypoxic lesion. At present, there is no clinical evidence that the rebound phenomenon is a result of anti-angiogenic therapy or any adverse effects of the inherent nature of anti-angiogenic therapy. A recent review has proposed putative mechanisms of resistance to antiangiogenic therapy [80], which could uncover evasive or intrinsic changes within the tumor as resistance mechanisms of antiangiogenic therapy.

A key molecule involved in another angiogenic switch under conditions of antiangiogenic therapy is the hypoxia inducible factor (HIF) [81]. HIF induces a hepatocyte growth factor (HGF) [82] that subsequently activates a mesenchymal-epidermal transition factor receptor (MET). Activation of this HGF/MET pathway leads to GC cell proliferation, survival, and migration [83]; thus, the HIF and HGF/MET axis is another rational therapeutic target for overcoming the resistance to antiangiogenic therapy. Furthermore, a strategy of HGF/MET inhibition is important because MET solely [84] or its interaction with EGFR [85] or HER3 [86] may mediate resistance to anti-HER therapy.

3.5. HGF/MET inhibitors—rilotumumab and onartuzumab

A number of inhibitors of the HGF/MET pathway have been developed, including monoclonal antibodies, such as rilotumumab and onartuzumab, or small molecule RTK inhibitor such as foretinib.

Rilotumumab, a humanized monoclonal antibody against HGF, has been investigated by two first-line RCTs. RILOMET-1 is a comparison between rilotumumab plus ECX (epirubicin, cisplatin and capecitabine) and a placebo plus ECX [87], and RILOMET-2 aims to evaluate cisplatin plus capecitabine with or without rilotumumab [88]. A rilotumumab benefit was seen in MET-positive patients [89] or was rilotumumab concentration dependent [90]. A very recent pharmacokinetic study revealed a lack of drug-drug interaction between rilotumumab and ECX [91]; however, the results were negative, thereby recommending the early cessation of the RILOMET-1 study [87]. Onartuzumab is a recombinant, fully humanized, monoclonal anti-MET antibody. A randomized phase II study of FOLFOX with or without onartuzumab failed to gain positive results with regard to mPFS and mOS [92]. Foretinib, an oral small molecule multikinase inhibitor that targets MET and VEGFR-2, has been evaluated by a phase II study; however, the results are discouraging [93].

4. Future perspectives

GC and breast cancer have similarities with regard to HER2 positivity rate and molecularly targeted agents first used, such as trastuzumab. However, differences are apparent with regard to tumor response to another HER-inhibitor between the two tumors. The evidence obtained by the current clinical trials suggests that GC and breast cancer do not necessarily show the same response to the HER-2 targeted therapies even if both tumors are HER2 positive. Such similarities and differences also exist between GC and colorectal cancer. This is partly ascribed to the absence of a validated biomarker specific for GC, for which we are currently unable to select patients who may benefit most or those who may most likely suffer toxicities. The recruitment of molecularly unselected patients may be one reason why many clinical trials did not add benefits or show any superiority over the conventional chemotherapy. The molecular categorization according to which pathways are most activated and which molecules are predominantly involved, as well as which factors or genes are most predictive to response and toxicities highlights the most responsible therapeutic target(s) and the opportunity to explore the most cost-effective agents. These challenges could enable only molecularly selected patients to be treated and the benefit-to-toxicity ratio will likely improve as well. This will ultimately allow clinicians to administer the right treatment to the right patients. Clinical trials with unselected patients are nearing their end, and welcome to those recruiting only correctly selected patients. The innovation of new therapeutic agents designed under this concept will certainly emerge in the future to help oncologists improve the clinical management of GC.

5. Conclusions

Chemotherapy has reached a plateau of efficacy for GC, with an mOS of around 12 months. Unfortunately, progress in treating this disease with chemotherapy over the last years has lagged behind other malignancies such as breast and colorectal cancer. During this time, molecular targeting therapies for colorectal cancer have evolved and their clinical efficacy has been evaluated by various phase III trials, resulting in the mOS being at least doubled. In GC, the use of molecularly targeted therapies is still in the early stages, but more and more targeted drugs have begun to be developed to target each step of the signaling pathways. Disappointingly, however, both monoclonal antibodies and RTK inhibitors targeting signal transduction pathways failed to meet expectations or their efficacy was modest at best.

Such a painful slow advance is partly ascribed to either the lack of validated biomarkers to predict a therapeutic response or adverse events to molecular targeting therapy or to escape or resistance phenomena. Better therapeutic responses could sometimes be obtained at the expense of adverse events; however, drug-related severe adverse events might depress patient QOL. In addition, the blockade of a single signal transduction axis does not provide long-term efficacy due to escape or resistance phenomena. Research should be continued to bridge these adverse events and efficacy gaps or to circumvent resistance, but we are still far from any major breakthrough. Such a reality is challenging, but thanks to the accumulation of the knowledge of the mechanisms of RTK action and its downstream signal transduction cascade, there are several candidate surrogate biomarkers of response and adverse events, or multiple blockade strategies or kinases are being developed. New predictive biomarkers and the clarification of resistance mechanisms may hopefully lead to the selection of a potentially drug-sensitive cohort, to intensify drug efficacy, and to predict more accurately adverse events, holding promise for more tailored therapies. In this respect, both challenges and progress engender optimism as they unveil biological mechanisms underlying GC, ultimately identifying those patients most likely to benefit.

Author details

Shouji Shimoyama

Address all correspondence to: shimoyama@apost.plala.or.jp

Gastrointestinal Unit, Settlement Clinic, Adachi-ku, Tokyo, Japan

References

[1] Ferlay J, Soerjomataram I, Dikshit R, Eser S, Mathers C, Rebelo M, Parkin DM, Forman D, Bray F. Cancer incidence and mortality worldwide: sources, methods and major patterns in GLOBOCAN 2012. International Journal of Cancer. 2015;**136**:E359-E386. DOI: 10.1002/ijc.29210

[2] D'Angelica M, Gonen M, Brennan MF, Turnbull AD, Bains M, Karpeh MS. Patterns of initial recurrence in completely resected gastric adenocarcinoma. Annals of Surgery. 2004;**240**:808-816

[3] Wagner AD, Grothe W, Haerting J, Kleber G, Grothey A, Fleig WE. Chemotherapy in advanced gastric cancer: A systematic review and meta-analysis based on aggregate data. Journal of Clinical Oncology. 2006;**24**:2903-2909

[4] Shimoyama S. Chemotherapy for gastric cancer. What comes next? In: Rangel LBA, Silva V, editors. Updates on Cancer Treatment. In Tech, Croatia; 2015. pp. 103-117

[5] GASTRIC (Global Advanced/Adjuvant Stomach Tumor Research International Collaboration) Group, Oba K, Paoletti X, Bang YJ, Bleiberg H, Burzykowski T, Fuse N, Michiels S, Morita S, Ohashi Y, Pignon JP, Rougier P, Sakamoto J, Sargent D, Sasako M, Shitara K, Tsuburaya A, Van Cutsem E, Buyse M. Role of chemotherapy for advanced/recurrent gastric cancer: An individual-patient-data meta-analysis. European Journal of Cancer. 2013;**49**:1565-1577. DOI: 10.1016/j.ejca.2012.12.016

[6] Badiani B, Maratea D, Messori A. Second-line treatments for advanced gastric cancer: Interpreting outcomes by network meta-analysis. World Journal of Clinical Oncology. 2015;**6**:73-79. DOI: 10.5306/wjco.v6.i4.73

[7] Thuss-Patience PC, Kretzschmar A, Bichev D, Deist T, Hinke A, Breithaupt K, Dogan Y, Gebauer B, Schumacher G, Reichardt P. Survival advantage for irinotecan versus best supportive care as second-line chemotherapy in gastric cancer—A randomised phase III study of the Arbeitsgemeinschaft Internistische Onkologie (AIO). European Journal of Cancer. 2011;**47**:2306-2314. DOI: 10.1016/j.ejca.2011.06.002

[8] Kang JH, Lee SI, Lim DH, Park KW, Oh SY, Kwon HC, Hwang IG, Lee SC, Nam E, Shin DB, Lee J, Park JO, Park YS, Lim HY, Kang WK, Park SH. Salvage chemotherapy for pretreated gastric cancer: A randomized phase III trial comparing chemotherapy

plus best supportive care with best supportive care alone. Journal of Clinical Oncology. 2012;**30**:1513-1518. DOI: 10.1200/JCO.2011.39.4585

[9] Lemmon MA, Schlessinger J. Cell signaling by receptor tyrosine kinases. Cell. 2010; **141**:1117-1134. DOI: 10.1016/j.cell.2010.06.011

[10] Gravalos C, Jimeno A. HER2 in gastric cancer: A new prognostic factor and a novel therapeutic target. Annals of Oncology. 2008;**19**:1523-1529. DOI: 10.1093/annonc/mdn169

[11] Jorgensen JT, Hersom M. HER2 as a prognostic marker in gastric cancer—A systematic analysis of data from the literature. Journal of Cancer. 2012;**3**:137-144. DOI: 10.7150/jca.4090

[12] Matsusaka S, Nashimoto A, Nishikawa K, Miki A, Miwa H, Yamaguchi K, Yoshikawa T, Ochiai A, Morita S, Sano T, Kodera Y, Kakeji Y, Sakamoto J, Saji S, Yoshida K. Clinicopathological factors associated with HER2 status in gastric cancer: Results from a prospective multicenter observational cohort study in a Japanese population (JFMC44-1101). Gastric Cancer. 2016;**19**:839-851. DOI: 10.1007/s10120-015-0518-8

[13] Bang YJ, Van Cutsem E, Feyereislova A, Chung HC, Shen L, Sawaki A, Lordick F, Ohtsu A, Omuro Y, Satoh T, Aprile G, Kulikov E, Hill J, Lehle M, Rüschoff J, Kang YK; ToGA Trial Investigators. Trastuzumab in combination with chemotherapy versus chemotherapy alone for treatment of HER2-positive advanced gastric or gastro-oesophageal junction cancer (ToGA): A phase 3, open-label, randomised controlled trial. Lancet. 2010;**376**:687-697. DOI: 10.1016/S0140-6736(10)61121-X

[14] Satoh T, Bang YJ, Gotovkin EA, Hamamoto Y, Kang YK, Moiseyenko VM, Ohtsu A, Van Cutsem E, Al-Sakaff N, Urspruch A, Hill J, Weber HA, Chung HC; ToGA Trial Investigators. Quality of life in the trastuzumab for gastric cancer trial. The Oncologist. 2014;**19**:712-719. DOI: 10.1634/theoncologist.2014-0058

[15] Sawaki A, Ohashi Y, Omuro Y, Satoh T, Hamamoto Y, Boku N, Miyata Y, Takiuchi H, Yamaguchi K, Sasaki Y, Nishina T, Satoh A, Baba E, Tamura T, Abe T, Hatake K, Ohtsu A. Efficacy of trastuzumab in Japanese patients with HER2-positive advanced gastric or gastroesophageal junction cancer: A subgroup analysis of the Trastuzumab for Gastric Cancer (ToGA) study. Gastric Cancer. 2012;**15**:313-322. DOI: 10.1007/s10120-011-0118-1

[16] Shen L, Xu JM, Feng FY, Jiao SC, Wang LW, Li J, Guan ZZ, Qin SK, Wang JJ, Yu SY, Wang YJ, Jin YN, Tao M, Zheng LZ, Pan LX. Trastuzumab in combination with chemotherapy versus chemotherapy alone for first-line treatment of HER2-positive advanced gastric or gastroesophageal junction cancer: A Phase III, multi-center, randomized controlled trial, Chinese subreport. (In Chinese with English abstract) Zhonghua Zhong Liu Za Zhi. 2013;**35**:295-300. DOI: 10.3760/cma.j.issn.0253-3766.2013.04.012

[17] A Study of Herceptin (Trastuzumab) in Combination With Cisplatin/Capecitabine Chemotherapy in Participants With Human Epidermal Growth Factor Receptor 2 (HER2)-Positive Metastatic Gastric or Gastro-Esophageal Junction Cancer (HELOISE). https://clinicaltrials.gov [NCT 01450696]

[18] Van Cutsem E, Bang YJ, Feng-Yi F, Xu JM, Lee KW, Jiao SC, Chong JL, López-Sanchez RI, Price T, Gladkov O, Stoss O, Hill J, Ng V, Lehle M, Thomas M, Kiermaier A, Rüschoff J. HER2 screening data from ToGA: Targeting HER2 in gastric and gastroesophageal junction cancer. Gastric Cancer. 2015;**18**:476-484. DOI: 10.1007/s10120-014-0402-y

[19] Hofmann M, Stoss O, Shi D, Büttner R, van de Vijver M, Kim W, Ochiai A, Rüschoff J, Henkel T. Assessment of a HER2 scoring system for gastric cancer: Results from a validation study. Histopathology. 2008;**52**:797-805. DOI: 10.1111/j.1365-2559.2008.03028.x

[20] Shimoyama S. Unraveling trastuzumab and lapatinib in gastric cancer. Molecular and Clinical Oncology. 2014;**2**:175-181. DOI: 10.3892/mco.2013.218

[21] Slamon DJ, Leyland-Jones B, Shak S, Fuchs H, Paton V, Bajamonde A, Fleming T, Eiermann W, Wolter J, Pegram M, Baselga J, Norton L. Use of chemotherapy plus a monoclonal antibody against HER2 for metastatic breast cancer that overexpresses HER2. The New England Journal of Medicine. 2001;**344**:783-792

[22] Wong H, Leung R, Kwong A, Chiu J, Liang R, Swanton C, Yau T. Integrating molecular mechanisms and clinical evidence in the management of trastuzumab resistant or refractory HER-2^{+} metastatic breast cancer. The Oncologist. 2011;**16**:1535-1546. DOI: 10.1634/theoncologist.2011-0165

[23] Serra V, Markman B, Scaltriti M, Eichhorn PJ, Valero V, Guzman M, Botero ML, Llonch E, Atzori F, Di Cosimo S, Maira M, Garcia-Echeverria C, Parra JL, Arribas J, Baselga J. NVP-BEZ235, a dual PI3K/mTOR inhibitor, prevents PI3K signaling and inhibits the growth of cancer cells with activating PI3K mutations. Cancer Research. 2008;**68**:8022-8030. DOI: 10.1158/0008-5472.CAN-08-1385

[24] Nahta R, Yuan LX, Zhang B, Kobayashi R, Esteva FJ. Insulin-like growth factor-I receptor/human epidermal growth factor receptor 2 heterodimerization contributes to trastuzumab resistance of breast cancer cells. Cancer Research. 2005;**65**:11118-11128

[25] Nagata Y, Lan KH, Zhou X, Tan M, Esteva FJ, Sahin AA, Klos KS, Li P, Monia BP, Nguyen NT, Hortobagyi GN, Hung MC, Yu D. PTEN activation contributes to tumor inhibition by trastuzumab, and loss of PTEN predicts trastuzumab resistance in patients. Cancer Cell. 2004;**6**:117-127

[26] Cho HS, Mason K, Ramyar KX, Stanley AM, Gabelli SB, Denney DW Jr, Leahy DJ. Structure of the extracellular region of HER2 alone and in complex with the Herceptin Fab. Nature. 2003;**421**:756-760

[27] Baselga J, Swain SM. Novel anticancer targets: Revisiting ERBB2 and discovering ERBB3. Nature Reviews Cancer. 2009;**9**:463-475. DOI: 10.1038/nrc2656

[28] Zhang XL, Yang YS, Xu DP, Qu JH, Guo MZ, Gong Y, Huang J. Comparative study on overexpression of HER2/neu and HER3 in gastric cancer. World Journal of Surgery. 2009;**33**:2112-2118. DOI: 10.1007/s00268-009-0142-z

[29] Tang D, Liu CY, Shen D, Fan S, Su X, Ye P, Gavine PR, Yin X. Assessment and prognostic analysis of EGFR, HER2, and HER3 protein expression in surgically resected gastric adenocarcinomas. OncoTargets and Therapy. 2014;**8**:7-14. DOI: 10.2147/OTT.S70922

[30] Ema A, Yamashita K, Ushiku H, Kojo K, Minatani N, Kikuchi M, Mieno H, Moriya H, Hosoda K, Katada N, Kikuchi S, Watanabe M. Immunohistochemical analysis of RTKs expression identified HER3 as a prognostic indicator of gastric cancer. Cancer Science. 2014;**105**:1591-1600. DOI: 10.1111/cas.12556

[31] Nahta R, Hung MC, Esteva FJ. The HER-2-targeting antibodies trastuzumab and pertuzumab synergistically inhibit the survival of breast cancer cells. Cancer Research. 2004;**64**:2343-2366

[32] Lee-Hoeflich ST, Crocker L, Yao E, Pham T, Munroe X, Hoeflich KP, Sliwkowski MX, Stern HM. A central role for HER3 in HER2-amplified breast cancer: Implications for targeted therapy. Cancer Research. 2008;**68**:5878-5887. DOI: 10.1158/0008-5472.CAN-08-0380

[33] Scheuer W, Friess T, Burtscher H, Bossenmaier B, Endl J, Hasmann M. Strongly enhanced antitumor activity of trastuzumab and pertuzumab combination treatment on HER2-positive human xenograft tumor models. Cancer Research. 2009;**69**:9330-9336. DOI: 10.1158/0008-5472.CAN-08-4597

[34] Swain SM, Kim SB, Cortés J, Ro J, Semiglazov V, Campone M, Ciruelos E, Ferrero JM, Schneeweiss A, Knott A, Clark E, Ross G, Benyunes MC, Baselga J. Pertuzumab, trastuzumab, and docetaxel for HER2-positive metastatic breast cancer (CLEOPATRA study): Overall survival results from a randomised, double-blind, placebo-controlled, phase 3 study. The Lancet Oncology. 2013;**14**:461-471. DOI: 10.1016/S1470-2045(13)70130-X

[35] Swain SM, Baselga J, Kim SB, Ro J, Semiglazov V, Campone M, Ciruelos E, Ferrero JM, Schneeweiss A, Heeson S, Clark E, Ross G, Benyunes MC, Cortés J; CLEOPATRA Study Group. Pertuzumab, trastuzumab, and docetaxel in HER2-positive metastatic breast cancer. The New England Journal of Medicine. 2015;**372**:724-734. DOI: 10.1056/NEJMoa1413513

[36] Tabernero J, Hoff PM, Shen L, Ohtsu A, Yu R, Eng-Wong J, Kang Y-K. Pertuzumab (P) with trastuzumab (T) and chemotherapy (CTX) in patients (pts) with HER2-positive metastatic gastric or gastroesophageal junction (GEJ) cancer: An international phase III study (JACOB). Journal of Clinical Oncology. 2013;**31**:TPS 4150

[37] Kang Y-K, Shah MA, Ohtsu A, Van Cutsem E, Ajani JA, van der Horst T, Harle-Yge M-L, Piao Y, Betsy Althaus B, Thuss-Patience PC. A randomized, open-label, multicenter, adaptive phase 2/3 study of trastuzumab emtansine (T-DM1) versus a taxane (TAX) in patients (pts) with previously treated HER2-positive locally advanced or metastatic gastric/gastroesophageal junction adenocarcinoma (LA/MGC/GEJC). Journal of Clinical Oncology. 2016;**34**:abs5

[38] Amir E, Ocaña A, Seruga B, Freedman O, Clemons M. Lapatinib and HER2 status: Results of a meta-analysis of randomized phase III trials in metastatic breast cancer. Cancer Treatment Reviews. 2010;**36**:410-415. DOI: 10.1016/j.ctrv.2009.12.012

[39] Hecht JR, Bang YJ, Qin SK, Chung HC, Xu JM, Park JO, Jeziorski K, Shparyk Y, Hoff PM, Sobrero A, Salman P, Li J, Protsenko SA, Wainberg ZA, Buyse M, Afenjar K, Houé V, Garcia A, Kaneko T, Huang Y, Khan-Wasti S, Santillana S, Press MF, Slamon D. Lapatinib in combination with capecitabine plus oxaliplatin in human epidermal growth factor receptor 2-positive advanced or metastatic gastric, esophageal, or gastroesophageal adenocarcinoma: TRIO-013/LOGiC—A randomized phase III trial. Journal of Clinical Oncology. 2016;**34**:443-451. DOI: 10.1200/JCO.2015.62.6598

[40] Satoh T, Xu RH, Chung HC, Sun GP, Doi T, Xu JM, Tsuji A, Omuro Y, Li J, Wang JW, Miwa H, Qin SK, Chung IJ, Yeh KH, Feng JF, Mukaiyama A, Kobayashi M, Ohtsu A, Bang YJ. Lapatinib plus paclitaxel versus paclitaxel alone in the second-line treatment of HER2-amplified advanced gastric cancer in Asian populations: TyTAN—A randomized, phase III study. Journal of Clinical Oncology. 2014;**32**:2039-2049. DOI: 10.1200/JCO.2013.53.6136

[41] Lordick F, Kang YK, Chung HC, Salman P, Oh SC, Bodoky G, Kurteva G, Volovat C, Moiseyenko VM, Gorbunova V, Park JO, Sawaki A, Celik I, Götte H, Melezínková H, Moehler M; Arbeitsgemeinschaft Internistische Onkologie and EXPAND Investigators. Capecitabine and cisplatin with or without cetuximab for patients with previously untreated advanced gastric cancer (EXPAND): A randomised, open-label phase 3 trial. The Lancet Oncology. 2013;**14**:490-499. DOI: 10.1016/S1470-2045(13)70102-5

[42] Waddell T, Chau I, Cunningham D, Gonzalez D, Okines AF, Okines C, Wotherspoon A, Saffery C, Middleton G, Wadsley J, Ferry D, Mansoor W, Crosby T, Coxon F, Smith D, Waters J, Iveson T, Falk S, Slater S, Peckitt C, Barbachano Y. Epirubicin, oxaliplatin, and capecitabine with or without panitumumab for patients with previously untreated advanced oesophagogastric cancer (REAL3): A randomised, open-label phase 3 trial. The Lancet Oncology. 2013;**14**: 481-489. DOI: 10.1016/S1470-2045(13)70096-2

[43] [43]. Du F, Zheng Z, Shi S, Jiang Z, Qu T, Yuan X, Sun Y, Song Y, Yang L, Zhao J, Wang J, Chi Y. S-1 and cisplatin with or without nimotuzumab for patients with untreated unresectable or metastatic gastric cancer: A randomized, open-label phase 2 trial. Medicine (Baltimore). 2015;**94**:e958. DOI: 10.1097/MD.0000000000000958

[44] Satoh T, Lee KH, Rha SY, Sasaki Y, Park SH, Komatsu Y, Yasui H, Kim TY, Yamaguchi K, Fuse N, Yamada Y, Ura T, Kim SY, Munakata M, Saitoh S, Nishio K, Morita S, Yamamoto E, Zhang Q, Kim JM, Kim YH, Sakata Y. Randomized phase II trial of nimotuzumab plus irinotecan versus irinotecan alone as second-line therapy for patients with advanced gastric cancer. Gastric Cancer. 2015;**18**:824-832. DOI: 10.1007/s10120-014-0420-9

[45] Park SR, Kook MC, Choi IJ, Kim CG, Lee JY, Cho SJ, Kim YW, Ryu KW, Lee JH, Lee JS, Park YI, Kim NK. Predictive factors for the efficacy of cetuximab plus chemotherapy as salvage therapy in metastatic gastric cancer patients. Cancer Chemotherapy and Pharmacology. 2010;**65**:579-587. DOI: 10.1007/s00280-009-1067-9

[46] Lordick F, Luber B, Lorenzen S, Hegewisch-Becker S, Folprecht G, Wöll E, Decker T, Endlicher E, Röthling N, Schuster T, Keller G, Fend F, Peschel C. Cetuximab plus

oxaliplatin/leucovorin/5-fluorouracil in first-line metastatic gastric cancer: A phase II study of the Arbeitsgemeinschaft Internistische Onkologie (AIO). British Journal of Cancer. 2010;**102**:500-505. DOI: 10.1038/sj.bjc.6605521

[47] Moehler M, Mueller A, Trarbach T, Lordick F, Seufferlein T, Kubicka S, Geissler M, Schwarz S, Galle PR, Kanzler S; German Arbeitsgemeinschaft Internistische Onkologie. Cetuximab with irinotecan, folinic acid and 5-fluorouracil as first-line treatment in advanced gastroesophageal cancer: A prospective multi-center biomarker-oriented phase II study. Annals of Oncology. 2011;**22**:1358-1366. DOI: 10.1093/annonc/mdq591

[48] Stella G, Llimpe FR, Barone C, Falcone A, Di Fabio F, Martoni A, Lamba S, Ceccarelli C, Siena S, Bardelli A, Pinto C. KRAS and BRAF mutational status as response biomarkers to cetuximab combination therapy in advanced gastric cancer patients. Journal of Clinical Oncology. 2009;**27**:abs e15503

[49] Bjornsti MA, Houghton PJ. The TOR pathway: A target for cancer therapy. Nature Reviews Cancer. 2004;**4**:335-348

[50] Ohtsu A, Ajani JA, Bai YX, Bang YJ, Chung HC, Pan HM, Sahmoud T, Shen L, Yeh KH, Chin K, Muro K, Kim YH, Ferry D, Tebbutt NC, Al-Batran SE, Smith H, Costantini C, Rizvi S, Lebwohl D, Van Cutsem E. Everolimus for previously treated advanced gastric cancer: Results of the randomized, double-blind, phase III GRANITE-1 study. Journal of Clinical Oncology. 2013;**31**:3935-3943. DOI: 10.1200/JCO.2012.48.3552

[51] Hurwitz H, Fehrenbacher L, Novotny W, Cartwright T, Hainsworth J, Heim W, Berlin J, Baron A, Griffing S, Holmgren E, Ferrara N, Fyfe G, Rogers B, Ross R, Kabbinavar F. Bevacizumab plus irinotecan, fluorouracil, and leucovorin for metastatic colorectal cancer. The New England Journal of Medicine. 2004;**350**:2335-2342

[52] Miller K, Wang M, Gralow J, Dickler M, Cobleigh M, Perez EA, Shenkier T, Cella D, Davidson NE. Paclitaxel plus bevacizumab versus paclitaxel alone for metastatic breast cancer. The New England Journal of Medicine. 2007;**357**:2666-2676

[53] Reck M, von Pawel J, Zatloukal P, Ramlau R, Gorbounova V, Hirsh V, Leighl N, Mezger J, Archer V, Moore N, Manegold C. Phase III trial of cisplatin plus gemcitabine with either placebo or bevacizumab as first-line therapy for nonsquamous non-small-cell lung cancer. AVAil. Journal of Clinical Oncology. 2009;**27**:1227-1234. DOI: 10.1200/JCO.2007.14.5466

[54] Kim SE, Shim KN, Jung SA, Yoo K, Lee JH. The clinicopathological significance of tissue levels of hypoxia-inducible factor-1alpha and vascular endothelial growth factor in gastric cancer. Gut Liver. 2009;**3**:88-94. DOI: 10.5009/gnl.2009.3.2.88

[55] Lieto E, Ferraraccio F, Orditura M, Castellano P, Mura AL, Pinto M, Zamboli A, De Vita F, Galizia G. Expression of vascular endothelial growth factor (VEGF) and epidermal growth factor receptor (EGFR) is an independent prognostic indicator of worse outcome in gastric cancer patients. Annals of Surgical Oncology. 2008;**15**:69-79

[56] Ohtsu A, Shah MA, Van Cutsem E, Rha SY, Sawaki A, Park SR, Lim HY, Yamada Y, Wu J, Langer B, Starnawski M, Kang YK. Bevacizumab in combination with chemotherapy as first-line therapy in advanced gastric cancer: A randomized, double-blind, placebo-controlled phase III study. Journal of Clinical Oncology. 2011;**29**:3968-3976. DOI: 10.1200/JCO.2011.36.2236

[57] Shen L, Li J, Xu J, Pan H, Dai G, Qin S, Wang L, Wang J, Yang Z, Shu Y, Xu R, Chen L, Liu Y, Yu S, Bu L, Piao Y. Bevacizumab plus capecitabine and cisplatin in Chinese patients with inoperable locally advanced or metastatic gastric or gastroesophageal junction cancer: Randomized, double-blind, phase III study (AVATAR study). Gastric Cancer. 2015;**18**:168-176. DOI: 10.1007/s10120-014-0351-5

[58] Van Cutsem E, de Haas S, Kang YK, Ohtsu A, Tebbutt NC, Ming Xu J, Peng Yong W, Langer B, Delmar P, Scherer SJ, Shah MA. Bevacizumab in combination with chemotherapy as first-line therapy in advanced gastric cancer: A biomarker evaluation from the AVAGAST randomized phase III trial. Journal of Clinical Oncology. 2012;**30**:2119-2127. DOI: 10.1200/JCO.2011.39.9824

[59] Miles DW, de Haas SL, Dirix LY, Romieu G, Chan A, Pivot X, Tomczak P, Provencher L, Cortés J, Delmar PR, Scherer SJ. Biomarker results from the AVADO phase 3 trial of first-line bevacizumab plus docetaxel for HER2-negative metastatic breast cancer. British Journal of Cancer. 2013;**108**:1052-1060. DOI: 10.1038/bjc.2013.69

[60] Lambrechts D, Claes B, Delmar P, Reumers J, Mazzone M, Yesilyurt BT, Devlieger R, Verslype C, Tejpar S, Wildiers H, de Haas S, Carmeliet P, Scherer SJ, Van Cutsem E. VEGF pathway genetic variants as biomarkers of treatment outcome with bevacizumab: An analysis of data from the AViTA and AVOREN randomised trials. The Lancet Oncology. 2012;**13**:724-733. DOI: 10.1016/S1470-2045(12)70231-0

[61] Bronte G, Galvano A, Cicero G, Passiglia F, Rolfo C, Bazan V, Russo A. Ramucirumab and its use in gastric cancer treatment. Drugs of Today (Barcelona, Spain). 2014;**50**:613-621. DOI: 10.1358/dot.2014.50.9.2207198

[62] Fuchs CS, Tomasek J, Yong CJ, Dumitru F, Passalacqua R, Goswami C, Safran H, dos Santos LV, Aprile G, Ferry DR, Melichar B, Tehfe M, Topuzov E, Zalcberg JR, Chau I, Campbell W, Sivanandan C, Pikiel J, Koshiji M, Hsu Y, Liepa AM, Gao L, Schwartz JD, Tabernero J; REGARD Trial Investigators. Ramucirumab monotherapy for previously treated advanced gastric or gastro-oesophageal junction adenocarcinoma (REGARD): An international, randomised, multicentre, placebo-controlled, phase 3 trial. Lancet. 2014;**383**:31-39. DOI: 10.1016/S0140-6736(13)61719-5

[63] Wilke H, Muro K, Van Cutsem E, Oh SC, Bodoky G, Shimada Y, Hironaka S, Sugimoto N, Lipatov O, Kim TY, Cunningham D, Rougier P, Komatsu Y, Ajani J, Emig M, Carlesi R, Ferry D, Chandrawansa K, Schwartz JD, Ohtsu A; RAINBOW Study Group. Ramucirumab plus paclitaxel versus placebo plus paclitaxel in patients with previously treated advanced gastric or gastro-oesophageal junction adenocarcinoma (RAINBOW): A double-blind, randomised phase 3 trial. The Lancet Oncology. 2014;**15**:1224-1235. DOI: 10.1016/S1470-2045(14)70420-6

[64] Shitara K, Muro K, Shimada Y, Hironaka S, Sugimoto N, Komatsu Y, Nishina T, Yamaguchi K, Segawa Y, Omuro Y, Tamura T, Doi T, Yukisawa S, Yasui H, Nagashima F, Gotoh M, Esaki T, Emig M, Chandrawansa K, Liepa AM, Wilke H, Ichimiya Y, Ohtsu A. Subgroup analyses of the safety and efficacy of ramucirumab in Japanese and Western patients in RAINBOW: A randomized clinical trial in second-line treatment of gastric cancer. Gastric Cancer. 2016;**19**:927-938. DOI: 10.1007/s10120-015-0559-z

[65] Hofheinz RD, Lorenzen S. Ramucirumab as second-line treatment for patients with metastatic esophagogastric adenocarcinoma. Expert Review of Anticancer Therapy. 2015;**15**:607-614. DOI: 10.1586/14737140.2015.1052412

[66] Yoon HH, Bendell JC, Braiteh FS, Firdaus I, Philip PA, Cohn AL, Lewis N, Anderson DM, Arrowsmith E, Schwartz JD, Gao L, Hsu Y, Xu Y, Ferry D, Alberts SR, Wainberg ZA. Ramucirumab combined with FOLFOX as front-line therapy for advanced esophageal, gastroesophageal junction, or gastric adenocarcinoma: A randomized, double-blind, multicenter Phase II trial. Annals of Oncology. 2016;**27**: 2196-2203. DOI: 10.1093/annonc/mdw423

[67] Li J, Qin S, Xu J, Xiong J, Wu C, Bai Y, Liu W, Tong J, Liu Y, Xu R, Wang Z, Wang Q, Ouyang X, Yang Y, Ba Y, Liang J, Lin X, Luo D, Zheng R, Wang X, Sun G, Wang L, Zheng L, Guo H, Wu J, Xu N, Yang J, Zhang H, Cheng Y, Wang N, Chen L, Fan Z, Sun P, Yu H. Randomized, double-blind, placebo-controlled phase III trial of apatinib in patients with chemotherapy-refractory advanced or metastatic adenocarcinoma of the stomach or gastroesophageal junction. Journal of Clinical Oncology. 2016;**34**: 1448-1454. DOI: 10.1200/JCO.2015.63.5995

[68] Erber R, Thurnher A, Katsen AD, Groth G, Kerger H, Hammes HP, Menger MD, Ullrich A, Vajkoczy P. Combined inhibition of VEGF and PDGF signaling enforces tumor vessel regression by interfering with pericyte-mediated endothelial cell survival mechanisms. FASEB Journal. 2004;**18**:338-340. DOI: 10.1096/fj.03-0271fje

[69] Fischer C, Jonckx B, Mazzone M, Zacchigna S, Loges S, Pattarini L, Chorianopoulos E, Liesenborghs L, Koch M, De Mol M, Autiero M, Wyns S, Plaisance S, Moons L, van Rooijen N, Giacca M, Stassen JM, Dewerchin M, Collen D, Carmeliet P. Anti-PlGF inhibits growth of VEGF(R)-inhibitor-resistant tumors without affecting healthy vessels. Cell. 2007;**131**:463-475. DOI: 10.1016/j.cell.2007.08.038

[70] Wilhelm SM, Adnane L, Newell P, Villanueva A, Llovet JM, Lynch M. Preclinical overview of sorafenib, a multikinase inhibitor that targets both Raf and VEGF and PDGF receptor tyrosine kinase signaling. Molecular Cancer Therapeutics. 2008;**7**:3129-3140. DOI: 10.1158/1535-7163.MCT-08-0013

[71] Wilhelm S, Carter C, Lynch M, Lowinger T, Dumas J, Smith RA, Schwartz B, Simantov R, Kelley S. Discovery and development of sorafenib: A multikinase inhibitor for treating cancer. Nature Reviews Drug Discovery. 2006;**5**:835-844

[72] Mendel DB, Laird AD, Xin X, Louie SG, Christensen JG, Li G, Schreck RE, Abrams TJ, Ngai TJ, Lee LB, Murray LJ, Carver J, Chan E, Moss KG, Haznedar JO, Sukbuntherng J, Blake

RA, Sun L, Tang C, Miller T, Shirazian S, McMahon G, Cherrington JM. In vivo antitumor activity of SU11248, a novel tyrosine kinase inhibitor targeting vascular endothelial growth factor and platelet-derived growth factor receptors: Determination of a pharmacokinetic/pharmacodynamic relationship. Clinical Cancer Research. 2003;**9**:327-337

[73] Moehler M, Gepfner-Tuma I, Maderer A, Thuss-Patience PC, Ruessel J, Hegewisch-Becker S, Wilke H, Al-Batran SE, Rafiyan MR, Weißinger F, Schmoll HJ, Kullmann F, von Weikersthal LF, Siveke JT, Weusmann J, Kanzler S, Schimanski CC, Otte M, Schollenberger L, Koenig J, Galle PR. Sunitinib added to FOLFIRI versus FOLFIRI in patients with chemorefractory advanced adenocarcinoma of the stomach or lower esophagus: A randomized, placebo-controlled phase II AIO trial with serum biomarker program. BMC Cancer. 2016;**16**:699. DOI: 10.1186/s12885-016-2736-9

[74] Wilhelm SM, Dumas J, Adnane L, Lynch M, Carter CA, Schütz G, Thierauch KH, Zopf D. Regorafenib (BAY 73-4506): A new oral multikinase inhibitor of angiogenic, stromal and oncogenic receptor tyrosine kinases with potent preclinical antitumor activity. International Journal of Cancer. 2011;**129**:245-255. DOI: 10.1002/ijc.25864

[75] Demetri GD, Reichardt P, Kang YK, Blay JY, Rutkowski P, Gelderblom H, Hohenberger P, Leahy M, von Mehren M, Joensuu H, Badalamenti G, Blackstein M, Le Cesne A, Schöffski P, Maki RG, Bauer S, Nguyen BB, Xu J, Nishida T, Chung J, Kappeler C, Kuss I, Laurent D, Casali PG; GRID study investigators. Efficacy and safety of regorafenib for advanced gastrointestinal stromal tumours after failure of imatinib and sunitinib (GRID): An international, multicentre, randomised, placebo-controlled, phase 3 trial. Lancet. 2013;**381**:295-302. DOI: 10.1016/S0140-6736(12)61857-1

[76] Pavlakis N, Sjoquist KM, Martin AJ, Tsobanis E, Yip S, Kang YK, Bang YJ, Alcindor T, O'Callaghan CJ, Burnell MJ, Tebbutt NC, Rha SY, Lee J, Cho JY, Lipton LR, Wong M, Strickland A, Kim JW, Zalcberg JR, Simes J, Goldstein D. Regorafenib for the Treatment of Advanced Gastric Cancer (INTEGRATE): A multinational placebo-controlled phase II trial. Journal of Clinical Oncology. 2016;**34**:2728-2735. DOI: 10.1200/JCO.2015.65.1901

[77] Ebos JM, Lee CR, Cruz-Munoz W, Bjarnason GA, Christensen JG, Kerbel RS. Accelerated metastasis after short-term treatment with a potent inhibitor of tumor angiogenesis. Cancer Cell. 2009;**15**:232-239. DOI: 10.1016/j.ccr.2009.01.021

[78] Mancuso MR, Davis R, Norberg SM, O'Brien S, Sennino B, Nakahara T, Yao VJ, Inai T, Brooks P, Freimark B, Shalinsky DR, Hu-Lowe DD, McDonald DM. Rapid vascular regrowth in tumors after reversal of VEGF inhibition. The Journal of Clinical Investigation. 2006;**116**:2610-2621

[79] Johannsen M, Flörcken A, Bex A, Roigas J, Cosentino M, Ficarra V, Kloeters C, Rief M, Rogalla P, Miller K, Grünwald V. Can tyrosine kinase inhibitors be discontinued in patients with metastatic renal cell carcinoma and a complete response to treatment? A multicentre, retrospective analysis. European Urology. 2009;**55**:1430-1438. DOI: 10.1016/j.eururo.2008.10.021

[80] Sennino B, McDonald DM. Controlling escape from angiogenesis inhibitors. Nature Reviews Cancer. 2012;**12**:699-709. DOI: 10.1038/nrc3366

[81] Salceda S, Caro J. Hypoxia-inducible factor 1alpha (HIF-1alpha) protein is rapidly degraded by the ubiquitin-proteasome system under normoxic conditions. Its stabilization by hypoxia depends on redox-induced changes. Journal of Biological Chemistry. 1997;**272**:22642-22647

[82] Yu F, Lin Y, Zhan T, Chen L, Guo S. HGF expression induced by HIF-1α promote the proliferation and tube formation of endothelial progenitor cells. Cell Biology International. 2015;**39**:310-317. DOI: 10.1002/cbin.10397

[83] Lordick F. Targeting the HGF/MET pathway in gastric cancer. The Lancet Oncology. 2014;**15**:914-916. DOI: 10.1016/S1470-2045(14)70273-6

[84] Bardelli A, Corso S, Bertotti A, Hobor S, Valtorta E, Siravegna G, Sartore-Bianchi A, Scala E, Cassingena A, Zecchin D, Apicella M, Migliardi G, Galimi F, Lauricella C, Zanon C, Perera T, Veronese S, Corti G, Amatu A, Gambacorta M, Diaz LA Jr, Sausen M, Velculescu VE, Comoglio P, Trusolino L, Di Nicolantonio F, Giordano S, Siena S. Amplification of the MET receptor drives resistance to anti-EGFR therapies in colorectal cancer. Cancer Discovery. 2013;**3**:658-673. DOI: 10.1158/2159-8290.CD-12-0558

[85] Troiani T, Martinelli E, Napolitano S, Vitagliano D, Ciuffreda LP, Costantino S, Morgillo F, Capasso A, Sforza V, Nappi A, De Palma R, D'Aiuto E, Berrino L, Bianco R, Ciardiello F. Increased TGF-α as a mechanism of acquired resistance to the anti-EGFR inhibitor cetuximab through EGFR-MET interaction and activation of MET signaling in colon cancer cells. Clinical Cancer Research. 2013;**19**:6751-6765. DOI: 10.1158/1078-0432.CCR-13-0423

[86] Engelman JA, Zejnullahu K, Mitsudomi T, Song Y, Hyland C, Park JO, Lindeman N, Gale CM, Zhao X, Christensen J, Kosaka T, Holmes AJ, Rogers AM, Cappuzzo F, Mok T, Lee C, Johnson BE, Cantley LC, Jänne PA. MET amplification leads to gefitinib resistance in lung cancer by activating ERBB3 signaling. Science. 2007;**316**:1039-1043

[87] Cunningham D, Tebbutt NC, Davidenko I, Murad AM, Al-Batran SE, Ilson DH, Tjulandin S, Gotovkin E, Karaszewska B, Bondarenko I, Tejani MA, Udrea AA, Tehfe MA, Baker N, Oliner KS, Zhang Y, Hoang T, Sidhu R, Catenacci DVT. Phase III, randomized, double-blind, multicenter, placebo (P)-controlled trial of rilotumumab (R) plus epirubicin, cisplatin and capecitabine (ECX) as first-line therapy in patients (pts) with advanced MET-positive (pos) gastric or gastroesophageal junction (G/GEJ) cancer: RILOMET-1 study. Journal of Clinical Oncology. 2015;**33**:abs4000

[88] A Phase 3 Study of Rilotumumab (AMG 102) With Cisplatin and Capecitabine (CX) as First-line Therapy in Gastric Cancer. https://clinicaltrials.gov [NCT 02137343]

[89] Zhu M, Tang R, Doshi S, Oliner KS, Dubey S, Jiang Y, Donehower RC, Iveson T, Loh EY, Zhang Y. Exposure-response analysis of rilotumumab in gastric cancer: The role of tumour MET expression. British Journal of Cancer. 2015;**112**:429-437. DOI: 10.1038/bjc.2014.649

[90] Doshi S, Gisleskog PO, Zhang Y, Zhu M, Oliner KS, Loh E, Perez Ruixo JJ. Rilotumumab exposure-response relationship in patients with advanced or metastatic gastric cancer. Clinical Cancer Research. 2015;**21**:2453-2461. DOI: 10.1158/1078-0432.CCR-14-1661

[91] Zhang Y, Kuchimanchi M, Zhu M, Doshi S, Hoang T, Kasichayanula S. Assessment of pharmacokinetic interaction between rilotumumab and epirubicin, cisplatin and capecitabine (ECX) in a Phase 3 study in gastric cancer. British Journal of Clinical Pharmacology. 2017;**83**:1048-1055. DOI: 10.1111/bcp.13179

[92] Shah MA, Bang YJ, Lordick F, Alsina M, Chen M, Hack SP, Bruey JM, Smith D, McCaffery I, Shames DS, Phan S, Cunningham D. Effect of fluorouracil, leucovorin, and oxaliplatin with or without onartuzumab in HER2-negative, MET-positive gastroesophageal adenocarcinoma: The METGastric randomized clinical trial. JAMA Oncology. 2017;**3**: 620-627. DOI: 10.1001/jamaoncol.2016.5580

[93] Shah MA, Wainberg ZA, Catenacci DV, Hochster HS, Ford J, Kunz P, Lee FC, Kallender H, Cecchi F, Rabe DC, Keer H, Martin AM, Liu Y, Gagnon R, Bonate P, Liu L, Gilmer T, Bottaro DP. Phase II study evaluating 2 dosing schedules of oral foretinib (GSK1363089), cMET/VEGFR2 inhibitor, in patients with metastatic gastric cancer. PLoS One. 2013; **8**:e54014. DOI: 10.1371/journal.pone.0054014

Gastric Cancer with Liver Metastasis (GCLM) and the Importance of Dormant Cancer Stem Cells

Vitězslav Marek and Štefan Durdik

Additional information is available at the end of the chapter

http://dx.doi.org/10.5772/intechopen.69829

Abstract

Surgical treatment of gastric cancer with liver metastasis (GCLM) is even more interested for oncologists. Liver resection or RFA (radiofrequency ablation) is not commonly indicated in gastric cancer with liver metastasis (GCLM). There is no direct marker defining the degree of biological aggressiveness of the tumor (indicating or contraindicating the surgical treatment), therefore we are left to rely on indirect prognostic factors: 1. cancerous invasion in the gastric wall serosa; 2. the presence of three and more liver metastases; 3. the size of metastasis exceeding 50 mm. Clarification of the nature of biological behavior of gastric cancer is a turning point of this treatment. Small light in explanation of the above problem is cancer stem cells (CSCs) theory. This theory proposes that CSCs serve not only as the basis for the development and progression of tumors, but also as the primary reason for tumor recurrence and metastasis. A better understanding of CSCs' contribution to clinical tumor dormancy and metastasis will provide new therapeutic revenues to eradicate metastatic tumors and significantly reduce the mortality of cancer patients.

Keywords: gastric cancer with liver metastasis (GCLM), radiofrequency ablation (RFA), cancer stem cells (CSCs), metastasis, tumor dormancy, cell dormancy, epithelial-mesenchymal transition (EMT)

1. Introduction

Gastric cancer is the fourth most common cancer worldwide [1]. The stage of gastric cancer at diagnosis determines treatment options and has a strong influence on the length of the patient's survival.

Early diagnosis of earlier stages of the disease with adequate treatment/R0 resection of stomach + D2 lymphadenectomy + suitable perioperative chemotherapy/bring a better outlook [3] (**Figure 1**).

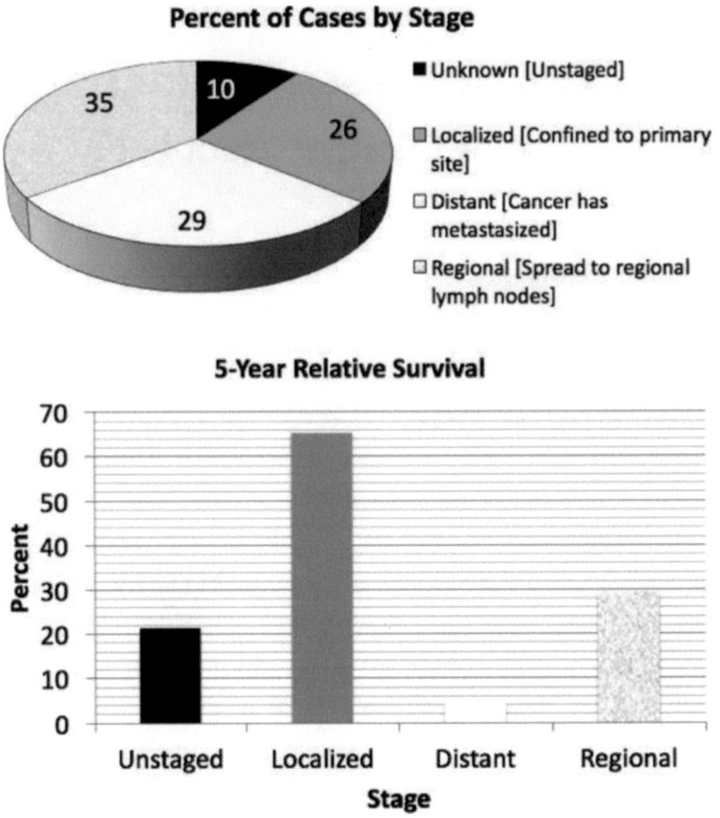

Figure 1. Percentage of cases and 5-year relative survival by stage at diagnosis: gastric cancer. The earlier gastric cancer is diagnosed, the better chance a patient has of surviving 5 years after diagnosis. For gastric cancer, 26.0 and 29.0% of cases are diagnosed at the local and distant stage, respectively. Of note, the stage of disease is unknown at diagnosis in more than one-third of cases. The 5-year survival for localized gastric cancer is 65.4%, compared with 4.5% for distant stomach cancer [2].

Remote metastases as a sign of systemic disease reduce the overall patient survival. The most common site for gastric cancer metastasis is the liver [4].

For the sake of comparison, at present, the liver resection is currently accepted as a treatment for liver metastases of colorectal cancer with referred 5-year survival in 40–56% of patients [5]. Thanks to advances in surgical techniques and perioperative chemotherapy, the indication range keeps expanding.

Compared with colorectal cancer, the gastric cancer represents a more aggressive cancer disease with heterogenic nature [6].

Other metastatic lesions associated with gastric cancer such as peritoneal carcinomatosis or extensive involvement of the regional lymph nodes significantly deteriorates the patient's outcome, contraindicating the surgical treatment.

GCLM is considered a systemic disease with adverse outcome and systemic chemotherapy is indicated as the first line of treatment [7].

Thanks to the effort on the part of some of the surgeons to reverse the adverse outcome in resectable GCLM, who performed resection or RFA surgery on the liver, we were able to collect interesting outcomes—5-year survival of 0–45% of patients [8, 9].

These studies are greatly handicapped by the low number of patients, mostly from a single center [8].

However, over 90% of mortality in cancer patients is described to the subsequent spread of cancer cells to distant tissues [10]. In patients, the threat of tumor can return after chemotherapy and radiation remains terrifying and painfully real.

This phenomenon is described as tumor or cell dormancy. The experimental models have revealed that cancer patients may have hundreds to thousands of disseminated cancer cells in circulation but only a small portion of these cells progresses to form clinically overt metastases [11].

Metastasis is a multistep process. The metastatic cancer cells acquire epithelial-mesenchymal transition (EMT)-like phenotype allowing them to disseminate from the primary tumor into circulation; the early step of metastasis (intravasate, survival, arrest, and extravasation) is a very complicated and complex process [12].

However, only a small subset of these cells (~2%) can initiate growth as micrometastases, and an even smaller fraction of these cells (~0.02%) is able to persist and forms macrometastases [12].

The sub-population of cancer cells has stem-like properties and is capable of initiating tumor, invasive growth, and spread to distant organs [13]. These cancer stem cells (CSCs) have the ability to self-renew, to produce more cancer cells, as well as undergo differentiation to give rise to phenotypically diverse nontumorigenic cancer cells.

2. Gastric cancer with liver metastasis (GCLM) and surgery

Liver resection/RFA is not a frequent treatment modality for gastric cancer with liver metastasis (GCLM).

This is well documented by a Korean study, where in 10% of the 100,000 GCLM patients, only 4% had hepatic surgery. At present, there is no clear consensus supporting liver resection in this type of tumor [14].

In this respect, the study of Kinoshita et al. has become a breakthrough [15]. It describes a 5-year disease-free survival in 30% of carefully selected patients. This confirmed that a small sub-population of patients with GCLM may benefit from liver resection or RFA. The median recurrence-free survival time was 9 months.

Half of the patients had recurrence within 1 year, in spite of R0 resection and careful selection. On the other hand, there was sufficient number of patients with long-term survival. This can be explained by varying tumor sub-populations with differing biological behavior [15, 72].

The question is: Which GCLM patients are suitable for surgical intervention?

At present, there is no direct marker available, defining the degree of biological aggressiveness of the tumor (indicating or contra-indicating the surgical treatment), therefore we are left to rely on indirect prognostic factors—number of liver metastases, size of metastatic lesion [8, 72].

Several studies have attempted to identify the prognostic factors defining adverse outlook for patients and contraindicating surgical intervention.

Among these studies, a multicenter study by Japanese authors stands out [15]. This study defines three adverse prognostic factors:

1. Invasion of serosa by primary tumor
2. Three and more liver metastases
3. Size of liver metastasis exceeding 50 mm.

The study noted a significant difference in survival between patients without a prognostic factor and patients with one of the three prognostic factors. The authors recommend to consider surgical intervention in the presence of any of the three risk factors.

Patients with lower number of risk factors had better 3- and 5-year survival following liver resection [15].

The indication for surgical intervention in GCLM is subject to overall clinical condition of the patient, but liver resection should definitely be contraindicated in the presence of all three adverse prognostic factors (no long-term survival was noted) [15].

Repeated hepatectomy was performed only in 14.4% of patients, which is significantly lower number of hepatectomies compared to patients with colorectal cancer. This is caused by different pathophysiological course of gastric cancer relapse [16].

Hepatic resection is presently considered and justified only in case of solitary relapsing metastasis of GCLM [16].

The role of chemotherapy in GCLM is not clearly defined. Neo-adjuvant chemotherapy is being brought forward that can be used to differentiate responders from nonresponders. Surgical intervention is contraindicated in nonresponders [17].

GCLM patients treated by systemic chemotherapy alone have 1.7% 5-year survival [17].

Several studies assessed the use of RFA in GCLM, recommending it for solitary lesions up to 30 mm in size, located in the periphery of the liver. No clear advantage of RFA compared to surgical resection has been shown [18, 72].

Surgical treatment is not able to provide patients with GCLM a complete cure. Half of the patients had recurrence within 1 year, in spite of R0 resection and careful selection. On the other hand, there was sufficient number of patients with long-term survival. This can be explained by varying tumor sub-populations with differing biological behavior [15].

The number of studies aimed to clarify the explanation of the process invasive gastric cancer growth, metastasis, and particularly its biological aggressiveness essentially failed.

We do not differentiate the varying degrees of biological aggressiveness of gastric cancer.

A small light in explanation of the above problem is cancer stem cells (CSCs) theory.

This theory proposes that CSCs serve not only as the basis for the development and progression of primary tumors, but also as the primary reason for tumor recurrence and metastasis (theory of minimal residual disease).

Micrometastases involving dormant cancer stem cells are mistaken for small macrometastases. These are distinct disease entities responsible for late recurrence (months, years) with high resistance to current chemotherapy.

The combined use of traditional therapies with targeted CSC-specific agents may target the whole cancer and offer a promising strategy for lasting treatment and even its cure.

3. Gastric cancer stem cells (CSCs) theory

3.1. Minimal residual disease—definition

Minimal residual diseases are remnant tumor cells that are left after treatment and that cannot be detected by conventional clinical studies. These cells can persist in the primary site or as disseminated tumor cells in proliferative and/or dormant phases [19].

A source of minimal residual disease is considered systemic micrometastatic diseases caused by early dissemination of cancer cells from the primary tumor. These cells have the ability of dormancy [17].

In gastric cancer patients, minimal residual disease is defined as micrometastases and isolated tumor cells (ITC). First, micrometastasis is defined as tumor cell clusters between 0.2 and 2.0 mm in the greatest dimension, whereas ITC are defined as single tumor cells or small clusters of tumor cells less than 0.2 mm in size (seventh Tumour-Node-Metastasis Classification classification) [20].

Cancer stem cells (CSCs) are the cornerstone of micrometastases and define their characteristics and behavior. The clinical implications and/or prognostic significance of the micrometastases are still a matter of debate.

3.2. Definition of cancer stem cells (CSCs)

As defined by the American Association for Cancer Research Workshop on Cancer Stem Cells, a cancer stem cell (CSC) is a cell within a tumor that possesses the capacity to self-renew and to give rise to the heterogeneous lineages of cancer cells that comprise the tumor. Because they have an intrinsic ability to propagate tumor cells, CSCs are also referred to as "tumor-initiating cells" or "tumorigenic cells" [21]. The ability of stem cells to self-renew and give rise to multiple cell lineages is termed as "stemness" [22] (**Table 1**).

Self-renewal	CSCs serially transplant through multiple generations
Differentiation	CSCs generate symmetrical and asymmetrical cells
Tumorigenicity	CSCs can propagate tumor cells
Specific surface markers	Allow for separation of CSCs from nonstem cells

Table 1. Characteristics of the cancer stem cells [21].

3.3. Brief history of cancer stem cells (CSCs)

History of cancer stem cells dates back to the nineteenth century. A hypothesis of cancer stem cells (CSCs) that have similar properties to stem cells (SCs) was first described by Rudolf Virchow and Julius Conheim in 1855 [23]. Virchow suggested that cancers arise from the activation of dormant cells present in mature tissue, which are remainders of embryonic cells (perhaps similar to cells now known as stem cells) [23]. Virchow believed that cancer is caused by severe irritation in the tissues, and his theory came to be known as chronic irritation theory. However, Conheim had suspected that the remaining embryonic cells from which cancers form during organogenesis were "lost."

In 1997, Bonnet and Dick described a subpopulation of cells with the presence of a specific surface marker CD34 ($CD34^+$) and the absence of a CD38 marker ($CD38^-$) in patients with acute myeloid leukemia capable of inducing a cancerous disease after transplanting those cells to mice with an altered immunological system—leukemic-initiating cells [24, 25].

CSCs have already been identified in breast, lung, ovarian, prostate, gastric, colorectal cancer, and brain tumors [26].

It is estimated that in these malignancies, CSCs constitute <5% of all tumor cells [26].

3.4. Origin of the gastric cancer stem cells (CSCs)

The origin of gastric cancer stem cells (CSCs) is described as follows:

1. CSCs are derived from progenitor and normal stem cells [27].
2. Dedifferentiated gastric cells, via nuclear factor-kappa-B (NF-κB) modulation of Wnt signaling [27].
3. Bone marrow-derived progenitor cells progressing through metaplasia and dysplasia to cancer (**Figure 2**) [29].

Helicobacter pylori infection triggers inflammation and changes the local gastric microenvironment. This change might affect the differentiation of gastric stem cells and could induce gastric cancer. Helicobacter pylori colonizes and manipulates both progenitor and leucine-rich repeat containing G protein-coupled receptor-5 ($Lgr5^+$) stem cells, which then change gland turnover and cause hyperplasia [28].

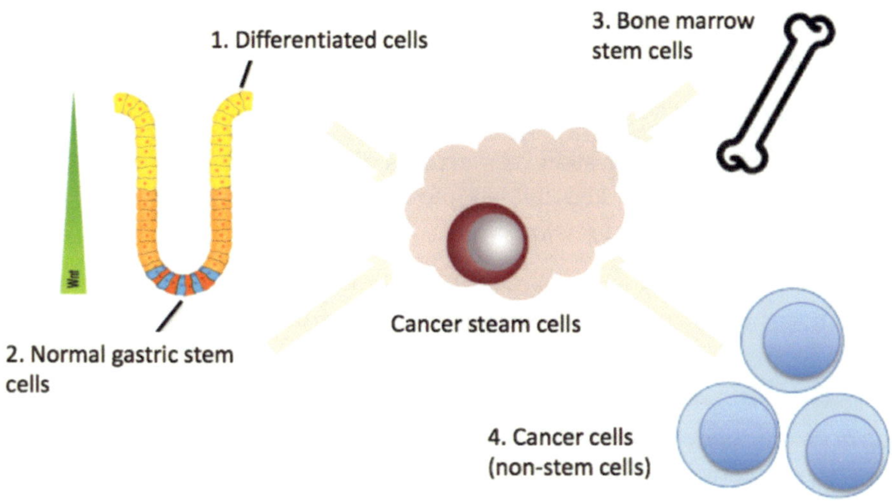

Figure 2. Gastric cancer stem cells formation [28].

Chronic infection with Helicobacter felis caused inflammation and induced the reconstruction of gastric tissue with bone marrow-derived cells, whereas acute inflammation does not lead to bone marrow-derived cell recruitment [29].

3.5. Cancer stem cells (CSCs) properties

Within both primary and metastasized tumors, cell subpopulations can differ on the basis of such factors as morphology, expression of surface antigens, specific alterations of the genome, and patterns of gene expression [30]. Likewise, CSCs are heterogeneous with varying degrees of self-renewal capacity, development potential, and expression of cellular markers. Like normal stem cells, CSCs exist in a hierarchy [31–33]. Their capacity for self-renewal and differentiation places CSCs at the top of a cellular hierarchy from which all other cells within a tumor are derived (**Table 2**) [32].

Using glioma stem cells, research has shown that CSCs can divide symmetrically, producing new CSC progeny, or asymmetrically, producing nonstem cell and stem cell progeny [34]. Intratumoral heterogeneity likely derives from asymmetrical division and differentiation of CSCs [33]. Over time, unrestrained differentiation and proliferation produces the heterogeneous

Characteristic	Normal stem cells	CSCs
Self-renewal	✓	✓✓
Differentiation	✓	✓✓
Plasticity	–	✓
Quiescence	✓✓	✓

Table 2. Characteristics of normal stem cells and cancer stem cells [32].

populations of primary and metastatic tumor cells that contribute to tumor properties, such as recurrence, resistance to therapy, and metastasis [30].

The manifestation of CSCs heterogeneity:

First, different subsets of cancer stem cells express different surface markers. Wright et al. described that breast CSCs could be divided into $CD44^+/CD24^-$ and $CD133^+$ subsets based on differences in surface marker expression [35].

Second, the heterogeneity of CSCs is manifested in the differences of the cell properties. Specifically, some cancer stem cell subsets possess a strong invasive capability, whereas other cancer stem cell subsets are in a quiescent (dormant) state and do not differentiate [36, 37].

Third, the dormant state of cancer stem cells is not permanent. Under the influence of appropriate external or internal stimuli, dormant cancer stem cells may undergo invasive transformation and become invasive cancer stem cells [38]. Therefore, an investigation of the factors that promote quiescent stem cell transformation is of great clinical significance.

3.6. Cancer stem cells (CSCs) dormancy

Many solid tumors undergo an extended period of "dormancy," characterized by the presence of minimal residual disease over many years before overt metastases may eventually arise.

Gastric CSCs consisted of both quiescent gastric CSCs and invasive gastric CSCs (increased metastatic activity). Invasive gastric CSCs are defined as $CD26^+$ $CXCR4^+$ double-positive cells and the $CD26^-$ $CXCR4^-$ double-negative cells as quiescent gastric CSCs based on surface marker expression [39].

In 2007, Aquirre-Ghiso postulated two different states of "cancer dormancy," tumor-cell dormancy, and tumor mass dormancy [19, 40, 41].

Tumor mass dormancy (micrometastasis) occurs when cancer cell proliferation is counterbalanced by apoptosis owing to poor vascularization (angiogenic dormancy) or by an immune response. In this case, the cancer cells are never truly inactive, but rather are incapable of expanding beyond a certain number (**Figure 3**).

Tumor-cell dormancy is defined as the condition in which cancer cells enter the G0 phase of the cell cycle and have low metabolism. This form of dormancy is clinically asymptomatic.

However, this conceptual framework is still under debate. At present, little is known about the factors that might have a role in the "awakening" of dormant tumor cells that leads them into the dynamic phase of macrometastatic formation.

CSCs exist within a microenvironment of surrounding vasculature, stromal cells, immune cells, and secreted factors produced by these cells. These create a niche wherein the CSCs can survive and thrive in order to propagate and differentiate into the cells that make up the tumor mass. In essence, the niche is a regulatory microenvironment that nurtures the stem-cell–like

http://dx.doi.org/10.5772/intechopen.69829

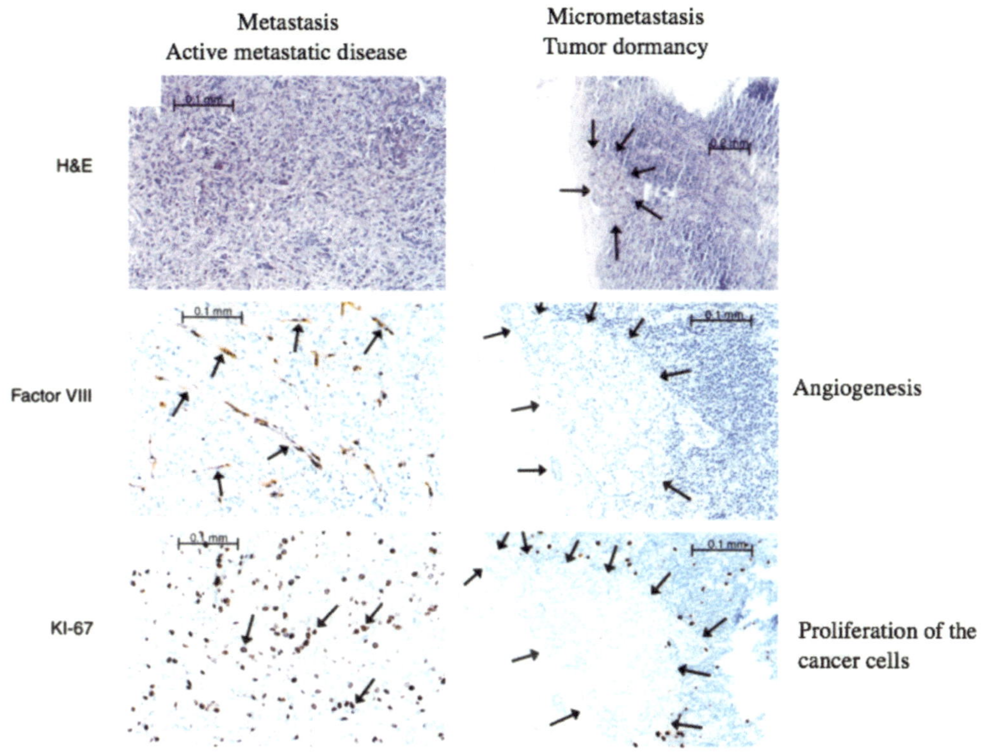

Figure 3. Metastasis vs. micrometastasis. H&E staining of breast cancer lymph node macrometastases (*A*, ×400) and micrometastases (*B*, *arrows*, tumor-lymph node interface, ×200). Immunohistochemical analysis of vascularization of human breast cancer lymph node metastases (*C*, ×400) and micrometastases (*D*, ×400). Tumor vascularization was analyzed by staining with polyclonal antibody against factor VIII, an endothelial-speci c marker. In breast cancer metastases (*C*), there was marked neovascularization (brown stain; arrows, representative blood vessels). In contrast, breast cancer micrometastases (*D*) had a marked decrease in tumor microvessel density. *Arrows*, tumor-lymph node interface. Immunohistochemical analyses of proliferation of breast cancer metastases (*E*, ×400) and micrometastases (*F*, ×400). Tumor proliferation was analyzed by staining with antibody against Ki-67. In breast cancer metastases, there was a much higher rate of proliferation (*E*, red/brown stain; arrows, representative proliferating cells) compared with micrometastases (*F*, *arrows*, tumor-lymph node interface) [71].

characteristics of CSCs so that they can generate or regenerate the tumor bulk and maintain their self-renewing potential. Intracellular and intercellular signals operate within CSC microenvironments and support CSC activities. The internal signals include molecular pathways that regulate stemness, whereas extracellular signals consist of cells designed to anchor CSCs within the microenvironment, and cell receptors and secreted factors that are necessary for maintaining CSCs in their quiescent state [42].

Signaling pathways are key components in all cells. They stimulate a wide variety of cell processes—from cell growth, proliferation, and differentiation to invasion and apoptosis. Well-known internal signals or pathways that function in normal stem cell niches include the Wnt, Notch, Hedgehog (Hh), and Janus kinase/signal transducer and activator of transcription (JAK/STAT) pathways [42]. Several intracellular signaling pathways may be altered in the process of malignant transformation of stem cells. For example:

1. The evolutionarily conserved *Wnt family* of proteins is cysteine-rich, secreted glycoproteins that control tissue homeostasis, and regulate diverse processes during development. Wnt pathway dysregulation has been identified in several hereditary diseases and is associated with gastrointestinal cancers [43].

2. *The Notch pathway* has crucial roles in stem cell control and cell-fate determination. Research has found that a signature of the Notch pathway is found in CSCs identified patients with poorly differentiated lung adenocarcinoma, and was prognostic for poorer overall survival. By inhibiting the Notch pathway, CSCs were prevented from forming tumors when implanted into mice [44].

3. *The Hedgehog (Hh) protein family members* turn on the genes that regulate the cell cycle and determine cell fate. They are also known to be key regulators of carcinogenesis. Hh and downstream factors have been shown to have significant roles in pancreatic cancer, gastric cancer, glioma, and basal cell carcinoma. Inhibition of the Hh pathway in pancreatic cancer depressed the self-renewal of CSCs and impaired their resistance to chemotherapy [45].

4. *The Hippo pathway* and its related mediators Yes/Yap regulate several tumor suppressor genes to control cellular processes such as survival, proliferation, differentiation, apoptosis, and stem or progenitor cell expansion [46]. Dysregulation of the Hippo pathway has been identified in multiple cancers including liver, lung, colorectal, gastric, ovarian, and prostate [46]. Researchers also found that the expression levels of Yes/Yap genes were prognostic for survival in patients receiving certain types of chemotherapy [46].

5. *NANOG* is a transcription factor involved in the self-renewal and maintenance of pluripotency in normal stem cells. Experimental inhibition of NANOG or related transcription factors has been shown to decrease stem-cell–like activities in breast cancer, colorectal cancer, gastric, prostate cancer, and melanoma [47].

6. *The STAT family* of transcriptional factors cooperates with NANOG to transcribe stemness genes that are required for modulating pluripotency [33]. The STATS are upstream signals activated by interleukin-6 (IL-6).

Activated STAT3 has been found in leukemia, squamous cell carcinoma of the head and neck, multiple myeloma, breast cancer, and prostate cancer. Blocking the STAT3 signaling pathway has been shown to inhibit the clonogenic and tumorigenic potential of CSCs in prostate cancer [26]. In addition, it has been shown that blockade of STAT3 activity inhibits both tumor growth and tumor-initiating potential in colon CSCs [48].

Cancer-associated cells in the microenvironment may secrete growth factors and cytokines to support CSCs. Examples of these include cytokines such as stromal cell-derived factor-1, IL-6, and IL-8, all of which function to regulate CSC activity [49].

During dormancy, micrometastases are somehow able to evolve and acquire a full complement of metastasis-colonization functions that they did not express before. It is difficult to envision how this progression could occur in CSCs (section of micrometastasis) that remain in a state of replicative quiescence. Although CSCs in bone marrow look quiescent, the overall CSCs population is not static. Circulating cancer cells can be detected in blood in the apparent absence of active metastatic disease. If not in the bone marrow, at least in other tissues, micrometastases may be constantly exiting and re-entering a dormant state, and become familiar with the environment, undergoing further selection for colonization traits during the active interludes. Transition between quiescent and proliferative states is a property of adult stem cells that may be hijacked by CSCs [49].

3.7. Epithelial-mesenchymal transition (EMT): the source of cancer stem-like cells

Elizabeth Hay first described an "epithelial-mesenchymal transformation" [50].

The term "transformation" has been replaced with "transition," pointing to reversibility of the process and the fact that it is different from neoplastic transformation [51].

An epithelial-mesenchymal transition (EMT) is defined as the process that allows a polarized epithelial cell, which normally interacts with basement membrane via its basal surface, to undergo multiple biochemical changes that enable it to assume a mesenchymal cell phenotype, which includes enhanced migratory capacity, invasiveness, elevated resistance to apoptosis, and greatly increased production of extracellular matrix (ECM) components [51].

These processes are consistent with the acquisition of a "cancer stem-like cell" phenotype that is also known as "stemness" or cancer stem cell (CSCs) characteristics [52, 53, 37].

EMTs are encountered in three distinct biological settings that carry very different functional consequences:

1. EMTs associated with implantation, embryo formation, and organ development;
2. EMTs associated with wound healing, tissue regeneration, and organ fibrosis;
3. EMTs associated with cancer progression and metastasis.

While the specific signals that delineate the EMTs in the three discrete settings are not yet clear, it is now well accepted that functional distinctions are apparent.

Pathologists have accepted the hypothesis of EMT in carcinogenesis albeit skeptically.

However, increasing evidence have demonstrated that the process of EMT is vitally important in cancer progression and metastasis, where cancer cells acquire a more invasive and metastatic phenotype [54].

Metastatic cancer cells with a mesenchymal phenotype are believed to undergo reverse transition, i.e., mesenchymal-to-epithelial transition (MET) at the site of metastasis to gain the pathology of their corresponding primary tumors [55].

This process is an important step by which metastatic tumor cells grow at the metastatic site.

Epithelial-mesenchymal transition is associated with carcinogenesis, invasion, metastasis, recurrence, and chemoresistance, which have been shown to be tightly linked with the function of CSCs. However, the direct relationship between CSCs and EMT in terms of molecular mechanisms remains to be elucidated.

3.8. The cancer stem cells phenomenon and the clinical course of the disease

Gastric cancer is usually diagnosed at later stages. This may be because patients often do not exhibit symptoms until their disease has progressed, or their symptoms have been vague and attributed initially to cause other than cancer.

Dormant CSCs (micrometastases) cannot be detected by current imaging examination methods and are overlooked.

When the primary tumor is treated, whether with preoperative chemotherapy and/or chemoradiation followed by surgery, we observe several phenomena. The primary tumor is often resistant to therapy. We know from our experience that the more resistant the primary tumor is, the more metastatic potential it has. In other words, this aggressive biology, which is probably related to the number of CSCs (and evolved species of CSCs) present in the primary tumor or volume of the tumor, dictates metastatic potential. In addition, although it may appear that local treatment has been successful, highly resistant metastatic disease often becomes apparent very quickly.

We distinguish three patterns of response and resistance observed in patients with advanced and metastatic gastric cancer following first-line therapy (docetaxel, cisplatin, and 5-FU).

A first pattern involves patients with gastric cancer, where there is almost a 50% chance they will experience some reduction in tumor volume and improvement in their symptoms for a short time, but, after a few months, the cancer starts to grow. Second-line therapy produces less reduction in tumor volume and for a shorter duration response. Between these patients, it can be seen that the CSCs population is enriched by cancer treatments, making the tumor more resistant.

A second pattern involves patients whose tumors exhibit primary resistance. These patients never experience tumor shrinkage even with the initial treatment option.

A third resistance pattern is one in which the patient has a mixed treatment response. Metastatic lesions in the liver, for example, will become smaller, while those in abdominal lymph nodes increase in size. This phenomenon is intrapatient tumor heterogeneity. Not only can tumors in different organs exhibit different molecular characteristics, but multiple metastases in the same organ can have different somatic profiles.

While an anti-HER2–targeted therapy is showing efficacy, only about 20% of gastric cancers overexpress HER2 [56]. In a review of first-line therapy in patients with metastatic disease, the inclusion of an anti-HER2–targeted agent provided a modest increase in survival to slightly more than 1 year [56]. Patients receiving anti-HER2 therapy develop resistance immediately after treatment. Recently, the mechanism of acquired resistance to the anti-HER2–targeted agent trastuzumab in gastric cancer has been explored. Treatment of gastric cancer cells for 20 weeks with trastuzumab resulted in epithelial-mesenchymal transition (EMT) induction in drug-resistant cells. This EMT induction was characterized by loss of E-cadherin and ZO1, as well as overexpression of claudin-1, vimentin, β-catenin, ZEB1, Slug, and Snail 22. These drug-resistant cells also exhibited an aggressive tumor phenotype, including higher motility, invasion potential, tumor formation potential, and metastatic capacity [56]. Furthermore, the drug-resistant cells exhibited other CSC properties, including higher sphere-forming capacity and expression of the CSC markers Oct4, CD133, and CD44 [56]. The increase in CSC potential was accompanied by downregulation of the AKT signaling pathway and upregulation of the STAT3 pathway. The STAT3 pathway was activated by Notch-dependent autocrine secretion of interleukin 6 [56].

These are real problems in the clinic, which are difficult to control. In solving this problem, it is necessary to penetrate into the cellular or molecular basis of gastric cancer and speculate whether different clinical outcomes reflect different CSC populations or molecular characteristics.

Gastric cancer is a heterogeneous disease with diverse molecular characteristics. Multiple experimental and clinical investigations have implicated a wide range of germ line and somatic alterations that drive tumor progression [57]. Recently, the Cancer Genome Atlas Research Network analyzed nearly 300 samples of previously untreated gastric and gastro-esophageal cancer and grouped them into four major molecular subtypes [58]:

1. The Epstein-Barr Virus (EBV)–positive group, which made up 9% of gastric cancers. This group displays high prevalence of DNA hypermethylation, including promoter methylation of the tumor suppressor CDKN2A (p16INK4A). There is a high incidence of PIK3CA mutations, amplifications of several oncogenes, including ERBB2, and recurrent amplifications of chromosome p9 (leading to overexpression of PD L1/2 and JAK2) [58].
2. The microsatellite instability (MSI) group, which made up 22% of gastric cancers. This group is characterized by enrichment for microsatellite instability (MSI), including hypermethylation at the MLH1 promoter. The MSI subgroup exhibits mutations in many cancer "hotspots," such as PIK3CA, ERBB3, ERBB2, EGFR, and overexpresses mitotic pathway components [58].
3. The genomically stable subgroup, which made up 20% of gastric cancers. This group exhibited mutations in CDH1 and in RHOA, a protein important in cell motility and the STAT3 signaling pathway [58].
4. The high chromosomal instability (CIN) group, which made up about 50% of gastric cancers. This subgroup is concentrated at the gastroesophageal junction. The CIN group exhibited hyperactivation of EGFR and other RAS-driven receptor tyrosine kinases, mutation of the tumor suppressor TP53, and high levels of aneuploidy. Chromosomal instability has been shown to be prevalent in several solid tumors, including those of the head and neck, testes, lung, and liver, as well as in gastric and gastroesophageal cancers. Fewer CINs are seen in melanoma, and even fewer in Wilms' tumors [59].

3.9. Identifying CSCs

Cancer stem cells in solid tumors were first reported in breast cancer ($CD44^{+}CD24^{-}$/low fraction) [60].

The first report of gastrointestinal CSCs was in the $CD133^{+}CD44^{+}ALDH1^{+}$ fraction of colorectal cancer [61].

Subsequently, gastrointestinal CSCs have been detected in cancers of esophagus, stomach, liver, and pancreas [62].

To distinguish CSCs from other cancer cells, researchers have developed profiles of unique cellular markers. These profiles allow detection of CSCs within a tumor and enable the separation of CSCs from nonstem cancer cells for ***research purposes***.

Markers and characteristics of the cancer stem cells:

1. surface markers (e.g., CD24, CD26, CD44, CD90, CD133, and CD166) [63].
2. high aldehyde dehydrogenase (ALDH) activity [63].
3. formation of the spheres when cultured in nonadherent conditions [63].
4. high tumorigenic potential when xenografted into immunocompromised mice.

The existence of CSCs in gastric cancer was first revealed by analyzing a panel of gastric cancer cell lines [64, 65]. Cancer stem cells from either gastric cancer cell lines or resected tumors were isolated using cell surface markers, such as CD44 and epithelial cell adhesion molecule (EpCAM) [65]. Moreover, gastric CSCs can even be isolated from the peripheral blood of gastric cancer patients using CD44 and CD54.

Leucine-rich repeat containing G protein-coupled receptor-5 (Lgr5) is a gastric CSC marker and $Lgr5^{+}$ stem cells in the stomach could be the origin of gastric CSCs [66]. Patients with gastric cancer containing $Lgr5^{+}$ cells have a short median survival [66].

Stem cells that express villin exist in the pyloric gland and villin + gastric stem cells might be converted to gastric cancer cells [66]. Kruppel-like factor-4 (KLF4) might play a critical role in gastric cancer initiation and progression in villin + gastric stem cells [66].

In addition, ALDH1, CD90, CD71, and CD133 could be candidate markers of gastric CSCs. MicroRNAs might regulate the properties of gastric CSCs by inducing epithelial-mesenchymal transition [67].

It must be noted, however, that no set of markers are exclusive to CSCs, and also that CSC phenotypes vary over time and between individual patients' tumors of the same subtype. These facts have caused researchers to speculate whether different clinical outcomes reflect different CSC populations [63].

3.10. Treatment of the cancer stem cells

Multiple research findings indicate that conventional therapies, which target the rapidly dividing cells in tumors, have limited efficacy or even adverse effects on CSCs [30] and lead to treatment failure, chemoresistance, and recurrence.

Consequently, two types of cancer therapies targeting CSCs have been investigated: first, to induce and/or maintain dormancy of tumor cells, and second, to induce cell death in residual dormant cancer cells by targeting their markers. Consequently, gastric cancer therapies targeting CSCs have been investigated (**Table 3**) [70].

Target molecules/pathways		Target tumors	Therapeutic agents
Surface markers	CD44	Gastric cancer	Sulfasalazine
Signaling pathways	JAK/STAT signaling	Gastric cancer	Napabucasin (BBI-608), fedratinib, pacritinib
Microenvironment	VEGF/VEGF-R	Gastric cancer	Bevacizumab, cediranib, ziv-aflibercept
Epigenetic system	Histone deacetylases	Gastric cancer	Entinostat, vorinostat, mocetinostat, romidepsin, belinostat, panobinostat
	EZH2 inhibitor	Gastric cancer	Tazemetostat (EPZ-6438)
Others	ABC transporters	Gastric cancer	Zosuquidar, tariquidar, laniquidar
	Immune-mediated antitumor effect, insulin resistance	Gastric cancer	Metformin

JAK, Janus-activated kinase; VEGF-R, VEGF receptor; EZH2, enhancer of zeste homolog 2; ABC, ATP-binding cassette.

Table 3. Target molecules and pathways for gastric cancer stem cells.

3.11. The risks of anticancer stem cells (CSCs) therapy

1. Many markers for CSCs are also found on normal stem cells, which is a disadvantage in terms of their use as therapeutic targets. Thus, the best way to eradicate CSCs is to discover the molecules responsible for the specific properties of CSCs, but not of normal cells, such as variants of stem cell surface markers, such as CD44v8–10 in gastric cancer [68].

2. The second challenge is the need to rethink the use of traditional endpoints of tumor regression in clinical trials. Because CSC-targeting agents do not cause tumor regression, investigators must determine how to demonstrate conclusively that these agents provide a benefit. The circulating tumor cells are highly enriched in stem cell markers in patients. Whereas 1–5% of cells are CSCs in primary cancers, studies have shown that closer to 30–50% of circulating tumor cells express stem cell markers [25]. Circulating tumor cells may prove useful as biomarkers for patients in clinical trials. Isolating and measuring circulating tumor cells may be a way to monitor patients and determine the efficacy of potential treatments [69].

4. Conclusion

Surgical treatment is not able to provide patients with GCLM a complete cure.

Advanced gastric cancer is one of the most difficult challenges in clinical practice. Research has shown that CSCs can initiate tumor development and play a significant role in tumor relapse and metastasis. Indeed, evidence is accumulating that treatments, such as chemotherapy and radiation, can increase the proliferation of CSCs. Investigations are underway into the molecular signaling pathways involved in tumor cell repopulation. The small subpopulation of CSCs in gastric cancer may be a rational treatment target.

Acknowledgements

I thank Roman Zahorec, MD PhD for control and revision of the manuscript.

Author details

Vitězslav Marek* and Štefan Durdik

*Address all correspondence to: vitezslav.marek@gmail.com

Department of Surgical Oncology, St. Elizabeth Hospital, Medical School of Comenius University, Bratislava, Slovak Republic

References

[1] International Agency for Research on Cancer. GLOBOCAN 2012: Estimated Cancer Incidence, Mortality and Prevalence Worldwide in 2012 [Internet]. Available form: http://globocan.iarc.fr/Pages/fact-sheets-population.aspx

[2] National Cancer Institute. Surveillance, Epidemiology, and End Results Program (SEER). SEER Stat Fact Sheets: Stomach Cancer [Internet]. Available form: http://seer.cancer.gov/statfacts/html/stomach.html. [Accessed: August 3, 2015]

[3] Tanaka M, Ma E, Tanaka H, Ioka A, Nakahara T, Takahashi H. Trends of stomach mortality in Eastern Asia in 1950-2004: Comprehensive study of Japan, Hong Kong and Singapore using age, period and cohort analysis. International Journal of Cancer. 2012;**130**:930-936

[4] Sakamoto Y, Ohyama S, Yamamoto J, Yamada K, Seki M, Ohta K, et al. Surgical resection of liver metastases of gastric cancer: Analysis of a 17-year experience with 22 patients. Surgery. 2003;**133**:507-511

[5] de Jong MC, Pulitano C, Ribero D, Sturb J, Mentha G, Schulick RD, et al. Rates and patterns of recurrence following curative intent surgery for colorectal liver metastasis an international multi-institutional analysis of 1669 patients. Annals of Surgery. 2009;**250**:440-448

[6] Kodera Y, Fujinati K, Fujinati N, Ito S, Muro K, Ohashi N, et al. Surgical resection of hepatic metastasis from gastric cancer: A review and new recommendation in the Japanese gastric cancer treatment guidelines. Gastric Cancer. 2014;**17**:206-212

[7] Japanese Gastric Cancer Association. Japanese gastric cancer treatment guidelines (Ver.3). Gastric Cancer. 2011;**14**:113-123

[8] Takemura N, Saiura A, Koga R, Arita J, et al. Long term outcomes after surgical resection for gastric cancer liver metastasis: An analysis of 64 macroscopically complete resections. Langenbeck's Archives of Surgery. 2012;**397**:951-957

[9] Schildberg CW, Croner R, Merkel S, Schellerer V, et al. Outcome of operative therapy of hepatic metastasis stomach carcinoma: A retrospective analysis. World Journal of Surgery. 2012;**36**:872-878

[10] Jemal A, Siegel R, Ward E, Murray T, Xu J, Smigal C, et al. Cancer statistics. CA Cancer Journal of Clinicians. 2006;**56**:106-130

[11] Weiss L. Metastatic inefficiency. Advances in Cancer Research. 1990;**54**:159-211

[12] Suzuki M, Mose ES, Montel V, Tarin D. Dormant cancer cells retrieved from metastasis-free organs regain tumorigenic and metastatic potency. The American Journal of Surgical Pathology. 2006;**169**:673-681

[13] Liu H, Patel MR, Prescher JA, Patsialou A, Qian D, Lin J, et al. Cancer stem cells from human breast tumors are involved in spontaneous metastases in orthotopic mouse models. Proceedings of the National Academy of Sciences of the United States of America. 2010;**107**:18115-18120

[14] Cheon SH, Rha SY, Jeung HC, Im CK, Kim SH, Kim HR, et al. Survival benefit of combined curative resection of the stomach/D2 resection/and liver in gastric cancer patients with liver metastases. Annals of Oncology. 2008;**19**:1146-1153

[15] Kinoshita T, Kinoshita T, Saiura A, Esaki M, Sakamoto H, Yamanaka T, et al. Multicentre analysis of long-term outcome after surgical resection for gastric cancer liver metastases. British Journal of Surgery. 2015;**102**:102-107

[16] Takemura N, Saiura A, Koga R, Yoshioka R, Yamamoto J, Kokudo N, et al. Repeat hepatectomy for recurrent liver metastasis from gastric carcinoma. World Journal of Surgery. 2013;**37**:2664-2670

[17] Yoshida M, Ohtsu A, Boku N, Miyata Y, Shirao K, Shimada Y, et al. Long –term survival and prognostic factors in patients with metastatic gastric cancer treated with chemotherapy in the Japan Clinical Oncology Group (JCOG) study. Japanese Journal of Clinical Oncology. 2004;**34**:654-659

[18] Chen J, Tang Z, Dong X, Gao S, Fang H, Wu D, et al. Radiofrequency ablation for liver metastasis from gastric cancer. European Journal of Surgical Oncology. 2013;**39**:701-706

[19] Aguirre-Ghiso JA. Models, mechanisms and clinical evidence for cancer dormancy. Nature Reviews Cancer. 2007;**7**:834-846

[20] Sobin LH, Gospodarowicz MK, Wittekind C, editos. TNM Classification of Malignant Tumours. 7th ed. Singapore: Blackwell Publishing Ltd; 2010

[21] Clarke MF, Dick JE, Dirks PB, Eaves CJ, Jamieson CH, Jones DL, et al. Cancer stem cells—Perspectives on current status and future directions: AACR Workshop on cancer stem cells. Cancer Research. 2006;**66**:9339-9344

[22] Wong DJ, Segal E, Chang HY. Stemness, cancer and cancer stem cells. Cell Cycle. 2008; **7**:3622-3624

[23] Huntly BJP, Gilliland DG. Leukemia stem cells and the evolution of Cancer Stem Cells. Nature Reviews Cancer 2005;**5**:311-321

[24] Bonnet D, Dick JE. Human acute myeloid leukemia is organized as a hierarchy that originates from a primitive hematopoetic cell. Nature Medicine. 1997;**3**:730-737

[25] Al-Hajj M, Wicha MS, Benito-Hernandez A, Morrison SJ, Clarke MF. Prospective identification of tumorigenic breast cancer cells. Proceedings of the National Academy of Sciences of the United States of America. 2003;**100**:3983-3988

[26] Costa FF, Le Blanc K, Brodin B. Cancer/Testis antigens, stem cells and cancer [Internet]. 2006. Available from: Http://www. StemCells.com

[27] Jordan CT, Guzman ML, Noble M. Cancer stem cells. New England Journal of Medicine. 2006;**355**:1253-1261

[28] Sigal M, Rothenberg ME, Logan CY, et al. Helicobacter pylori activates and expands Lgr5+ stem cells through direct colonization of the gastric glands. Gastroenterology. 2015;**148**:1392-1404

[29] Houghton J, Stoicov C, Nomura S, et al. Gastric cancer originating from bone marrow-derived cells. Science. 2004;**306**:1568-1571

[30] Bao B, Ahmad A, Azmi AS, Ali S, Sarkar FH. Overview of cancer stem cells (CSCs) and mechanisms of their regulation: Implications for cancer therapy. Current Protocols in Pharmacology. 2013;**14**:Unit-14.25

[31] Wicha MS, Liu S, Dontu G. Cancer stem cells: An old idea—A paradigm shift. Cancer Research. 2006;**66**(4):1883-1890. discussion 1895-1886

[32] Visvader JE. Cells of origin in cancer. Nature. 2011;**469**(7330):314-322

[33] Carrasco E, Alvarez PJ, Prados J, et al. Cancer stem cells and their implication in breast cancer. European Journal of Clinical Investigation. 2014;**44**(7):678-687

[34] Lathia JD, Hitomi M, Gallagher J, et al. Distribution of CD133 reveals glioma stem cells self-renew through symmetric and asymmetric cell divisions. Cell Death and Disease. 2011;**2**:e200

[35] Wright MH, Calcagno AM, Salcido CD, Carlson MD, Ambudkar SV, Varticovski L. Brca1 breast tumors contain distinct CD44+/CD24− and CD133+ cells with cancer stem cell characteristics. Breast Cancer Research. 2008;**10**:R10

[36] Qiao B, Gopalan V, Chen Z, Smith RA, Tao Q, Lam AK. Epithelial-mesenchymal transition and mesenchymal-epithelial transition are essential for the acquisition

of stem cell properties in hTERT-immortalised oral epithelial cells. Biology Cell. 2012;**104**:476-489

[37] Mani SA, Guo W, Liao MJ, Eaton EN, Ayyanan A, Zhou AY, et al. The epithelial-mesenchymal transition generates cells with properties of stem cells. Cell. 2008;**133**: 704-715

[38] Hermann PC, Huber SL, Herrler T, Aicher A, Ellwart JW, Guba M, et al. Distinct populations of cancer stem cells determine tumor growth and metastatic activity in human pancreatic cancer. Cell Stem Cell. 2007;**1**:313-323

[39] Bleau AM, Agliano A, Larzabal L, de Aberasturi AL, Calvo A. Metastatic dormancy: A complex network between cancer stem cells and their microenvironment. Histology and Histopathology. 2014;**29**:1499-1510

[40] Gao D, et al. endothelial progenitor cells control the angiogenic switch in mouse lung metastasis. Science. 2008;**319**:195-198

[41] Mahnke YD, Schwendemann J, Beckhove P, Schirrmacher V. Maintenance of long-term tumour-specific T-cell memory by residual dormant tumour cells. Immunology. 2005;**115**:325-336

[42] Pajonk F, Vlashi E. Characterization of the stem cell niche and its importance in radiobiological response. Seminars in Radiation Oncology. 2013;**23**(4):237-241

[43] Herr P, Basler K. Porcupine-mediated lipidation is required for Wnt recognition by Wls. Developmental Biology. 2012;**361**(2):392-402

[44] Hassan KA, Wang L, Korkaya H, et al. Notch pathway activity identifies cells with cancer stem cell-like properties and correlates with worse survival in lung adenocarcinoma. Clinical Cancer Research. 2013;**19**(8):1972-1980

[45] Wang ML, Chiou SH, Wu CW. Targeting cancer stem cells: Emerging role of Nanog transcription factor. OncoTargets and Therapy. 2013;**6**:1207-1220

[46] Mo JS, Park HW, Guan KL. The Hippo signaling pathway in stem cell biology and cancer. EMBO Report. 2014;**15**(6):642-656

[47] Bourguignon LY, Earle C, Wong G, Spevak CC, Krueger K. Stem cell marker (Nanog) and Stat-3 signaling promote microRNA-21 expression and chemoresistance in hyaluronan/CD44-activated head and neck squamous cell carcinoma cells. Oncogene. 2012;**31**(2):149-160

[48] Lin L, Liu A, Peng Z, et al. STAT3 is necessary for proliferation and survival in colon cancer-initiating cells. Cancer Research. 2011;**71**(23):7226-7237

[49] Ablett MP, Singh JK, Clarke RB. Stem cells in breast tumours: Are they ready for the clinic? European Journal of Cancer. 2012;**48**(14):2104-2116

[50] Hay ED. An overview of epithelio-mesenchymal transformation. Acta Anatomica. (Basel). 1995;**154**:8-20

[51] Kalluri R, Neilson EG. Epithelial-mesenchymal transition and its implications for fibrosis. Journal of Clinical Investigation. 2003;**112**:1776-1784

[52] Brabletz T, Jung A, Spaderna S, Hlubek F, Kirchner T. Opinion: Migrating cancer stem cells—An integrated concept of malignant tumour progression. Nature Reviews Cancer. 2005;**5**:744-749

[53] Kasper S. Stem cells: The root of prostate cancer? Journal of Cellular Physiology. 2008;**216**:332-336

[54] Brabletz T, Jung A, Reu S, Porzner M, Hlubek F, Kunz-Schughart LA, Knuechel R, Kirchner T. Variable beta-catenin expression in colorectal cancers indicates tumor progression driven by the tumor environment. Proceedings of the National Academy of Sciences of the United States of America. 2001;**98**:10356-10361

[55] Thompson EW, Newgreen DF, Tarin D. Carcinoma invasion and metastasis: A role for epithelial-mesenchymal transition? Cancer Research. 2005;**65**:5991-5995

[56] Elimova E, Shiozaki H, Wadhwa R, et al. Medical management of gastric cancer: A 2014 update. World Journal of Gastroenterology. 2014;20:13637-13647

[57] Wadhwa R, Song S, Lee JS, Yao Y, Wei Q, Ajani JA. Gastric cancer: Molecular and clinical dimensions. Nature Reviews Clinical Oncology. 2013;**10**:643-655

[58] Cancer Genome Atlas Research Network. Comprehensive molecular characterization of gastric adenocarcinoma. Nature. 2014;**513**:202-209

[59] Rooney PH, Murray GI, Stevenson DAJ, Haites NE, Cassidy J, McLeod HL. Comparative genomic hybridization and chromosomal instability in solid tumours. British Journal of Cancer. 1999;**80**:862-873

[60] Al-Hajj M, Wicha MS, Benito-Hernandez A, et al. Prospective identification of tumorigenic breast cancer cells. Proceedings of the National Academy of Sciences of the United States of America. 2003;**100**:3982-3988

[61] Ricci-Vitiani L, Lombardi DG, Pilozzi E, et al. Identification and expansion of human colon-cancer-initiating cells. Nature. 2007;**445**:111-115

[62] Mikhail S, Zeidan A. Stem cells in gastrointestinal cancers: The road less travelled. World Journal of Stem Cells. 2014;**6**:606-613

[63] Visvader JE, Lindeman GJ. Cancer stem cells in solid tumours: Accumulating evidence and unresolved questions. Nature Reviews Cancer. 2008;**8**:755-768

[64] Vermeulen L, Todaro M, de Sousa Mello F, et al. Single-cell cloning of colon cancer stem cells reveals a multi-lineage differentiation capacity. Proceedings of the National Academy of Sciences of the United States of America. 2008;**105**:13427-13432

[65] Barker N, Huch M, Kujala P, et al. Lgr5(+ve)stem cells drive self–renewal in the stomach and build long–lived gastric units in vitro. Cell Stem Cell. 2010;**6**:25-36

[66] Li Q, Jia Z, Wang L, et al. Disruption of Klf4 in villin–positive gastric progenitor cells promotes formation and progression of tumors of the antrum in mice. Gastroenterology. 2012;**142**:531-542

[67] Lee MS, Hsu CC, Wahlqvist ML, et al. Type-2 diabetes increases and metformin reduces total, colorectal, liver and pancreatic cancer incidences in Taiwanese: A representative population prospective cohort study of 800,000 individuals. BMC Cancer. 2011;**11**:20

[68] Ishimoto T, Nagano O, Yae T, et al. CD44 variant regulates redox status in cancer cells by stabilizing the xCT subunit of system xc(–) and thereby promotes tumor growth. Cancer Cell. 2011;**19**:387-400

[69] Lianidou ES, Markou A. Circulating tumor cells in breast cancer: Detection systems, molecular characterization, and future challenges. Clinical Chemistry. 2011;**57**:1242-1255

[70] Taniguchi H, Moriya C, Igarashi H, Saitoh A, Yamamoto H, Adachi Y, Imal K. Cancer stem cells in human gastrointestinal cancer. Cancer Science. 2016;**107**(11):1556-1562

[71] Klauber-DeMore N, Van Zee KJ, Linkov I, Borgen PI, Gerald WL. Biological behavior of human breast cancer micrometastases. Clinical Cancer Research. 2001;**2434**:2434-2439

[72] Marek V, Zahorec R, Palaj J, Durdik S. Gastric cancer with liver metastasis. Bratislavske Lekarske Listy. 2016;**117**(1):59-61

Section 6

Key-role of Pathologists in the Diagnosis and in the Therapeutic Decisions in Patients with Gatric Cancer

Chapter 12

Malignant Gastric Tumours: The Role of Pathologist in the Diagnosis and for Therapeutic Decisions

Alexander Quaas

Additional information is available at the end of the chapter

http://dx.doi.org/10.5772/intechopen.69838

Abstract

This chapter gives an overview about the most important malignant gastric tumours from the perspective of the pathologist. The first focus is the systematic classification of gastric carcinoma, neuroendocrine tumours, mesenchymal tumours and malignant lymphoma with related histomorphology-based and molecular-based diagnosis criteria including differential diagnosis pathologists have to consider when dealing with gastric tumours. The second focus addresses the issues of personalized therapy options in gastric tumours pathologists have to bear in mind. Currently, some subtypes of gastric adenocarcinomas have been proposed with therapeutic implications like microsatellite-instable carcinoma and checkpoint-inhibition or Her2/neu positive adenocarcinoma of intestinal-type and specific tyrosine-receptor blockade. Mesenchymal tumours are rare and can morphologically be quite variable. Mucosa-associated lymphoid tissue (MALT)-related marginal zone lymphoma is the most frequent gastric lymphoma but all other B-and T-cell lymphoma can occur in the stomach as well, and an exact subcharacterisation is very important due to different treatment decisions (e.g. eradication of helicobacter-pylori in MALT-lymphoma as first choice treatment vs. chemotherapy in Burkitt-lymphoma). Pathologists have to consider a large spectrum of differential diagnosis and conflicting immunohistochemical and molecular results. It will become more and more important to find out therapeutically relevant tumour subtypes and to use biomarkers to predict a successful individualized treatment.

Keywords: classification systems, diagnosis criteria, tumour subtyping, personalized treatment options

1. Introduction

The pathologist who deals with gastric tumours is responsible for the determination of the following factors:

- Dignity
- Main tumour differentiation (e.g. epithelial, mesenchymal, lymphatic)
- Treatment options
- Consider differential diagnosis (main differential diagnosis of gastric adenocarcinoma include neuroendocrine carcinoma, malignant lymphoma, metastasis of lobular breast carcinoma, epithelioid angiosarcoma or malignant melanoma)
- Morphology-based subtyping of gastric carcinoma (according to WHO or Lauren)
- Grading
- Staging (according to TNM-classification)
- Surgery resection status (R0-R2)
- Treatment relevant biomarkers: Her2/neu in gastric adenocarcinoma or in gastrointestinal stromal tumour (GIST), mutational analysis of c-kit or PDGFR)
- Regression scores after neoadjuvant treatment

Adenocarcinoma (including different subtypes) is the most common malignant gastric tumours of epithelial origin. In Western countries, declining incidence of gastric carcinoma is found; nevertheless, it remains the second most common cause of cancer-related death in the world [3]. In Germany, we expect about 9200 men and 6400 women with a newly diagnosed gastric carcinoma per year, and 70% of them will die carcinoma-related in the following 5

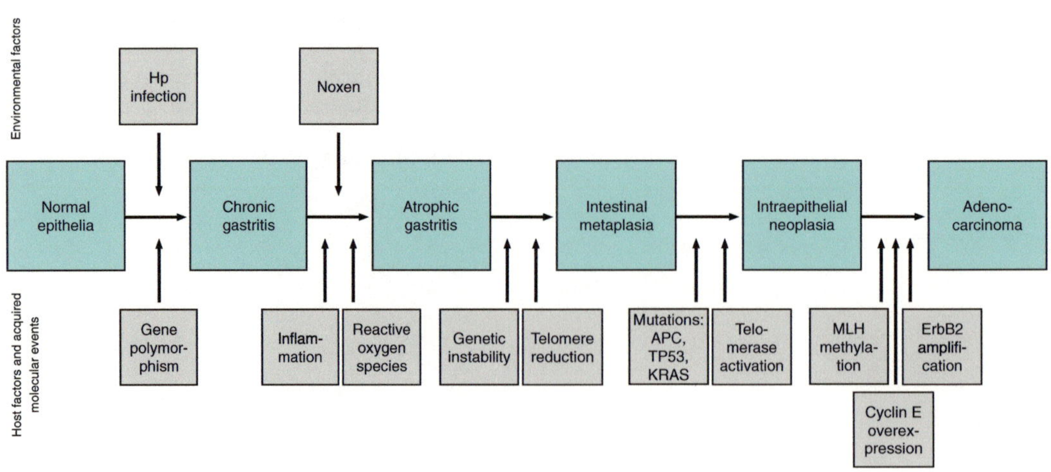

Figure 1. Pathogenesis of intestinal-type gastric adenocarcinoma.

years. Particularly, if metastases/recurrences occur, the prognosis is still dismal with a median survival of 8 months (krebsdaten.de—Robert-Koch-Institut, Berlin 2015). Particularly, in Northern Europe and the United States, the distribution of carcinomas within the stomach changed in the past decades. The distal-located tumours (typically from the diffuse type of adenocarcinoma) are decreasing and the proximal tumours (typically from the intestinal type of adenocarcinoma) are increasing [1, 2].

From the pathophysiological point of view, main features of the intestinal type of gastric adenocarcinoma are (a) chronic inflammation of the mucosa (typically due to an infection of helicobacter pylori) with related mucosa damage and atrophy, (b) intraepithelial neoplasia and (c) fully invasive adenocarcinoma (**Figure 1**).

2. Classification of primary gastric carcinomas

In the past 90 years, there have been some different proposals for classification systems (**Table 1**). Especially in Western countries, the classification of Lauren (from 1965) and the current World Health Organisation (WHO) (from 2010) are accepted and of practical importance.

In general, gastric adenocarcinomas are built of (a) cohesive tumour cells forming tubular or papillary structures or (b) poorly cohesive (and often but not always) single carcinoma cells. It is not uncommon to see different growth pattern in the same tumour (morphology-based tumour heterogeneity).

2.1. WHO classification

The current WHO classification system describes four main subtypes of gastric adenocarcinoma and some rare entities [3].

2.1.1. *Tubular adenocarcinoma*

Cohesive tumour cells form slit-like, branching or someone dilated tubules or acinar structures. The individual carcinoma cells typically are columnar or cuboidal (**Figure 2A**).

2.1.2. *Papillary adenocarcinoma*

Papillary adenocarcinoma is usually a well-differentiated exophytic (finger-like) tumour. Fibrovascular tissue cores support the cohesive cylindrical or cuboidal tumour cells. Especially in superficial tumour biopsies, it is easy to miss an infiltrating growth pattern or desmoplastic stroma response (**Figure 2B**).

2.1.3. *Mucinous adenocarcinoma*

The main feature of this subtype is the dominance of extra-cellular mucinous pools—by definition, mucinous adenocarcinoma shows more than 50% extra-cellular mucin (**Figure 2C**). It is not uncommon to see some signet-ring cells scattered in the mucin.

WHO (2010)	Lauren (1965)	Goseki (1992)	Ming (1992)	Molecular (2014)
Papillary adenocarcinoma	Intestinal type		(Expanding type)	Chromosomal instable, MSI*
Tubular adenocarcinoma		Type 1 (type 2, type 3)	(Infiltrating type)	
Mucinous adenocarcinoma				
Signet-ring cell carcinoma	Diffuse type	type 4		Genomic stable
And other poorly cohesive carcinoma				
Mixed carcinoma	Indeterminate-type			
Adenosquamous carcinoma				
Squamous cell carcinoma				
Hepatoid adenocarcinoma				
Carcinoma with lymphoid stroma				EBV-related; MSI*
Choriocarcinoma				
Carcinosarcoma				
Parietal cell carcinoma				
Malignant rhabdoid tumour				
Mucoepidermoid carcinoma				
Paneth cell carcinoma				
Undifferentiated carcinoma				
Mixed adeno-neuroendocrine carcinoma				
Endodermal sinus tumour				
Embryonal carcinoma				
Pure gastric yolk sac tumour				
Oncocytic adenocarcinoma				

Notes: The correlation between the different classification systems is relative. The Ming classification cannot be assigned to the other classifications.

*MSI, microsatellite instable.

Table 1. Classification systems of adenocarcinoma.

2.1.4. Signet-ring cell and other poorly cohesive adenocarcinoma

Non-cohesive, isolated single tumour cells or carcinoma cells arranged in only small aggregates of few cells (**Figure 2D**).

Signet-ring cell carcinoma is composed of more than 50% signet-ring cells. The classic form of signet-ring cells is usually a single cell and has a central droplet of cytoplasmic mucin (optically clear in HE-staining). The atypical, hyperchromatic nucleus is eccentrically placed. Sometimes signet-ring cells can form lace-like glands.

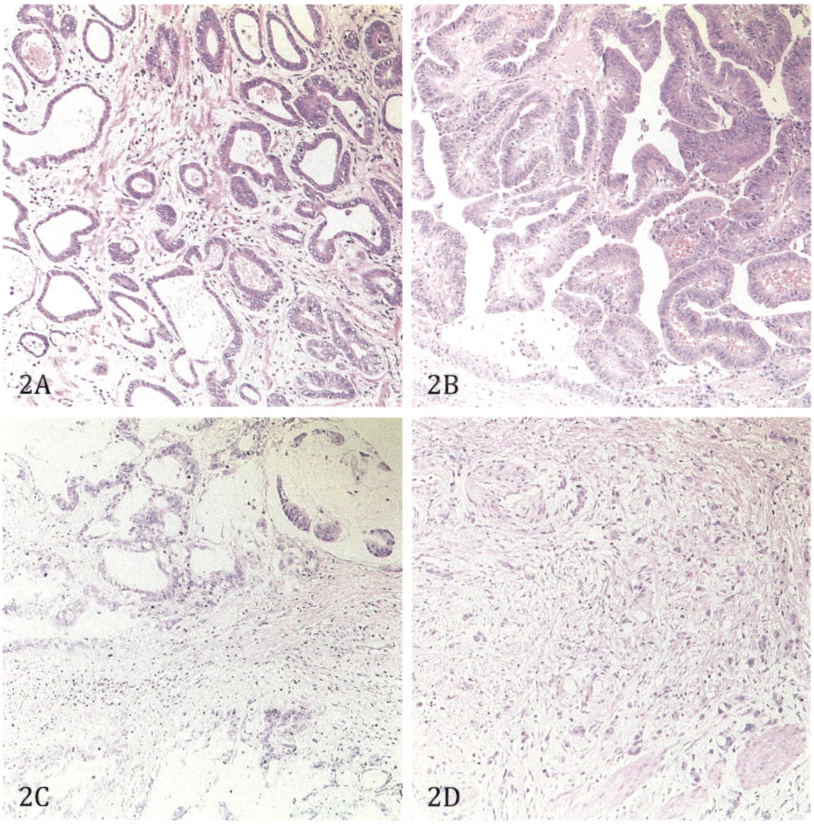

Figure 2. Four main histological subtypes of gastric adenocarcinoma (WHO): (A) tubular adenocarcinoma, (B) papillary adenocarcinoma, (C) mucinous adenocarcinoma and (D) poorly differentiated non-cohesive adenocarcinoma.

Other variants of poorly cohesive adenocarcinomas include (it is important to recognize that signet-ring cell carcinoma is just one subtype in the group of poorly cohesive adenocarcinoma): single cells with deeply eosinophilic cytoplasm, bizarre nuclei, histiocytic-like or accompanied with prominent lymphatic stroma.

2.1.5. Mixed adenocarcinoma

As described above, gastric carcinoma is highly heterogeneous (from the morphological as well as molecular point of view). The 'mixed' subtype is composed of different cohesive or poorly cohesive tumour components of the main four subtypes described above (for example tubular and signet-ring cell components). It is recommended to describe any histological component.

2.1.6. Rare carcinoma variants (to see all: compare **Table 1***)*

2.1.6.1. Adenocarcinoma with lymphoid stroma (lymphoepithelioma-like or medullary carcinoma)

Typically, poorly cohesive or vague tubular-forming tumour cells are associated with prominent lymphoid stroma. Often small lymphocytes are scattered between tumour cells. Poorly cohesive tumour cells can be misinterpreted as lymphatic blasts. Typically, this subtype is EBV-related and it is easy to detect EBV-RNA using *in-situ*-test like EBER. Furthermore, carcinoma cells are often immunohistochemically strong PD-L1 positive. Nevertheless, not all EBV-related adenocarcinomas show the typical medullary morphological features. Some carcinomas of this subtype are microsatellite-instable easy and cost-effective detectable using immunohistochemistry for MLH1 (MSH2, MLH6 and PMS2). The loss of one (or more) of these DNA-repair proteins in tumour cell nuclei is in keeping with microsatellite-instability.

2.1.6.2. Squamous cell carcinoma

A pure gastric squamous cell carcinoma is very rare and is suspicious for a metastasis. Sometimes a mixed adeno-squamous cell carcinoma can be seen.

2.2. Classification according to Lauren (established 1965)

2.2.1. Intestinal type

Cohesive tumour cells form tubular, papillary or solid structures. The tumour typically shows well-demarcated pushing borders and it is associated with chronic gastritis (usually w Hp-infection) including intestinal metaplasia and pre-cancerogenous epithelial lesions like flat intraepithelial neoplasia/dysplasia. Abundant intracytoplasmic mucin production is not a feature.

2.2.2. Diffuse type

Poorly or non-cohesive tumour cells include signet-ring cells. The tumour typically shows infiltrating margins. Usually intestinal metaplasia of the gastric mucosa or classic dysplasia is absent. Probably a signet-ring cell carcinoma *in situ* develops from the proliferative foveolar zone and directly invades into the lamina propria.

2.2.3. Indeterminate type

Mix of intestinal type and diffuse type tumour cells.

2.3. Goseki classification (established 1992)

According to the degree of tubular differentiation and the amount of intracellular mucin, this classification separates four subtypes.

1. Tubular differentiation, mainly (just a few tumour cells with intracellular mucin allowed)

2. Tubular differentiation accompanied by abundant intracellular mucin

3. Minor components of both: few tubular differentiations and few intracellular mucin

4. Abundant intracellular mucin and no/very few tubular differentiation

2.4. Ming classification (established 1997)

According to the infiltration zone, tumours with expanding, pushing border and tumours with infiltrating margins have separated. Types and architecture of tumour cells are not included.

1. Expanding type
2. Infiltrating type

2.5. Molecular subtypes

Most recently, molecular-based classification systems were introduced. According to the results of the cancer genome atlas research network [4], four subtypes exist (including their distribution):

1. Chromosomal instable (49.8%)
2. Microsatellite instable (21.7%)
3. Genomic stable (19.6%)
4. Epstein-Barr virus related (8.9%)

According to the results of Cristescu et al., four subtypes exist associated with distinct clinical outcomes [5].

1. Microsatellite stable TP53 inactivated
2. Microsatellite stable TP53 activated
3. Microsatellite stable with epithelial-mesenchymal-transposition (EMT)
4. Microsatellite instable

2.5.1. Clinical significance

Her2/neu (ERBB2) is a well-known receptor tyrosine kinase in breast carcinoma and currently, it is the only established therapeutically important tyrosine kinase in gastric adenocarcinoma. According to the results of the TOGA study, patients show a statistically significant benefit when using the Her2-specific tyrosine kinase inhibitor trastuzumab in Her2/neu positive gastric cancer. About 20% of gastric carcinomas are Her2/neu positive–most of them are located in the proximal part of the stomach and have an intestinal tumour differentiation. The role of the pathologists is the determination of the Her2-status on gastric carcinoma cells using immunohistochemistry or fluorescence-*in situ* (FISH). The criteria of Her2-positivity are different from that of breast carcinoma (compare **Table 2**).

	Gastric carcinoma	Breast carcinoma
Cut-off	Positive tumour cells biopsy: ≥5 cells resection: ≥10%	Positive tumour cells ≥10%
Pattern of expression	(Baso-)lateral expression sufficient	Circular expression required

Source: Modified according to Rüschoff et al. [6].

Table 2. Immunohistochemical Her2/neu criteria.

Gastric carcinomas are highly heterogeneous tumours and Her2/neu is usually not diffusely expressed in most of carcinoma cells (like it is commonly the case in breast carcinoma).

2.5.2. Molecular-based classification systems and prediction of treatment options

The molecular-based classification systems can be correlated to classical morphology-based divisions. The pathologist can use both to predict treatment options. The chromosomal instable/microsatellite stable subtype is more likely to belong to the intestinal type of adenocarcinoma or to the tubuloacinar-subtype and these tumours are more often correlated with a Her2/neu overexpression/amplification. The genomic stable/microsatellite stable with pithelial-mesenchymal-transposition (EMT) subtype is typically related to the diffuse type of adenocarcinoma or to the poorly cohesive adenocarcinoma including signet-ring cell carcinoma nearly never show Her2/neu positivity.

On the other hand, the microsatellite unstable or EBV-related subtypes can show different morphological patterns (sometimes associated with prominent lymphatic stroma) and are probably associated with better prognosis (Cristescu et al. described a better outcome in patients with microsatellite-instable tumours) and good treatment response to checkpoint-inhibitors (currently subject of clinical trials). In view of the above, pathologists should consider both traditional morphology-based and molecular-based classifications to find out the most reliable statement about prognosis and treatment options.

Cost-effective molecular-based classifications are possible using traditional morphology, immunohistochemistry (using antibodies against TP53, Her2/neu and MLH1) and *in-situ* technics (like EBER) [7, 8].

In surgical specimens, the determination of tumour stage is the most important prognostic factor in gastric carcinoma. In Western countries, the UICC-based TNM-classification system is well established (compare **Table 3**).

T	Primary tumour
T1	Tumour invades lamina propria, muscularis mucosae or submucosa
T1a	Tumour invades lamina propria or muscularis mucosa
T1b	Tumour invades submucosa
T2	Tumour invades muscularis propria
T3	Tumour invades subserosa
T4	Tumour perforates serosa or invades adjacent structures

T	Primary tumour
T4a	Tumour perforates serosa
T4b	Tumour invades adjacent structures
N	**Regional lymph nodes**
NX	Regional lymph nodes cannot be assessed
N0	No regional lymph node metastasis
N1	Metastasis in 1–2 regional lymph nodes
N2	Metastasis in 3–6 regional lymph nodes
N3	Metastasis in 7 or more regional lymph nodes
N3a	Metastasis in 7–15 regional lymph nodes
N3b	Metastasis in 16 or more regional lymph nodes
M	**Distant metastasis**
M0	No distant metastasis
M1	Distant metastasis

Source: Modified according to Brierley et al [9].

Table 3. TNM classification.

The determination of tumour regression and estimation of the percentage of residual tumour after neoadjuvant chemo or radio-chemotherapy treatment is possible using standardized regression scores. Especially in Western countries, the regression score according to Becker et al. is well established (compare **Table 4**).

1a	No residual tumour (incl. treatment effect)
1b	<10% residual tumour (incl. treatment effect)
2	10–50% residual tumour (incl. treatment effect)
3	>50% residual tumour (incl. treatment effect)

Sources: Becker et al [10].

Table 4. Regression score.

3. Pre-cancerogenous epithelial lesions

3.1. Adenoma

Gastric adenomas are polypoid and typically solitary lesions. They commonly arise in a background of chronic atrophic gastritis with accompanied intestinal metaplasia. By definition, the epithelia of adenomas are neoplastic (intraepithelial neoplasia/dysplasia). Most of them show an intestinal differentiation (including goblet cells, Paneth cells) and look like a colon adenoma. According to the classification of colon adenoma, they can be subdivided into tubular, villous or mixed adenomas and into low-grade or high-grade intraepithelial neoplasia. A minor group of gastric adenomas shows gastric gland differentiation like foveolar (so-called type II dysplasia) or pyloric gland differentiation, a mixture of foveolar/intestinal like differentiation or (very rare) a predominant Paneth-cell differentiation.

3.2. Pyloric gland-adenoma

Pyloric gland-adenoma usually arises in women and has a background of atrophic autoimmune-gastritis. This type of adenoma is polypoid and show closely packed pyloric gland-like tubuli. The epithelia are cuboidal with round nuclei and pale cytoplasm. Immunohistochemically pyloric gland-adenoma shows common gastric mucin (MUC 5A/C and MUC6).

3.2.1. Clinical significance

Adenomas must be removed with clear margins. Large adenomas (more than 2 cm) show a higher risk of malignancy.

3.3. Flat intraepithelial neoplasia

Especially in the stomach, intraepithelial neoplasia is flat and demonstrates endoscopically with only slight, uncharacteristic abnormalities. Frequently flat intraepithelial neoplasia arises in a background of chronic gastritis later in life (beyond the fifth decade). By convention, the intraepithelial neoplasia has to divide into either low grade or high grade.

Microscopically, the main characteristics of intraepithelial neoplasia consider cytology and architecture (like in adenoma):

Low-grade intraepithelial neoplasia preserves more or less the normal glandular differentiation, the epithelia show enlarged hyperchromatic nuclei, the nucleoli are not prominent, and cell pleomorphism and cell stratification are limited.

High-grade intraepithelial neoplasia demonstrates with crowding of glands, including budding and branching of some glands. The nucleoli are prominent and often intense eosinophilic.

3.3.1. Clinical significance

Flat low-grade intraepithelial neoplasia: re-endoscopy to exclude concurrent carcinoma is suggested. The risk of carcinoma is low (about 25%). Re-endoscopy twice a year and annual after two negative endoscopies is suggested.

Flat high-grade intraepithelial neoplasia: the risk of accompanied carcinoma is high (about 85%). An excision of the whole lesion/region is necessary [2, 11].

3.3.2. Vienna classification of gastrointestinal epithelial neoplasia

Geographic differences in interpretation of gastric epithelial tumours exist (generally between Western pathologists and Japanese pathologists). The Vienna classification of (pre-)cancerous lesions of the GI-tract tries to harmonize both interpretations (**Table 5**).

Category 1	Negative for neoplasia/dysplasia
Category 2	Indefinite for neoplasia/dysplasia
Category 3	Non-invasive low-grade neoplasia (low-grade adenoma/dysplasia)
Category 4	Non-invasive high-grade neoplasia
4.1.	High-grade adenoma/dysplasia
4.2.	Non-invasive carcinoma (carcinom *in situ*)
4.3.	Suspicion of invasive carcinoma
Category 5	Invasive neoplasia
5.1.	Intramucosal carcinoma
5.2.	Submucosal carcinoma or beyond

Source: From Schlemper et al. [12].

Table 5. Vienna classification of gastrointestinal epithelial neoplasia.

4. Classification of neuroendocrine gastric tumours

According to WHO, tumours with neuroendocrine differentiation are separated into the following:

- well-differentiated neuroendocrine tumours (NETs) (grade 1 and grade 2)
- neuroendocrine carcinoma (NEC; subdivided into either small- and large-cell neuroendocrine carcinoma)

4.1. Neuroendocrine tumours (NETs)

NETs in total represent about 2% of all gastric malignancies.

Gastric neuroendocrine tumours (formerly 'carcinoid tumours') are mostly asymptomatic small 'polyps' on a background of hypergastrinemia-associated hyperplasia of endocrine cells in the gastric corpus of middle age adults (the 'classical' type 1 gastric NET, compare **Table 6**). But rarely they also can be associated with syndromes or unrelated to hypergastrinemia —these rare manifestations are usually correlated to unusual locations (e.g. antrum, more aggressive behaviour) [2, 16].

According to clinico-pathophysiological characteristics, three types of gastric NETs have been proposed (**Table 6**). These types share the same histological pattern. The great majority are tumours of enterochromaffin-like (ECL) cells induced by hypergastrinemia and caused by chronic atrophic corpus gastritis due to autoimmune gastritis and consecutive hypochlorhydria (type 1 NET) [3, 13, 17, 18].

Pathophysiologically, NETs start with ECL-cell hyperplasia (scattered or linear ECL-hyperplasia), which may confluent to micronodules. More than five micronodules in a group are called adenomatoid ECL-hyperplasia. Enlargement of adenomatoid ECL-hyperplasia with

	Type 1	Type 2	Type 3	Indicators of behaviour
Background mucosa	Chronic atrophic corpus gastritis—*usually autoimmune*	Hypertrophic with hyperplastic, intense eosinophilic parietal cells due to Zollinger-Ellison syndrome—*usually MEN1*	Normal (sporadic tumour)	Benign <1 cm mucosa or submucosa no angioinvasion
ECL-hyperplasia	Yes	Yes	No	Low-grade malignant beyond sumucosa angioinvasion >2 cm any endocrine functioning tumour Ki67 > 2–20%
Size	<1.5 cm multiple	<1.5 cm multiple > 1.5 cm in 20%	>1.5 cm, solitary rare < 1.5 cm multiple	High-grade malignant smaller or large cell neuroendocrine carcinoma Ki67 > 20%
Outcome	Never fatal	Rarely fatal	25% mortality	

Sources: Modified from Abraham et al. [13]; Capella et al. [14], and Klöppel et al. [15].

Table 6. Typing of gastric neuroendocrine tumours.

invasion and accompanied stroma reaction, the term dysplastic ECL-hyperplasia can be used. If the dysplastic ECL-nodules exceed 0.5 mm or invade the submucosa, the correct term is NET [2].

NETs of all types are composed of uniform cuboidal cells with round nuclei with stippled ('salt and pepper-like') chromatin and eosinophilic, granular cytoplasm. Nuclear pleomorphism, nucleoli and mitosis are unusual/infrequent in typical NETs (unlike neuroendocrine carcinoma). Growth pattern of NETs can be quite different and even quite heterogeneous in the same tumour forming nests, trabecular, tubules, rosettes or solid structures of tumour cells. Immunohistochemically, gastric NETs are consistent chromogranin A positive and have by definition a low Ki67 (up to 2%) [19, 20].

4.2. Neuroendocrine carcinomas (NECs)

Gastric neuroendocrine carcinomas are very rare (separated into small-cell and large-cell NECs). These poorly differentiated tumours are highly proliferative active (>20 mitosis/10 hpf or Ki67 >20%) and show an aggressive biological behaviour [3, 21].

Rare (atypical), NETs coexist with adenocarcinoma ('adenocarcinoid)—so-called MANEC (mixed adeno-neuroendocrine carcinoma, according to WHO). MANECs have the similar prognosis to that of conventional adenocarcinoma [2].

Clinical significance:

- NET, type 1: usually endoscopic polypectomy
- NET, type 2: usually endoscopic polypectomy
- NET, type 3: Surgery (e.g. gastrectomy); polypectomy in small tumours [2]

http://dx.doi.org/10.5772/intechopen.69838

5. Classification of malignant non-epithelial gastric tumours

5.1. Mesenchymal tumours

5.1.1. Gastrointestinal stromal tumour (GIST)

GISTs represent the great majority of mesenchymal tumour of the stomach and arise from the GI-pacemaker cells of Cajal; nearly all of gastric GISTs have a close contact to the gastric muscle wall (muscularis propria). Due to the wide morphological differences in the appearances of GIST: every mesenchymal tumour in the gastric wall is a GIST—until proven otherwise (compare differential diagnosis in Section 5.1.2.).

GISTs are usually tumours of adults with equal sex distribution but can affect children as well. Most of GISTs are solitary (rarely multiple) sporadic tumours but in some predisposing conditions like neurofibromatosis type 1, Carney-Stratakis syndrome (with paraganglioma and deficiency of succinate dehydrogenase) or associated with Carney triade (with extra-adrenal paraganglioma and pulmonary chondroma) tumours are more often multiple and show some other unusual features like epitheloid cell morphology or anatomical locations like oesophagus (compare **Table 7**) [22–28].

GISTs vary in size from very small only incidentally identified to very large bulky tumours. Particularly, the large tumours demonstrate with cysts, haemorrhage or necrosis. The histomorphology appearance is quite variable. Most GISTs show whorls, bundles or fascicle of monotonous spindle-cells with blunt-ended nuclei and eosinophilic cytoplasm (similar to tumours with muscle differentiation, compare **Figure 3**). Pleomorphism of tumour cells is not a typical feature (nevertheless some tumours can show striking pleomorphic nuclei). Sometimes paranuclear clear vacuoles or GISTs with small and intense eosinophilc homogenous filamentous material between tumour cells (skeinoid fibres; but usually seen in GIST of the small bowl) are seen. Some GISTs have an epitheloid cell appearance and these tumours are more often immunohistochemically CD117 negative. DOG1 ('discovered on GIST') is currently the protein with the highest sensitivity and specificity for GIST and is consistently positive in all epitheloid GISTs as well (compare **Tables 7** and **8**) [23, 29, 30].

The molecular basis for the CD117 protein-overexpression is an activating mutation of the c-kit gene (usually in the exons 9 or 11). A few tumours have mutations in platelet-derived growth factor receptor, alpha (PDGFRa), only.

Different mutations show different sensitivity to drug-related CD117 blockade (compare **Table 9**) [31]. Therefore, it is important to settle the exact underlying mutation.

Average age	60	40–50	<35	<25	50
Sex	1:1	1:1	w > m	1:1	1:1
Assoc. symptoms	None	Hyperpigmentation, Mastocytosis Urticaria	Extrarenal Paragan-glioma Chondroma	Extrarenal Paragan-glioma	Neurofibroma Cafe-au-lait

Source: Modified according to Agarwal et al. [28].

Table 7. Clinico-pathological characteristics in GIST.

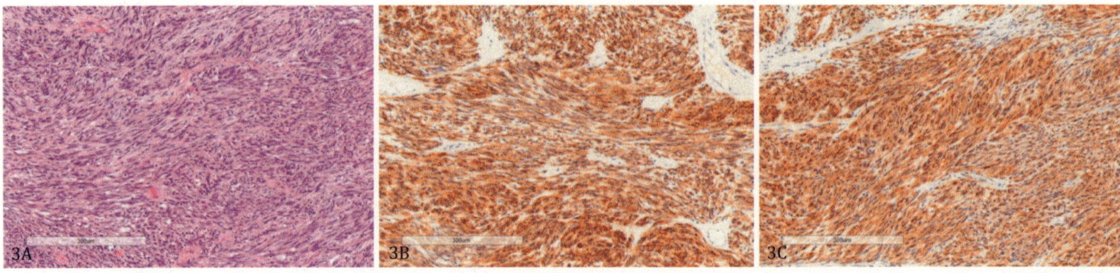

Figure 3. Spindle cell GIST (c-kit and DOG1 immunohistochemistry): (A) spindle cell GIST (HE), (B) DOG1 and (C) CD117.

Antibody	% of cases	Remarks
CD117(=c-kit)	90	Membrane staining; sometimes paranuclear dot; can be negative mainly in epitheloid GIST
DOG-1	≈100	Highest sensitivity and specificity
CD34	80	Low specificity
Vimentin	≈100	Very poor specificity; leiomyoma are negative for 'Vimentin'
SMA +h-Caldesmon	30	
Desmin	<5	Most GIST are completely negative, sometimes patchy
S100	1–5	Focally
MelanA	<1	Mainly in epitheloid GIST; DD: epitheloid PEComa

Table 8. Immunohistochemical markers in GIST.

Imatinib dosage in dependence of c-kit/PDGFRA-genotype	
Genotype	**Imatinib dosage per day**
c-kit Exon 11, 13, 17, wildtype	400 mg
c-kit Exon 9	800 mg
PDGFR-α-wild-type, Exon 12, 14	400 mg
PDGFR-α Exon 18 (D842V) mutation	Imatinib resistant
Source: Modified from onkopedia; GIST.	

Table 9. Imatinib dosage.

It is important to realize that all GISTs have the potential to metastasize. But most gastric GISTs follow a benign biological behaviour. The most important tumour characteristics associated with risk of progression are size, mitotic rate and anatomical location (but here we discuss gastric GIST, only) (compare **Tables 9** and **10**).

Risk of progression	Size (cm)	Mitotic activity (per 50 hpf*)
None	<2%	<5
1.9%	>2 to ≤5	<5
3.6%	>5 to ≤10	≤5
	≤2	≥5
10%	>10	≤5
16%	>2 to ≤5	>5
55%	>5 to ≤10	>5
86%	>10	>5

*high power field
Source: Modified from: Miettinen et al. [32].

Table 10. Risk of progression of gastric GIST.

5.1.2. Main differential diagnosis to GIST (including typical immunohistochemical/molecular findings)

- Leiomyoma/leiomyosarcoma—h-caldesmon, desmin
- Leiomyoma: usually small and related to muscularis mucosae. Very rare leiomyoma exist in the deeper gastric wall (usually located in the proximal part of the stomach). Diffuse positive for desmin, negative for dog1, CD117 (scattered mast cells between tumour cells are CD117 positive; mast-cell–rich leiomyoma can be challenging) and Vimentin
- Leiomyosarcoma: rare. Can look quite similar. Usually has much more cell pleomorphism
- Schwannoma—S100 and rim of lymphocytes in periphery of tumour
- Desmoid fibromatosis—ß-catenin nuclear expression
- Rhabdomyoma or rhabdomyosarcoma: Desmin, myogenin, MyoD1
- Haemangioma—ERG, CD31
- Calcifying fibrous tumour: paucillar, dense collagen, psammomatous calcification, patchy lymphocytes—factor XIIIa (in GI-tract usually adults, in soft tissue: usually children)
- Inflammatory fibroid polyp—CD34, PDGFRa
- Inflammatory myofibroblastic tumour—ALk1
- Solitary fibrous tumour (SFT)—STAT6
- Synovial sarcoma—TLE1
- Liposarcoma (well-/dedifferentiated or myxoid/roundcell)—mdm2 or FUS-CHOP-translocation
- Angiosarcoma (including: Kaposi-Sarcoma): ERG, CD31 (CAVE: macrophages)
- Clear cell sarcoma-like (malignant GI-neuroectodermal tumour): S100 (EWSR1 translocation)
- Glomustumour: SMA

- Gastroblastoma: benigne bi-phasic tumour in children. Epithelial component can be positive for CD117, mesenchymal component CD10 positive
- Granularcelltumour: S100
- Plexiform fibromyxoma: SMA, CD10 (very rare; multinodular, myxoid stroma, paucicellular, no atypia, prominent capillary network, just few mitosis, typically in wall of stomach)

5.2. Malignant lymphoma

5.2.1. Marginal zone lymphoma of mucosa-associated lymphoid tissue (MALT)

The great majority of gastric malignant lymphoma in Western countries belongs to the mucosa-associated lymphoid tissue (MALT) subtype. About 70–80% of MALT-lymphomas are associated with a chronic helicobacter pylori (Hp) infection. The Hp-infection is one of the main drivers of this type of lymphoma; eradication of Hp is the first choice of treatment and induces a regression of the MALT-lymphoma in about 75% of cases. Hp-negative MALT-lymphoma can be associated with some other infections (like Hepatitis C) or are related to immunosuppression (due to AIDS or post-transplant) or some autoimmune diseases. Prognosis is mainly related to stage (Ann Arbor staging). Gastric MALT lymphoma occurs frequently multifocal. It is noteworthy that some gastric MALT lymphoma can affect other MALT-bearing organs like gut, salivary glands and bronchial [2, 33].

Endoscopically, (MALT)-lymphoma imitates carcinoma (including mucosa-ulceration) and is usually located in distal parts of the stomach. Sometimes non-characteristic gastritis-like or nodular appearance dominates.

Histologically, MALT-lymphoma shows the characteristics of other marginal zone lymphomas like dense infiltrations of small to intermediate-sized more or less monomorphic lymphoid cells with clear cytoplasm. Some tumours show a striking plasmacytoid-like differentiation. Lympho-epithelial lesions (destruction of epithelial components of the mucosa) are highly characteristic for this type of lymphoma. Scattered blasts are typical [34, 35].

Immunohistochemically, MALT-lymphomas are positive for CD20 and half each for CD43. Negative for CD10, cyclin D1, CD5, CD23.

5.2.1.1. Clinical significance

Hp-eradication is the first choice of treatment (independent of Hp status at the surrounding mucosa). But tumours with nuclear BCL10 expression and positive translocation t (11;18) (q21;q21)) fail to response to Hp-eradication. This subtype is associated with a low risk of progression into an aggressive B-cell-lymphoma [36–38].

All other B- and T-cell-lymphomas and some other rare differential diagnosis can primary occur in the stomach, but are frequently an expression of a secondary infiltration (compare Sections 5.2.2–5.2.4) [39].

5.2.2. Small cell B-cell-lymphoma

- Follicular lymphoma (grade1/2): CD10, BCL6, HGAL
- Mantle cell lymphoma: CD5, Cyclin D1 (due to translocation t(11;14), Sox11
- Lymphocytic lymphoma: CD23, CD5

5.2.3. High-grade B-cell-lymphoma

- Diffuse large B-cell-lymphoma: CD20, CD79a, Mum1, BCL2 positive. Some MALT-lymphomas show a transformation into an aggressive large B-cell-lymphoma.
- Burkitt-lymphoma: CD20, CD79a, BCL2 negative, CD10 positive. C-Myc translocation by FISH.

5.2.4. Others

- Primary solitary gastric plasmacytoma
- T-cell-lymphoma
- Langerhans cell histiocytosis, myeloid leukaemia

6. Metastasis

About 2.6% of all gastric tumours are metastases to the stomach.

Malignant melanoma is the most frequent reason for metastases followed by some carcinoma: like lobular breast carcinoma (compare **Figure 4**) or colon, prostate, lung, pancreas, liver (mainly hepatocellular carcinoma) and very rare sarcoma (epithelioid angiosarcoma) [40–43].

The correct diagnosis can be quite challengingly—the following immunohistochemistry panel may help to find the correct answer:

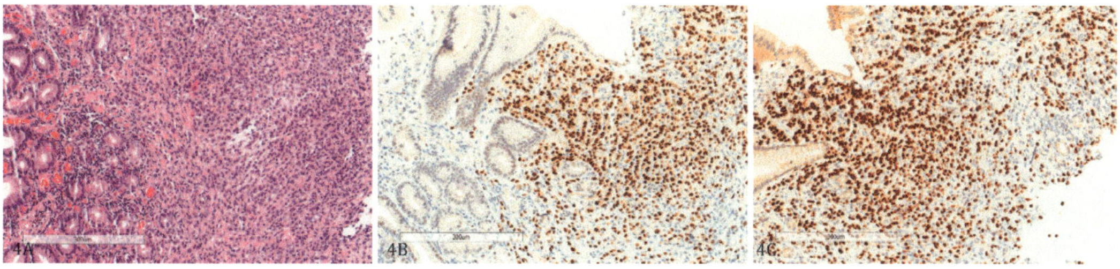

Figure 4. Metastasis lobular breast carcinoma: (A) metastasis lobular breast carcinoma (HE), (B) estrogen-receptor and (C) GATA3.

- AE1/AE3, GATA3, estrogen-receptor (progesterone -receptor, GCDFP): breast
- SOX10 (HMB45, MelanA, MITF): malignant melanoma
- SATB2, CDX2: colon
- Androgen-receptor (PSMA, NKX3.1, ERG): prostate

Author details

Alexander Quaas

Address all correspondence to: alexander.quaas@uk-koeln.de

Institute of Pathology, University of Cologne, Germany

References

[1] Henson DE, Dittus C, Younes M, Nguyen H, Albores-Saavedra J. Differential trends in the intestinal and diffuse types of gastric carcinoma in the United States, 1973-2000: Increase in the signet ring cell type. Archives of Pathology & Laboratory Medicine. 2004;**128**(7):765-770

[2] Fletcher CDM Diagnostic Histopathology of Tumours. 4 ed. chapter: In: Lauwers GY. Tumors of the Esophagus and Stomach; 2013. pp. 378-433

[3] Bosman FT, WHO, IAfRoC. WHO Classification of Tumours of the Digestive System. 2010

[4] Bass AJ, Thorsson V, Shmulevich I et al. Cancer Genome Atlas Research Network Comprehensive molecular characterization of gastric adenocarcinoma. Nature. 2014; **513**(7517):202-209

[5] Cristescu R, Lee J, Nebozhyn M, Kim KM, Ting JC, Wong SS, et al. Molecular analysis of gastric cancer identifies subtypes associated with distinct clinical outcomes. Nature Medicine. 2015;**21**(5):449-456

[6] Rüschoff J, et al. HER2 testing in gastric cancer: A practical approach. Modern Pathology. Official Journal of United States and Canadian Academy of Pathology. Inc. 2012;**25**:637-650

[7] Murphy A, Kelly RJ. From molecular classification to targeted therapeutics: The changing face of systemic therapy in metastatic gastroesophageal cancer. Gastroenterology Research and Practice. 2015;**2015**:896560

[8] Ahn S, Lee SJ, Kim Y, Kim A, Shin N, Choi KU, et al. High-throughput protein and mRNA expression-based classification of gastric cancers can identify clinically distinct subtypes, concordant with recent molecular classifications. The American Journal of Surgical Pathology. 2017;**41**(1):106-115

[9] Brierley JD, Gospodarowicz MK, Wittekind C. TNM Classification of Malignant Tumours. 8th ed.; 2017

[10] Becker K, Langer R, Reim D, Novotny A, Meyer zum Buschenfelde C, Engel J, Friess H, Hofler H. Significance of histopathological tumor regression after neoadjuvant chemotherapy in gastric adenocarcinomas: a summary of 480 cases. Annals of Surgery. 2011 May;**253**(5):934-9

[11] Tan DL, Gregory Y. Advances in surgical pathology. Gastric Cancer. Philadelphia: Wolters Kluwer Health/Lippincott Williams & Wilkins; 2011

[12] Schlemper RJ, Riddell RH, Kato Y, et al. The Vienna classification of gastrointestinal epithelial neoplasia. Gut. 2000;**47**:251-255

[13] Abraham SC, Carney JA, Ooi A, Choti MA, Argani P. Achlorhydria, parietal cell hyperplasia, and multiple gastric carcinoids: A new disorder. The American Journal of Surgical Pathology. 2005;**29**(7):969-975

[14] Capella C, Heitz P, Hofler H, et al. Revised classification of neuroendocrine tumours of the lung, pancreas and gut. Virchows Arch. 1995;**425**:547-560

[15] Klöppel G, Perren A, Heitz P. The gastroenteropancreatic neuroendocrine system and its tumors. Annals of the New York Academy of Sciences. 2004;**1014**:13-27

[16] Rindi G, Bordi C, Rappel S, La Rosa S, Stolte M, Solcia E. Gastric carcinoids and neuroendocrine carcinomas: Pathogenesis, pathology, and behavior. World Journal of Surgery. 1996;**20**(2):168-172

[17] Thomas RM, Baybick JH, Elsayed AM, Sobin LH. Gastric carcinoids: An immunohistochemical and clinicopathologic study of 104 patients. Cancer. 1994;**73**(8):2053-2058

[18] Borch K, Ahren B, Ahlman H, Falkmer S, Granerus G, Grimelius L. Gastric carcinoids: Biologic behavior and prognosis after differentiated treatment in relation to type. Annals of Surgery. 2005;**242**(1):64-73

[19] La Rosa S, Inzani F, Vanoli A, Klersy C, Dainese L, Rindi G, et al. Histologic characterization and improved prognostic evaluation of 209 gastric neuroendocrine neoplasms. Human Pathology. 2011;**42**(10):1373-1384

[20] Burkitt MD, Pritchard DM. Review article: Pathogenesis and management of gastric carcinoid tumours. Alimentary Pharmacology & Therapeutics. 2006;**24**(9):1305-1320

[21] Matsui K, Jin XM, Kitagawa M, Miwa A. Clinicopathologic features of neuroendocrine carcinomas of the stomach: Appraisal of small cell and large cell variants. Archives of Pathology & Laboratory Medicine. 1998;**122**(11):1010-1017

[22] Miettinen M, Lasota J. Gastrointestinal stromal tumors—Definition, clinical, histological, immunohistochemical, and molecular genetic features and differential diagnosis. Virchows Archiv: An International Journal of Pathology. 2001;**438**(1):1-12

[23] Miettinen M, Sobin LH, Lasota J. Gastrointestinal stromal tumors of the stomach: A clinicopathologic, immunohistochemical, and molecular genetic study of 1765 cases with long-term follow-up. The American Journal of Surgical Pathology. 2005;**29**(1):52-68

[24] Carney JA, Stratakis CA. Familial paraganglioma and gastric stromal sarcoma: A new syndrome distinct from the Carney triad. American Journal of Medical Genetics. 2002;**108**(2):132-139

[25] Pasini B, McWhinney SR, Bei T, Matyakhina L, Stergiopoulos S, Muchow M, et al. Clinical and molecular genetics of patients with the Carney-Stratakis syndrome and germline mutations of the genes coding for the succinate dehydrogenase subunits SDHB, SDHC, and SDHD. European Journal of Human Genetics. 2008;**16**(1):79-88

[26] Fuller CE, Williams GT. Gastrointestinal manifestations of type 1 neurofibromatosis (von Recklinghausen's disease). Histopathology. 1991;**19**(1):1-11

[27] Nishida T, Hirota S, Taniguchi M, Hashimoto K, Isozaki K, Nakamura H, et al. Familial gastrointestinal stromal tumours with germline mutation of the KIT gene. Nature Genetics. 1998;**19**(4):323-324

[28] Agarwal R, et al. Inherited predisposition to gastrointestinal stromal tumor. Hematology Oncology Clinics of North America. 2009;**23**:1-13

[29] Fletcher CD, Berman JJ, Corless C, Gorstein F, Lasota J, Longley BJ, et al. Diagnosis of gastrointestinal stromal tumors: A consensus approach. Human Pathology. 2002; **33**(5):459-465

[30] Liegl B, Hornick JL, Corless CL, Fletcher CD. Monoclonal antibody DOG1.1 shows higher sensitivity than KIT in the diagnosis of gastrointestinal stromal tumors, including unusual subtypes. The American Journal of Surgical Pathology. 2009;**33**(3):437-446

[31] Verweij J, Casali PG, Zalcberg J, LeCesne A, Reichardt P, Blay JY, et al. Progression-free survival in gastrointestinal stromal tumours with high-dose imatinib: Randomised trial. Lancet (London, England). 2004;**364**(9440):1127-1134

[32] Miettinen M, Lasota J, Sobin LH. Gastrointestinal stromal tumors of the stomach in children and young adults: A clinicopathologic, immunohistochemical, and molecular genetic study of 44 cases with long-term follow-up and review of the literature. The American Journal of Surgical Pathology. 2005;**29**:1373-1381

[33] Farinha P, Gascoyne RD. Helicobacter pylori and MALT lymphoma. Gastroenterology. 2005;**128**(6):1579-1605

[34] Wotherspoon AC, Doglioni C, Isaacson PG. Low-grade gastric B-cell lymphoma of mucosa-associated lymphoid tissue (MALT): A multifocal disease. Histopathology. 1992;**20**(1):29-34

[35] Isaacson PG. Lymphomas of mucosa-associated lymphoid tissue (MALT). Histopathology. 1990;**16**(6):617-619

[36] Bayerdorffer E, Neubauer A, Rudolph B, Thiede C, Lehn N, Eidt S, et al. Regression of primary gastric lymphoma of mucosa-associated lymphoid tissue type after cure of Helicobacter pylori infection. MALT Lymphoma Study Group. Lancet (London, England). 1995;**345**(8965):1591-1594

[37] Liu H, Ye H, Dogan A, Ranaldi R, Hamoudi RA, Bearzi I, et al. T(11;18)(q21;q21) is associated with advanced mucosa-associated lymphoid tissue lymphoma that expresses nuclear BCL10. Blood. 2001;**98**(4):1182-1187

[38] Liu H, Ye H, Ruskone-Fourmestraux A, De Jong D, Pileri S, Thiede C, et al. T(11;18) is a marker for all stage gastric MALT lymphomas that will not respond to H. Pylori eradication. Gastroenterology. 2002;**122**(5):1286-1294

[39] Kawamoto K, Nakamura S, Iwashita A, Watanabe J, Oshiro Y, Nakayama Y, et al. Clinicopathological characteristics of primary gastric T-cell lymphoma. Histopathology. 2009;**55**(6):641-653

[40] Attanoos R, Griffiths DF. Metastatic small cell melanoma to the stomach mimicking primary gastric lymphoma. Histopathology. 1992;**21**(2):173-175

[41] Campoli PM, Ejima FH, Cardoso DM, Silva OQ, Santana Filho JB, Queiroz Barreto PA, et al. Metastatic cancer to the stomach. Gastric Cancer: Official Journal of the International Gastric Cancer Association and the Japanese Gastric Cancer Association. 2006;**9**(1):19-25

[42] Green LK. Hematogenous metastases to the stomach. A review of 67 cases. Cancer. 1990;**65**(7):1596-1600

[43] Taal BG, Peterse H, Boot H. Clinical presentation, endoscopic features, and treatment of gastric metastases from breast carcinoma. Cancer. 2000;**89**(11):2214-2221